NURSING FOUNDATION

for

Post Basic BSc Nursing

NURSING FOUNDATION

for
Post Basic BSc Nursing

Suresh Sharma

PhD MSc (N) FNRS RN (USA)

Professor-cum-Principal
College of Nursing
All India Institute of Medical Sciences (AIIMS)
Jodhpur, Rajasthan, India

Shiv Kumar Mudgal

PhD MSc (N)

Associate Professor
College of Nursing
All India Institute of Medical Sciences (AIIMS)
Deoghar, Jharkhand, India

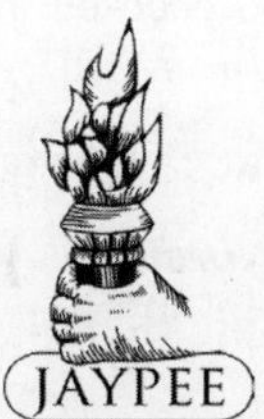

JAYPEE BROTHERS MEDICAL PUBLISHERS
The Health Sciences Publisher
New Delhi | London

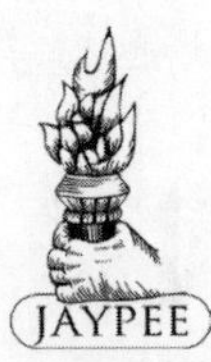

Jaypee Brothers Medical Publishers (P) Ltd.

Headquarters

Jaypee Brothers Medical Publishers (P) Ltd
EMCA House
23/23-B, Ansari Road, Daryaganj
New Delhi - 110 002, India
Landline: +91-11-23272143, +91-11-23272703
+91-11-23282021, +91-11-23245672
Email: jaypee@jaypeebrothers.com

Corporate Office

Jaypee Brothers Medical Publishers (P) Ltd
4838/24, Ansari Road, Daryaganj
New Delhi 110 002, India
Phone: +91-11-43574357
Fax: +91-11-43574314
Email: jaypee@jaypeebrothers.com

Overseas Office

J.P. Medical Ltd
83 Victoria Street, London
SW1H 0HW (UK)
Phone: +44 20 3170 8910
Fax: +44 (0)20 3008 6180
Email: info@jpmedpub.com

Website: www.jaypeebrothers.com

Website: www.jaypeedigital.com

Inquiries for bulk sales may be solicited at: jaypee@jaypeebrothers.com

Nursing Foundation for Post Basic BSc Nursing

First Edition: **2024**

ISBN: 978-93-5696-558-4

Printed in India by Rajkamal Electric Press, Kundli, Haryana.

Preface

This textbook is a comprehensive exploration of how the changing landscape of nursing practice is shaped by advancements in medical technology, new treatment methods, and a deeper understanding of patient-centered care. We invite educators, students, and healthcare professionals to join us on this transformative journey. In India, nursing is swiftly evolving due to influences from the West, shifts in disease patterns, healthcare systems, and government policies. Nurses play a multifaceted role, providing essential care and medications while requiring a deep understanding of scientific nursing principles. They employ evidence-based approaches to ensuring comprehensive care for patients, families, and communities, aiming to optimize healthcare outcomes.

Nurses must grasp the foundational concepts of nursing to swiftly build upon them for advanced practice. They are expected to function independently, collaboratively, and assertively to deliver high-quality, cost-effective, and evidence-based care. Amid dynamic changes and persistent challenges, nurses must adapt to the evolving healthcare landscape, focusing more on community-based care, health promotion, and catering to diverse patient demographics.

Despite these transformations, the fundamentals of nursing remain essential. Nurses must be knowledgeable, professional, technically adept, empathetic, and capable of synthesizing extensive knowledge and experience to provide top-notch patient care.

The *Nursing Foundation for Post Basic BSc Nursing* covers fundamental nursing concepts, skills, and techniques essential for students, addressing changes in practice and preparing nurses for various healthcare settings. Specifically tailored to Indian nursing faculty and students, it meets international standards of scientific nursing knowledge.

Throughout this exploration, we glean insights from trailblazing educators, researchers, and practitioners who have embraced the fusion of nursing education and practice. Their experiences serve as guiding lights, illuminating the path for others seeking innovative and effective nursing practices.

We hope this textbook serves as a valuable resource for the Post Basic BSc Nursing students and their teachers to reimagine the possibilities of nursing foundations within the context of real nursing practice. The journey of transformation commences here, and we eagerly welcome you to join us on this thrilling expedition and also anticipate suggestions that could enhance forthcoming editions.

Suresh Sharma
Shiv Kumar Mudgal

Contents

Section 6: Innovative Approaches in Nursing Practice

Syllabus

Placement: First Year   **Time Allotted: 45 Hours**

Course Description

This course will help students develop an understanding of the philosophy, objectives and responsibilities of nursing as a profession. The purpose of the course is to orient to the current concepts involved in the practices of nursing and developments in the nursing profession.

Objectives

At the end of the course, the student will:

- Identify professional aspects of nursing.
- Explain theories of nursing.
- Identify ethical aspects of nursing profession.
- Utilize steps of nursing process.
- Identify the role of the nurse in various levels of health services.
- Appreciate the significance of quality assurance in nursing.
- Explain current trends in health and nursing.

Course Contents

Unit I

- Development of nursing as a profession:
  - Its philosophy
  - Objectives and responsibilities of a graduate nurse.
- Trends influencing nursing practices.
- Expended role of the nurse.
- Development of nursing education in India and trends in nursing education.
- Professional organization, career planning.
- Code of ethics and professional conduct for nurse.

Unit II

- Ethical, legal and other issues in nursing.
- Concept of health and illness, effects on the person.
- Stress and adaptation.
- Healthcare concept and nursing care concept.
- Development concept, needs, roles and problems of the development stages of individual newborn, infant, toddler, pre-adolescent, adolescent, adulthood, middle age and old age.

Unit III

- Theory of nursing practices.
- Meta-paradigm of nursing—characterized by four central concepts, i.e., nurse, person (client/patient), health and environment.

Unit IV

- Nursing process.
- **Assessment:** Tools for assessment, methods, recording.
- **Planning:** Teaching for planning care, types of care plans.
- **Implementation:** Different approaches to care, organizations and implementation of care, record.
- **Evaluation:** Tools for evaluation, process of evaluation, types of evaluation.

Unit V

- **Quality assurance:** Nursing standards, nursing audit, total quality management.
- Role of council and professional bodies in maintenance of standards.

Unit VI

- Primary healthcare concept:
  - Community-oriented nursing
  - Holistic nursing
  - Primary nursing.
- Family-oriented nursing concept:
  - Problem-oriented nursing
  - Progressive patient care
  - Team nursing.

Nursing Profession

☞ **Learning Objectives**

- Clearly articulate the concept of nursing.
- Explain the characteristics that define nursing as a profession.
- Distinguish nursing from other profession.
- Develop a personal nursing philosophy statement that reflects one's beliefs, values, and priorities in nursing practice.
- Define the overarching goals and purposes of nursing services within the healthcare system.

■ INTRODUCTION

An individual who is ready to provide care for the sick, injured, and elderly is a nurse. A nurse is someone who nourishes, fosters, and protects. The Latin word "nutrix", which meaning "nursing mother," is the source of the noun "nurse" in this context. The word "nurse" is defined in dictionaries as someone who "suckles or nourishes," "to take care of a kid or children," and "to bring up; rear." In this sense, the verb "nurse," which comes from the Latin "nutrire", that means "to suckle and nourish," is used. With such a history, it is unsurprising that most people connect nursing with female.

Within the domain of health care, nursing is a profession that focuses on the care of individuals, families, and communities with the goal of helping these groups achieve, maintain, or regain the highest possible level of health and quality of life. By their approach to patient care, training, and scope of practice, nurses are distinguishable from other healthcare professionals.

■ DEFINITION OF NURSING

Nursing might be hard to define. Because of the nursing's fascinating history, nurses themselves are unable to agree on a single definition. There is not much information available regarding the role of the nurse in prehistoric times, although Donahue (1996, p. 2) states "From the dawn of civilization, evidence prevails to support the premise that nurturing has been essential to the preservation of life. Survival of the human race, therefore, is inextricably intertwined with the development of nursing."

The International Council of Nurses' nursing service committee requested Virginia Henderson, in 1958 to explain her idea of fundamental nursing. One of the nursing definitions that is still most frequently used is hers:

- "The unique function of the nurse is to assist the individual, sick or well, in the performance of those activities contributing to health or its recovery (or to peaceful death) that he would perform unaided if he had the necessary strength, will or knowledge. And to do this in such a way as to help him gain independence as rapidly as possible."

—Henderson, 1966, p. 15; ICN 1973

- Nursing is "essential components of professional nursing practice include care, cure, and coordination". *—ANA, 1965*
- Another definition was added by ANA to its Social Policy Statement stated: "Nursing is the diagnosis and treatment of human responses to actual or potential health problems". *—ANA, 1980*
- "Nursing is the protection, promotion, and optimization of health and abilities; prevention of illness and injury; alleviation of suffering through the diagnosis and treatment of human responses; and advocacy in health care for individuals, families, communities, and populations."

  —American Nurses Association
- "The use of clinical judgment in the provision of care to enable people to improve, maintain, or recover health, to cope with health problems, and to achieve the best possible quality of life, whatever their disease or disability, until death."

  —Royal College of Nursing, 2003
- "Nursing encompasses autonomous and collaborative care of individuals of all ages, families, groups and communities, sick or well, and in all settings. Nursing includes the promotion of health, prevention of illness, and the care of ill, disabled and dying people. Advocacy, promotion of a safe environment, research, participation in shaping health policy and in patient and health systems management, and education are also key nursing roles."

  —International Council of Nurses, 2010

PROFESSION

There are many educational courses available that can be opted after the school education such as academic programs and professional programs. The academic programs focus more on the theoretical aspects and referred to as liberal courses which includes Bachelor of Arts (BA), Bachelor of Commerce (BCom), etc. On the contrary, the professional programs such as medicine (Bachelor of Medicine and Bachelor of Surgery; MBBS), Engineering (Bachelor of Engineering; BE or BEng); Nursing (Bachelor of Nursing; BSc Nursing) aimed for the cultivation of practical skills that enables a person to work in a particular career which include. The professional courses prepare specialized experts in a specific field through intensive training that can be applied to a variety of job-related situations.

Meaning

The English word "profess", meaning " to proclaim something publicly," is the root of the noun "Profession." A profession is a job, occupation, or vocation in which an individual works and has received formal training. The occupations known as professions are those that need a certain set of qualities sometimes referred to as specialization, autonomy, commitment, and accountability.

A profession is a type of work that requires formal education and training in a certain field of knowledge in order to provide the public with a specific type of expert service.

Definition

- "An occupation whose core element is work based upon the mastery of a complex body of knowledge and skills. It is a vocation in which knowledge of some department of science or learning or the practice of an art founded upon it is used in the service of others." *—Sylvia RC, 2010*
- "Profession is any type of work that needs special training or a particular skill, often one that is respected because it involves a high level of education."

  —Cambridge Dictionary
- "Profession is a chosen, paid, occupation that requires a prolonged training and formal qualification."

  —Oxford Dictionary

- "An occupation in which an individual uses an intellectual skill based on an established body of knowledge and practice to provide a specialized service in a defined area, exercising independent judgement in accordance with a code of ethics and in the public interest."

   —The UK Inter-professional Group

In nutshell, profession can be viewed as an occupation with specialized study and training bounded by ethical standards to serve the mankind.

Differences between Occupation and Profession

Despite the fact that the terms "occupation" and "profession" are sometimes used interchangeably, the meanings of these terms in a more general sense are very different. Profession is an occupation, but all occupations are not professions. Understanding these differences, helps to easily identify and distinguish occupation and profession (**Table 1.1**).

Characteristics of a Profession

Characteristics refer to features that stand unique and differentiate from common things.

- **Based on a specialized body of knowledge:** Professionals render specialized services based on theory, knowledge, and skills that are most often peculiar to their profession. This provides the framework for the practice.
- **Based on professional standards and code of ethics:** A profession is based on a general body of core values and standards set by the concerned regulatory bodies of the profession.
- **Based on set of skills for specific services:** A profession stands to provide specialized services based on a set of skills distinct to that profession. Therefore, each profession is entrusted with great responsibilities and obligations towards the society.
- **Based on a standardized formal education:** Every profession is based on a standardized formal education controlled by various regulatory bodies. This helps in the preparation of competent members with practical experience in the protected environment that are typically required for a particular profession.
- **Autonomy and accountability:** Members of a profession has the freedom for making decisions and are answerable to their actions while rendering their services.

Criteria of a Profession

Criteria are the principles or standards for evaluating a profession. Many writers have explained the criteria of profession in different ways. Some of the major criteria which explain a profession are listed below:

According to Flexner's (1915)

Abraham Flexner has stated six criteria for a profession:

1. A profession is based on *intellectual* activities (as opposed to physical) and is accompanied by a high degree of individual responsibility.

Table 1.1: Differences between occupation and profession.

Aspects of comparison	*Occupation*	*Profession*
Meaning	Occupation refers to a person's regular activity that he or she does to earn a living	A profession is an occupation that needs a specialized knowledge and skill in a particular sector
Code of conduct	No	Yes
Formal training	It is not mandatory	It is essential
Regulated by statute	No	Yes
Values, beliefs and ethics	Not the most essential components of training	An essential component of training

2. The practice of a profession is founded on a body of knowledge that may be learnt and is expanded and improved via research.
3. In addition to focusing on theory, the professional activities emphasize practical application.
4. Techniques of a profession are taught through a highly specialized process of professional education.
5. The profession has a well-developed group consciousness and a robust internal organizational structure of members.
6. Practitioners in the profession are driven by altruism (a willingness to serve others) and are interested in public concerns.

According to Bixler and Bixler (1945)

- **Intellectual and body of knowledge:** The members practicing in the profession utilizes highly specialized knowledge and technical skill for their practice. The members in the profession are trained in all domains—cognitive, affective and psychomotor to develop competency.
- **Scientific:** A professional person's education is built on a foundation of scientific knowledge. Every profession has its own body of knowledge from which the members utilize the knowledge for their routine professional practice. A genuine profession will continue to research while also utilizing the developing amount of information and the expertise of its practitioners.
- **Requires higher education:** A professional person should be educated in a higher education institution, i.e., colleges which are regulated by the universities. Apart from it, higher qualification and specialization can be done to improve the professional practice.
- **Essential:** The services provided by profession should be a vital role in providing service to human and social welfare. The services are absolutely necessary for survival and it cannot be substituted by others.

- **Self-governing:** A genuine profession will give and cultivate leadership abilities among its members. They facilitate the establishment of policies and norms for professional activities.
- **Service-oriented:** Members of the profession are supposed to spend most of their energy on it for the rest of their lives.
- **Continuous professional growth:** The profession should offer its members with organized opportunities for continued professional growth. It can be done through continuing education, on-job training, seminars, workshops, conference, etc.
- **Personal development:** Professionals should be allowed to work with the confidence that they are free to enhance their job and implement new ideas and procedures. They have the right to question and assess what is being done. Professionals have a lot of opportunities to improve and develop their practice because of this freedom.
- **Economic security:** Economic security means having adequate amount of money to meet the daily expenses without any interruption which is important for an individual. A profession provides economic security to its members. The profession by their council or association supervises that its practitioners are paid adequately. This economic security is applicable during retirement time as well.

NURSING AS A PROFESSION

Nursing is considered as the "youngest of the professions". The practice of nursing has been elevated to the level of a learned profession, merging elements of science and art. As a science, nursing calls for a specialized education and a broad understanding of human nature. Art is a skill that is learned through study and practice and is developed while doing something. As an art consisting of a corpus of practical knowledge, nursing demands a compassionate heart and a willing hand. In addition to scientific knowledge and expert bedside skill, desirable attitudes are necessary in nursing. Therefore, the basic requirements for a nurse are knowledge of nursing science (Head), the desire to nurse, spirit of nursing (Heart), i.e., the attitude and the skill of nursing (Hand).

The Nursing fulfils most of the criteria of a profession. The following are the criteria that fulfils nursing as a profession.

- **Essential services:** Nursing services are critical to mankind and the well-being of society. Nursing is without a doubt a service that is essential to the well-being of both people and the larger community. Nursing promotes the maintenance and restoration of the health of people, groups, and society. Nursing's objective is to help others achieve the best level of well-being to which they are competent. Caring, which means nurturing and helping others, is a basic component of professional nursing.

- **Body of knowledge:** There is a unique body of knowledge that is continuously expanded through nursing research. Historically, nursing was founded on concepts derived from the social and physical sciences and other fields. But nowadays, nursing has its own body of knowledge. Nowadays, research is used as the foundation for nursing rather than task orientation, intuition, or trial and error.

- **Intellectual activities:** Individual accountability (responsibility) is a prominent aspect of the nursing services, which include intellectual activities. Nursing has evolved and polished its own distinct practice methodology, known as nursing process. The nursing process is primarily a cognitive (mental) effort that necessitates both analytical and innovative thinking and serves as the foundation for nursing care.

- **Accountability:** It is the process in which individuals are answerable for their action and have the obligation (duty) to act. Nurses are accountable not only to themselves but also to their patients and their families, the employers of the nursing profession, and the community at large.

- **Formal higher education:** Nursing practitioners are educated in institutes of higher education. The most of basic nursing education programs are now degree/baccalaureate programs or masters' programs offered by universities.

- **Autonomy:** Nursing professionals have a fair amount of independence and are in responsible of their own practices. Another controversial topic in nursing is how much freedom (autonomy) or control a nurse has over their work. Despite the fact that many nursing practices are independent, nurse practice acts vary from nation to nation and around the world.

- **Altruism:** Nursing practitioners are motivated by a desire to assist others (altruism) and consider their work to be a vital aspect of their lives. As a profession, nurses strongly support the idea of altruism, or serving others at the expense of their own needs.

- **Code of ethics:** The decisions and acts of nursing practitioners are governed by a code of ethics. An ethical code offers professional norms and a framework for decision-making, not instructions on how someone should behave in a particular circumstance. The public's faith in the nursing profession necessitates that nurses conduct honorably. Both the Indian nursing council (INC) and the International council of nurses (ICN) have developed codes of nursing ethics that establish, promote, and improve standards of practice to assist them in accomplishing this.

- **Professional associations:** There is an organization (association) that supports and promotes professional nursing practice standards. In order to enhance the nursing profession, numerous professional associations have been constituted. The purpose of which is to improve nursing care for all individuals by establishing high standards of nursing practice, promoting the professional and educational progress of nurses, and fostering the welfare of nurses. The organizations advocate for nursing concerns in general and serve as the official voice of nursing. In India, 'Trained Nurse Association of India' (TNAI) and State Government Nurses Association are the some of the professional associations in the Nursing.

Characteristics of Nursing Profession

Certain characteristics make nursing a unique profession as compared to other professions which are listed below:

- **Nursing is caring:** Caring is the dynamic core of nursing. Nursing's moral ideal is caring, and it's one of the most vital qualities for gaining others' trust. Caring is crucial in nursing since it aids in the process of healing. It allows nurses to demonstrate compassion and empathy for their clients. Being kind is a way people understand caring.
- **Nursing is service oriented:** Nursing is a call to service. Nursing services are those that consider persons as physiological, psychological, and sociological beings. Nursing services are rendered with dedication and commitment. Services are concentrated in preventive, promotive, curative and rehabilitative aspects.
- **Nursing is goal oriented:** Nursing is intended to help people achieve their personal, family, community, and universal healthcare goals in the most effective way possible. Nurses formulate specific and realistic goals that can be measured in real time to ensure patient progress is attained within a specified timeframe.
- **Nursing is impartial:** Nursing is dedicated to providing individualized care to all people, regardless of race, religion, economic or social position. All persons are treated with utmost respect and dignity without any discrimination.
- **Nursing requires personal contact:** It involves close personal contact with the recipient of care -patient, families, and communities. Care, cure and coordinated concept is applied in providing care
- **Nursing is bounded with ethical, legal, and political issues:** Ethics and ethical issues related to nursing are an important area of concern while dealing with human being. In ethical difficulties, the professional code of ethics in nursing serves as a set of norms for nurses' behavior and provides general recommendations for nursing actions.

PHILOSOPHY OF NURSING

In general, philosophy refers to the process of attempting to provide solutions to the most important question that people have faced throughout history. These inquiries deal with the existence of the universe (ontology), what may be known (epistemology), what is morally correct and seen as ethics, and whether there is an art to healthcare (aesthetics). Philosophizing in the West has its origins in ancient Greece, and the word's derivation derives from the two components of philosophy, "philo", which means love, and "Sophia", which means knowledge.

The literal definition of the phrase "philosophy" is "love of wisdom." In a broad sense, philosophy is the pursuit of understanding fundamental truths about oneself, the environment in which one lives, and one's connections with the world and other people. As a field of study, philosophy is essentially identical.

Philosophy of nursing describes our beliefs regarding the nature of the nursing profession and serves as a foundation for nursing. It supports the fundamental ethical norms we have and provides the theoretical foundation for our beliefs.

Meaning and Definition

A statement outlining a nurse's values, ethics, and beliefs as well as their reasons for choosing the profession serves as their nursing philosophy. It discusses the nurse's view on education, practice, and the ethics of patient care. A nursing philosophy enables you to identify the beliefs and theories that influence your daily decisions on the job.

- Nursing philosophy is a "statement of foundational and universal assumptions, beliefs, and principles about the nature of knowledge and truth (epistemology) and about the nature of the entities represented in the metaparadigm". *—Reed, 2012*
- Nursing philosophy is a "conceptual model or framework providing a frame of reference for nurses to guide their thinking, observations, interpretations and practices and it should include ideal about the person, the environment, health and illness, and the nurse". *—Seedhouse, 2000*

Components of a Personal Nursing Philosophy

A nursing philosophy has many different components, but the following are the essentials for any nursing philosophy or for developing a personal nursing philosophy (Fig. 1.1):

- **Role:** The term "role" refers to the individual who provides or manages care as well as their participation in the nursing profession. The role stresses the nurse's professional and patient responsibilities while offering and supervising patient care.

- **Knowledge:** Knowledge refers to the clinical and educational experiences of the nurse, as well as how such experiences pertain to the nurse's function.
- **Values:** Values are the guiding principles for a nurse's attitude, conduct, and moral reasoning. There are both personal and professional values. They are influenced by relationships, personal needs, and cultural and social factors. Additionally, the manner a nurse does her nursing duties is influenced by her professional values.
- **Process:** The nursing process is the method by which nurses carry out their interventions and make any necessary adjustments when required. The philosophy of nursing as a process takes into account the nurse's accountability for consistently applying the nursing process in service of better patient outcomes.

Principles of Nursing Philosophy

- The pursuit of reality and truth that results in ideas and aspirations is referred to as nursing philosophy.
- It is dynamic and evolves over time in accordance with societal, educational, professional, and environmental developments.
- It is affected by the setting in which it is used.
- It may be unique and reflect the values, beliefs, reasoning, morality, and ethics of the nurse particularly.
- It may exist on a global scale, be a part of a nursing organization or institution, etc.
- It expands the nursing profession's scope of practice.

How to Develop Your Own Personal Philosophy of Nursing

Creating your own nursing philosophy can be a little frightening, especially if you have never done it before. Remember that even if you have never thought of it or written down your nursing philosophy, you already have some notion of your own personal philosophy.

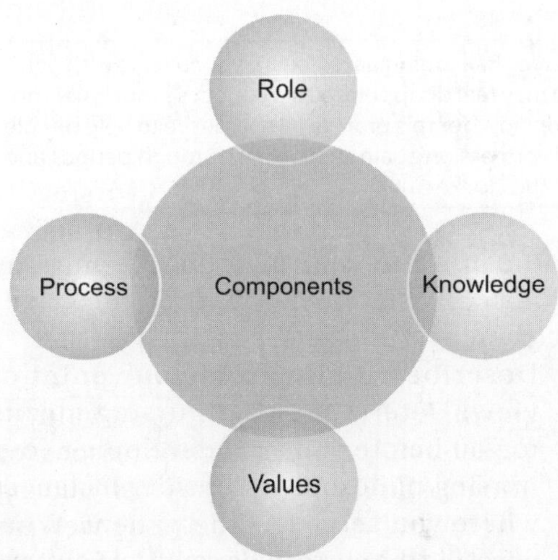

Fig. 1.1: Key components of nursing philosophy.

Table 1.2: Develop your own philosophy.

Question	How to find answer to this question
Why did I decide to become a nurse?	Understanding your motivation for wanting to become a nurse is the initial and most important step in creating a personal nursing philosophy. Tell yourself the truth about what motivated your choice. After that, you should be open to discussing your motivations for pursuing a career in nursing.
What do I believe about nursing personally?	As you start to formulate your own philosophy, you should consider what nursing signifies to you. What opinions do you have about nursing profession and your roles as a nurse? Do you think that being a nurse is just a job, or do you see it as a chance to change society, the healthcare system, and the lives of patients and their families?
What features made someone a successful nurse?	It is feasible to have the required clinical skills and academic background to become a nurse, but these are not the only characteristics of a successful nurse. Consider the characteristics you admire in others. What abilities would you look for in a nurse if you fell ill and need nursing care? One can consider honesty, morality, compassion, and the capacity to empathize with patients as desirable attributes.
What skills should every nurse possess?	Analyze the qualities you believe are crucial for nurses to possess and the reasons why. Consider how you might implement these abilities in your nursing practice. Effective communications, the ability to work well within a health team, critical thinking, and sound decision-making are abilities that nurses should aspire to acquire. Include the abilities you deem vital in your nursing philosophy statement as you identify them.
Why is nursing important to me?	To establish a personal nursing philosophy, it is crucial to comprehend why nursing is personally significant to you. Have you ever witnessed a nurse providing care for a friend or family member? Perhaps you were once a patient who required care and were drawn to the nurse who provided it. If you can identify a personal experience that sparked your passion in nursing, you can base your nursing philosophy on that experience and how it made you feel.
What theories do I hold towards nursing?	Nursing theories are concepts or ideas derived from knowledge that are used to define the scope of nursing practice. These theories serve as a foundation for nursing practice at all educational and understanding levels.
What values should nurses hold as paramount?	Typically, a person's personal philosophy is based on his or her conceptions about what values are essential or fundamental. What values should nurses possess, in your opinion, and why? To answer, consider how you would like to be treated as an individual. Do you want people to be truthful or manipulative with you? Are patience, compassion, and empathy essential? The qualities you admire in others are the same ones your patients would admire in you.
Would I select this profession again?	Nursing is a great profession, but there are challenging days. You may shed tears with or for patients and their family members. You may feel disappointed if a patient's prognosis is not favorable despite your best efforts. Is your love for this profession and desire to help people strong enough that you would pick this profession again in spite of the tough periods and the time you wish you could turn back the clock?

Your nursing philosophy is influenced by your thoughts, ideas, and beliefs. The following questions can help you establish your own unique nursing philosophy **(Table 1.2)**:

Write Your Own Personal Nursing Philosophy

Putting pen to paper to create a personal nursing philosophy could seem challenging. You can write your own unique nursing philosophy statement by using the stages below as a reference:

- **Describe nursing from your point of view:** Determine what nursing means to you before you start developing your nursing philosophy. Consider instances where you served as the patient. What effect did the nurses who cared for you have on your perspective on the profession?

- **Consider how your own experiences connect to your love of nursing:** Write a "narrative" about that encounter in which you elaborate on your ideas and offer insight into principles and characteristics important to nursing.
- **Think about the effect you want your work as a nurse to have on patients, families, and communities:** Think both little and big ideas simultaneously. Think about how you want to utilize nursing to encourage better patient outcomes or modifications to the way healthcare is delivered. Give some details about your goals for society and what those goals mean for you individually.
- **Emphasize your abilities:** Make a list of the talents that are most important to you and explain why you believe they are crucial. Consider how you might employ those abilities in nursing situations in the future.
- **Specify your values, both personally and professionally:** Be prepared to describe how you will use your ideals and expertise to advance your profession and bring about change.

Importance of Nursing Philosophy

It is crucial to have a personal nursing philosophy for a number of reasons. Here are seven explanations for why every nurse should think about creating a nursing philosophy.

- It acts as a guide to assist nurses in upholding the standards they have established for themselves.
- It enhances communication with patients, their families, and your fellow professionals.
- It directs the practice of nursing in an ethical, competent, evidence-based, and science-driven manner.
- It keeps you inspired when a professional difficulty arises.
- It enables nurses to recognize the theories and convictions required for regular decisions.

- Identifying strategies to demonstrate your innermost aspirations and beliefs is helpful.
- It aids in self-responsibility.

Philosophy of Nursing Examples

Florence Nightingale established a nursing concept that continues to be used today. She held that the practice of nursing should be done with the conviction that every patient has a personal, spiritual dimension and should be treated as a whole person since nursing is a spiritual calling. Florence Nightingale believed that nurses could assist patients experiencing spiritual distress since they were called to care for others and she believed in the spiritual dimension of persons.

The International Council of Nurses states nursing as "the unique function of the nurse is to assist the individual, sick or well, in the performance of those activities contributing to health or its recovery (or to peaceful death) that he would perform unaided if he had the necessary strength will or knowledge. And to do this in such a way as to help him gain independence as rapidly as possible". The International Council of Nurses has stated the following philosophy of nursing:

- We work as an interdisciplinary team to continuously enhance our own and the community's health and well-being.
- We respect and accept our patients' personal views about themselves and their environment.
- We support the professional nurse's participation in shared governance, and we include research and evidence-based practice in the formulation of care standards.

Nurses are expected to engage in interdisciplinary activities, be accountable for their profession, and pursue lifelong learning.

The Indian Nursing Council (INC) believes in the World Health Organization's (WHO) definition of health, i.e., "health is a state of complete physical, mental and social well-being and not merely the absence of disease or infirmity."

- The council acknowledged that basic nursing education is an officially accepted course of study that provides a sound, broad and basic foundation in the behavioral, life, and nursing sciences for the general practice of nursing, for a leadership role, and for the post basic education in specializations for advanced nursing practice.
- The council feels that this basic nursing course should enable nurses for entry-level nursing roles in all types of healthcare facilities.
- The council believes that nursing is affected by scientific and technological progress.
- The council believes that competence in all aspects of communication is also fundamental for nursing education and practice.
- The council also believes that, due to the nature of nursing, a substantial proportion of student learning occurs in clinical practice settings.
- The council further acknowledges the interdependence of nursing and other related professions and occupations in the promotion, prevention of diseases, diagnosis and treatment, as well as the recovery and restoration of health.
- The council considers it its obligation to assist students in nurturing a sense of pride in their profession, in addition to ensuring that they are up to date on the most recent information and trends in the profession, so that they can have a successful career in the future.

AIM AND OBJECTIVES OF NURSING SERVICING

Aims

In a broad sense, the aim of nursing practice can be summarized as the promotion of health, the prevention of illness, the restoration of health, and, last but certainly not least, the facilitation of coping with disability or death.

Promoting Health

Nursing practices can be looked at in terms of health promotion. When giving care, nurses take into account patients' level of self-awareness, health literacy, and willingness to utilize available resources. To improve health, a nurse carries out the following:

- Encouraging acceptance of personal responsibility for one's health.
- Facilitating decisions about improving their quality of life.
- Increasing health awareness by teaching certain behaviors and factors that can prevent deterioration in health.
- Encouraging health promotion by providing information and referrals.
- Teaching self-care activity to maximize achievement of goal.

Preventing Illness

- Nurse prevents illness primarily by teaching, which includes educational programs and community programs for promoting healthy habits, e.g., smoking cessation programs, stress reduction seminars, and physical fitness programs.
- Education through literatures, television, radio, and internet.

Restoring Health

The steps involved in restoring health are as follows:

- Emphasizing early disease detection for treatment and education throughout recovery.
- Promoting diagnostic measurements for early detection of disease, e.g., promotion of annual health check-ups.
- Providing direct care to person who is ill.
- Collaborating with other healthcare providers.

Facilitating Coping with Disability and Death

Altered function makes it harder for someone to perform their specific role and everyday activities. The patient's abilities and potentials can be maximized by the nurse by teaching and referring both the patient and his family to community resources during the last phase of life. Nurse prepares the patient's family for death and living as comfortably as possible until death occurs.

Objectives

Demonstrate competency in providing qualitative/comprehensive care to individual.

- Maximum comfort and happiness by way of pleasant surroundings.
- Assess the accurate nursing need of client.
- Offer high-quality nursing care to preserve the optimum level of overall health.
- Use communication skills effectively.
- Promote self-care in people under their care.
- Apply problem solving techniques in nursing practice.
- Take part in the delivery of nursing care that is promotive, preventive, curative, and rehabilitative as a member of the healthcare team.
- Mobilize community resources and their participation in community service.
- Demonstrate high ethical standards in their personal and professional conduct.
- Acknowledge the importance of lifelong learning, career advancement, and personal development.
- Demonstrate fundamental administrative and leadership abilities while collaborating with other members of the health team and the community.
- Actively involved or assist in research activities.

CHAPTER SUMMARY

1. Nursing is a profession that focuses on caring for the sick, injured, and elderly.
2. Nurses nourish, foster, and protect individuals, families, and communities.
3. A profession is characterized by specialized knowledge, professional standards, formal education, autonomy, and accountability.
4. Nursing fulfills the criteria of a profession, including essential services, a body of knowledge, intellectual activities, accountability, formal education, autonomy, altruism, and a code of ethics.
5. Philosophy refers to attempting to provide solutions to important questions about existence, knowledge, ethics, and aesthetics. Philosophy of nursing describes beliefs about the nursing profession and serves as a foundation.
6. Components of a personal nursing philosophy include role, knowledge, values, and process.
7. Developing a personal nursing philosophy involves reflecting on motivations, beliefs, values, skills, and experiences.
8. Objectives of nursing service include competency in care, assessment, communication, self-care promotion, problem-solving, collaboration, ethical conduct, lifelong learning, leadership, and research involvement.

REVIEW QUESTIONS

1. Define nursing. Discuss nursing as a profession.
2. Define philosophy of nursing'? How to develop your own personal philosophy of nursing?
3. Define Nursing philosophy and prepare your own philosophy with suitable example?
4. Enlist differences between profession and occupation. Explain characteristics of nursing profession.
5. Explains the objectives of nursing services.
6. Enlist the components of nursing philosophy.

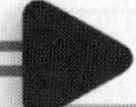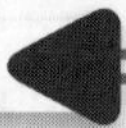

BIBLIOGRAPHY

1. 50 nursing philosophy examples + how to write your own. Available at: https://www.nursingprocess.org/nursing-philosophy-examples.html (Accessed: January 30, 2023).
2. American Association of Colleges of Nursing (AACN): Essentials of baccalaureate education for professional nursing, Washington, DC; 2008.
3. An international Electronic Journal for Exercise Physiologists, 4(5); ISSN 1099-5862. Available at: Http://www.Css.Edu/Users/Tboone2/Asep/ConstructingAprofession.Html
4. Blais KK, Hayes JS, Kozier B, Erb G. Professional nursing practice: Concepts and perspectives, 4th edition. New Jersey: Upper Saddle River, NJ; 2002.
5. Boone T. Constructing a profession, professionalization of exercise physiology; 2002.
6. Cheraghi F, Yousefzadeh MR, Goodarzi A. The role and status of philosophy in nursing knowledge, insight and competence. J Clin Res Paramed Sci. 2019;8(2):e90762.
7. Dahnke MD, Dreher HM. Philosophy of science for nursing practice: Concepts and applications, 2nd edition. New York, NY: Springer Publishing Company; 2016.
8. Doheny MO, Cook CB, Stopper MC. The discipline of nursing: An introduction, 4th edition. Stanford CT: Appleton and Lange; 1997.
9. Joel LA. Kelly's dimensions of professional nursing, 9th edition. New York: McGraw Hill/Appleton and Lange; 2003.
10. June FK, Helen SL. Developing a philosophy of nursing. New Delhi: Sage Publication, India Pvt. Ltd.; 1994.
11. Mass Medical Staffing. "How a personal philosophy of nursing can help your career." Available at: https://www.masmedicalstaffing.com/2018/03/15/personal-philosophy-of-nursing/ (March 15, 2018).
12. Mudgal SK. Assess learning needs of nursing students and effectiveness of workshop on knowledge regarding extended and expanded role of nurses. Intl J Nurs Edu. 2018; 10(3):109-13.
13. Potter PA, Perry AG, Stockert PA, Hall AM, Sharma SK. Potter and Perry's fundamentals of Nursing, 2nd edition. New Delhi: Elsevier; 2017.
14. The development of nursing as a profession. Available at: http://opac.fkik.uin-alauddin.ac.id/repository/Ch_05.pdf (Accessed: January 18, 2023).

Role and Responsibilities of a Nurse

- Articulate a comprehensive definition of what constitutes a high-quality nurse in terms of knowledge, skills, and attitudes.
- Summarize the core roles and responsibilities of a nurse upon graduating from nursing education.
- Examine how the role of a graduate nurse fits within the broader healthcare team and contributes to patient care.
- Define the concept of an expanded nursing role and its significance within the healthcare system.
- Explore specific examples of advanced nursing roles, such as nurse practitioners, clinical nurse specialists, and nurse educators.
- Identify and analyze current trends shaping the landscape of nursing practice in India.
- Examine how factors such as technological advancements, changing patient demographics, and healthcare policy reforms impact nursing care.

▮ INTRODUCTION

Nursing is a vital profession in the healthcare industry, and nurses play a crucial role in promoting and maintaining the health of individuals, families, and communities. The role of a nurse has evolved over time, and today, nurses are responsible for a wide range of tasks, including patient care, education, and advocacy. Nurses are responsible for a range of tasks, including assessing and monitoring patients, administering medications, providing wound care, and communicating with patients and their families. They also educate patients on disease prevention, health promotion, and treatment options, as well as provide emotional support and advocacy.

The primary goal of nursing practice is to provide holistic care that addresses the physical, emotional, and spiritual needs of patients. Nurses can be found in diverse work environments, ranging from hospitals and clinics to nursing homes, schools, and community settings. Nursing practice is guided by a set of ethical principles, including respect for patients' autonomy, beneficence, nonmaleficence, and justice. Nurses are also expected to practice evidence-based care, which involves using the best available research to guide clinical decision-making.

Overall, nursing is a challenging but rewarding profession that requires a high level of skill, compassion, and dedication. Nurses are an essential part of the healthcare team, and their role is critical to ensuring the well-being of patients and communities.

▮ QUALITIES OF A NURSE

There are some qualities that are generally considered important for nurses to have (**Fig. 2.1**):

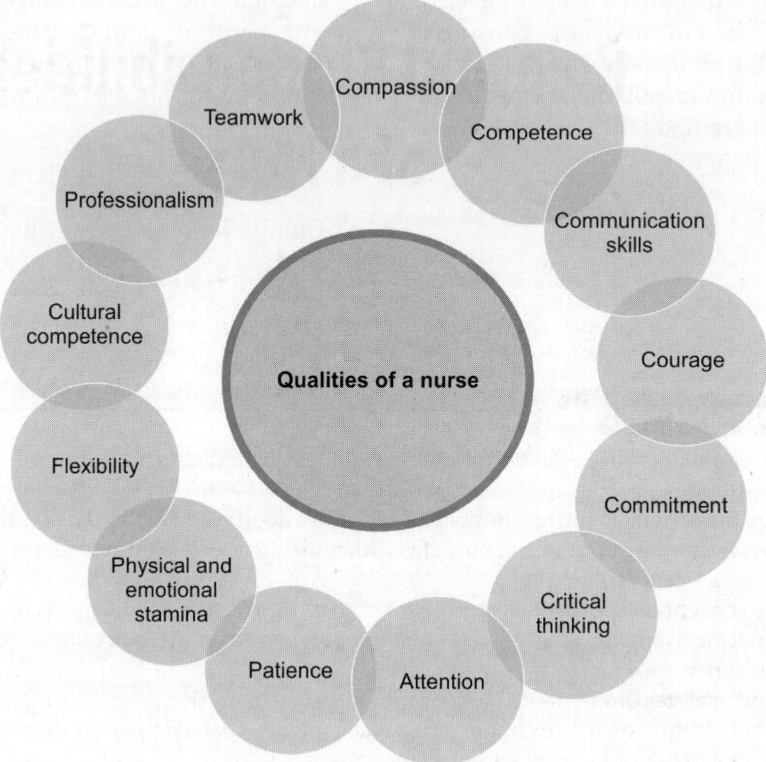

Fig. 2.1: Qualities of a nurse.

- **Compassion:** Nurses need to be able to empathize with their patients and provide them with emotional support during times of illness or distress.
- **Communication skills:** Nurses need to be able to communicate effectively with patients, their families, and other healthcare professionals.
- **Competence:** Ensuring that nursing practice is evidence-based and that nurses have the knowledge, skills, and experience to provide high-quality care.
- **Courage:** Speaking up and taking action when faced with situations that may compromise patient safety or dignity.
- **Commitment:** Being dedicated to delivering the best possible care and continually improving nursing practice through learning and development.
- **Critical thinking:** Nurses need to be able to analyze complex situations and make decisions quickly and effectively.
- **Attention to detail:** Nurses need to be detail-oriented to ensure that patient care is delivered accurately and safely.
- **Patience:** Nurses need to be patient and able to handle stress and long hours.
- **Physical and emotional stamina:** Nursing can be physically and emotionally demanding, so nurses need to have the stamina to work long hours and handle challenging situations.
- **Flexibility:** Nurses need to be flexible and adaptable to handle changes in patient conditions, staffing, and healthcare protocols.
- **Cultural competence:** Nurses need to understand and respect the cultural beliefs and values of their patients and provide care that is culturally sensitive.
- **Professionalism:** Nurses need to conduct themselves in a professional manner at all times and maintain patient confidentiality.

- **Teamwork:** Nurses need to work effectively as part of a healthcare team to ensure the best possible patient outcomes.

These qualities are all interconnected and essential for a graduate nurse to provide safe and effective patient care.

ROLE AND RESPONSIBILITIES OF A GRADUATE NURSE

Nurses hold a crucial position in the healthcare system, responsible for delivering top-notch care to patients across a diverse range of settings. The nature of a nurse's responsibilities can differ depending on their level of education, professional background, and the specific work environment they operate in. Nonetheless, some common duties and responsibilities that nurses generally undertake include:

- **Patient care:** Nurses are responsible for providing direct patient care, including assessing patient needs, developing care plans, administering medications, and monitoring vital signs.
- **Communication:** Nurses also function as intermediaries between patients, their families, and other healthcare professionals. By serving as a link between these parties, nurses ensure that patients receive the best possible care and that their needs are effectively communicated to physicians, nurse practitioners, social workers, and other healthcare providers to ensure coordinated care.
- **Health education:** One of the vital roles of nurses is to educate patients and their families about their medical conditions, treatment options, and self-care techniques that promote wellness and prevent disease. By imparting this knowledge, nurses empower patients to take an active role in their healthcare and make informed decisions that support their recovery and overall well-being.
- **Documentation:** Nurses bear the responsibility of ensuring that patient records are precise, comprehensive, and regularly updated. They must document assessments, interventions, and treatment outcomes, among other crucial patient information. By maintaining accurate records, nurses facilitate effective communication among healthcare professionals and promote quality care delivery.
- **Quality improvement:** Nurses participate in quality improvement initiatives to improve patient outcomes and promote best practices.
- **Advocacy:** Nurses advocate for their patients' needs, ensuring that they receive appropriate care and treatment and that their rights are protected.
- **Leadership:** Nurses may serve in leadership roles, overseeing the work of other nurses and providing guidance and support to less experienced staff.
- **Collaboration:** In order to deliver thorough and well-coordinated care to patients, nurses work in tandem with various healthcare personnel, including doctors, nurse practitioners, social workers, and pharmacists. Through this collaborative effort, patients receive comprehensive care that addresses their individual needs.
- **Crisis management:** Nurses are trained to identify and manage medical emergencies and crises, such as cardiac arrest, respiratory distress, and traumatic injuries.
- **Ethical decision making:** Nurses are responsible for making ethical decisions that promote patient autonomy, justice, beneficence, and nonmaleficence.
- **Counsellor:** Nurses can also serve as counsellors, offering emotional support and guidance to both patients and their loved ones. This aspect of their role helps patients cope with their medical conditions and eases the burden on their families.
- **Administrator:** Nurses can serve as administrators in healthcare organizations, managing the daily operations of healthcare facilities, managing budgets and resources, and overseeing the work of other healthcare staff.

Overall, nurses play a critical role in promoting the health and well-being of patients, advocating for their needs, and providing high-quality, evidence-based care. Nurses are essential members of the healthcare team, and their contributions are essential in ensuring optimal health outcomes for patients.

■ EXPANDED ROLE OF A NURSE

The role of a nurse has evolved significantly over time, from providing basic care to patients to taking on expanded responsibilities and roles that go beyond traditional patient care. Today, nurses play a crucial role in providing high-quality, patient-centered care, promoting health and wellness, and improving patient outcomes.

The expanded role of nurses reflects the increasing complexity of healthcare needs, as well as the recognition of the unique contributions that nurses can make to patient care and healthcare delivery. Nurses now work in a wide range of settings, from hospitals and clinics to community health centers, schools, and government agencies, and they are involved in a diverse array of activities and functions.

He expanded role of a nurse includes a range of responsibilities such as advanced clinical practice, nursing education and research, healthcare informatics, patient advocacy, healthcare administration and leadership, and more. Nurses in expanded roles are trained and equipped to provide comprehensive and holistic care that addresses the physical, emotional, social, and psychological needs of patients.

Definition of Expanded Role of a Nurse

The expanded role of a nurse refers to the range of activities and functions that nurses now perform beyond traditional patient care. This expanded role reflects the increasing complexity of healthcare needs and the recognition of the unique contributions that nurses can make to patient care and healthcare delivery.

Overall, the expanded role of a nurse reflects the ongoing evolution of healthcare and the important role that nurses play in promoting health and wellness, improving patient outcomes, and advancing the field of nursing. Some of the expanded roles of nurses include:

- **Nurse practitioner:** Nurse practitioners are skilled nurses with advanced training who offer essential healthcare services, encompassing the identification, treatment, and supervision of medical conditions. They are authorized to prescribe medications and order diagnostic tests, and they work independently or in collaboration with physicians.
- **Clinical nurse specialist (CNS):** Clinical nurse specialist is an advanced practice nursing role that involves providing specialized care to patients in a particular clinical area or specialty. Clinical nurse specialists are employed in diverse environments such as hospitals, clinics, private practices, and community. They are responsible for providing expert clinical care, consultation, education, and leadership to patients, families, and healthcare teams.
- **Nurse educator:** Nurse educators teach nursing students and healthcare professionals, developing and delivering training programs and educational materials. They may also contribute to the development of nursing curricula and conduct research in nursing education.
- **Nurse researcher:** Nurse researchers conduct scientific studies and clinical trials to advance nursing knowledge and improve patient outcomes. They may work in academic institutions, healthcare organizations, or government agencies.
- **Nurse informaticist:** Nurse informaticists are experts in healthcare information technology and data management. They design and implement electronic health records, develop data analytics tools, and ensure that healthcare data is accurate, secure, and accessible.

- **Nurse advocate:** Nurse advocates work to promote the rights and interests of patients, families, and communities. They might advocate for modifications in policies, engage in outreach initiatives within the community, or act as a go-between for patients and healthcare practitioners.
- **Nurse consultant:** Nurse consultants provide expertise and guidance to healthcare organizations, helping to develop policies, procedures, and programs that promote high-quality, patient-centered care. They may also provide advice and guidance to individual patients and families.
- **Nurse administrator:** Nurse administrators oversee the daily operations of healthcare organizations, managing budgets, staffing, and resources. They may also develop strategic plans, implement quality improvement initiatives, and ensure regulatory compliance.
- **Nurse as a change agent:** The role of nurses as change agents is critical to improving the quality of care within the healthcare system. By identifying areas for improvement, advocating for change, leading change initiatives, educating patients and families, and using technology to drive change, nurses can make a significant impact on patient outcomes and the overall quality of care.
- **Space nursing:** Involves providing healthcare services to astronauts who are in space.
- **Nurse liaisons:** Play a crucial role in serving as a connection between potential patients and rehabilitation facilities, with their responsibilities being varied.
- **Hospice nurses:** Focus on providing comprehensive physical, psychological, emotional, and spiritual care to individuals who are terminally ill, as well as their families, with the aim of promoting a high quality of life.
- **School health nurses:** Support the educational process by helping students maintain good health and teaching them preventive practices, both for themselves and their teachers.
- **Tele-nursing:** Involves providing nursing services to patients who are physically far away from the nurse, using telecommunications and information technology.
- **Cruise ship/resort nurses:** Work on ships or at resorts to provide emergency and general care to passengers, if required.
- **Nurse attorneys:** Engage in a range of legal activities, including providing legal consultation.
- **Disaster/bioterrorism:** Nurses work in disaster areas that result from bio-terrorist attacks or situations caused by natural or man-made disasters.
- **Epidemiology nurses:** Investigate trends in disease occurrence in specific areas, identifying populations at risk, monitoring disease progression, determining priorities, and identifying areas of healthcare need.
- **Sports nursing:** Which is a sub-specialty of orthopedic medicine, involves treating injuries or traumas that result from athletic training or competition.
- **Nurse authors:** Work in various areas of writing and produce material that may be used for research, education, training, and marketing purposes.
- **Nurse analysts:** They are involved in data analysis and interpretation related to the efficiency and effectiveness of data collection, entry, and utilization in healthcare facilities and hospitals.

TRENDS IN NURSING PRACTICES

The trends of nursing practice refer to the current developments, shifts, or patterns that are shaping the field of nursing and influencing how nurses deliver care. These trends can encompass a wide range of factors, including changes in healthcare policies, advancements in technology, evolving patient needs, and emerging research findings.

By understanding and adapting to these trends, nurses can enhance their practice, improve patient outcomes, and stay aligned with the evolving healthcare landscape. The trends of nursing practice provide insights into the direction in which the field is heading and highlight areas where nurses need to focus their attention and professional development.

It is essential for nurses to stay informed about these trends, as they can impact various aspects of their work, such as patient interactions, treatment approaches, documentation, collaboration with other healthcare professionals, and lifelong learning. By recognizing and embracing these trends, nurses can remain effective and responsive in providing quality care within the ever-changing healthcare environment.

Trends Influencing Nursing Practices in India

Several trends are influencing nursing practices in recent years. Here are some notable ones:

- **Increasing demand for healthcare services:** With a growing population and rising healthcare needs, there is an increasing demand for healthcare services in India. This trend puts pressure on the nursing workforce to deliver care efficiently and effectively, requiring nurses to adapt to evolving patient needs and healthcare delivery models.
- **Technological advancements:** India is witnessing rapid technological advancements in healthcare. Electronic health records (EHRs), telehealth, mobile health applications, and other digital platforms are being integrated into healthcare settings. Nurses need to embrace and leverage these technologies to enhance patient care, streamline documentation, and improve communication.
- **Emphasis on primary healthcare:** India is focusing on strengthening primary healthcare services to improve access and affordability. Nurses play a crucial role in primary healthcare, providing preventive care, health education, immunizations, and community-based services. This trend highlights the need for nurses to have a strong foundation in primary healthcare principles and skills.
- **Expansion of specialized nursing roles:** There is a growing recognition of specialized nursing roles in India. Advanced practice nursing, nurse practitioners, nurse anesthetists, and critical care nurses are being increasingly utilized in various healthcare settings. This trend offers nurses opportunities for career advancement and specialization, requiring them to acquire advanced skills and knowledge in their respective fields.
- **Quality improvement and patient safety:** There is an increased emphasis on quality improvement and patient safety in Indian healthcare. Nurses are actively involved in initiatives to enhance patient outcomes, reduce medical errors, and improve infection control practices. This trend highlights the importance of nurses' participation in quality improvement programs and their role in ensuring patient safety.
- **Evidence-based practice:** The use of evidence-based practice is gaining prominence in Indian nursing. Nurses are encouraged to incorporate the latest research evidence into their clinical decision-making and provide care based on best practices. This trend promotes a culture of lifelong learning and encourages nurses to stay updated with current research findings.
- **Global healthcare collaborations:** India is witnessing collaborations with international healthcare organizations, academic institutions, and nursing associations. These collaborations facilitate knowledge exchange, skill enhancement, and professional development opportunities for nurses. This trend opens doors for international exposure and collaboration with nurses from diverse backgrounds.
- **Chronic disease management:** The prevalence of chronic diseases such as diabetes, heart disease, and respiratory

conditions is increasing. Nurses play a vital role in managing these conditions, including patient education, lifestyle modification support, medication management, and monitoring. This trend highlights the importance of prevention, self-management, and long-term support for individuals with chronic illnesses.

- **Global health challenges:** Global health issues, such as pandemics, emerging infectious diseases, and natural disasters, have a significant impact on nursing practices. Nurses are at the forefront of responding to these challenges, providing direct patient care, infection control, vaccination campaigns, and community education. The ability to adapt to changing circumstances and implement effective public health measures is crucial in these situations.

- **Emphasis on education and training:** There is a growing emphasis on education and training in the nursing profession in India. Nurses are encouraged to pursue higher education and specialized training to improve their skills and knowledge.

- **Patient-centered care:** Patient-centered care is gaining importance in India, with an emphasis on providing care that is tailored to patients' unique needs, preferences, and values. Nurses are encouraged to involve patients in their care planning and promote patient autonomy.

- **Government initiatives:** The Indian government has launched several initiatives to improve healthcare access and quality, including the Ayushman Bharat program, which provides health insurance to vulnerable populations. Nurses play a vital role in implementing these initiatives and providing high-quality care to patients.

- **Increasing focus on mental health:** Mental health is an emerging healthcare concern in India, with rising rates of depression, anxiety, and other mental health disorders. Nurses are being trained to address these issues and provide mental health support to patients.

- **Aging population and complex care needs:** India's population is aging, leading to an increased demand for healthcare services for older adults. Nurses are facing the challenge of caring for a growing population with complex care needs, including managing multiple chronic conditions, promoting healthy aging, and addressing end-of-life care.

These trends in nursing practice in India reflect the need for nurses to adapt to changing healthcare dynamics, leverage technology, focus on primary healthcare, embrace specialized roles, promote quality improvement and patient safety, engage in evidence-based practice, and participate in global healthcare collaborations. By being aware of these trends, Indian nurses can contribute to providing high-quality, patient-centered care and positively impact the healthcare system.

CHAPTER SUMMARY

1. Nurses must have certain positive qualities such as commitment, knowledge, technical and interpersonal skills, problem-solving abilities, critical thinking, empathy, emotional strength, and advocacy, in addition to good personal characteristics.
2. Each role of a nurse involves a unique set of patterned behaviors and denotes their status or place within a specific context.

3. Defining the roles and responsibilities of nurses is important for achieving organizational objectives and meeting the needs of clients.
4. Professional nurses have multiple roles and responsibilities in various specialties, settings, and levels of nursing, including as care givers, educators, counselors, advocates, communicators, coordinators, leaders, managers, researchers, and administrators.
5. Nurses can also have expanded roles, such as clinical nurse specialists, primary care providers, partners in healthcare teams, change agents, researchers, and telenurses, which are not limited to traditional hospital settings.
6. Several trends reflect the changing healthcare landscape in India and the need for nurses to adapt to new technologies, patient-centered care, and emerging healthcare challenges. By staying informed and embracing these trends, nurses can provide high-quality care and contribute to positive patient outcomes in India.

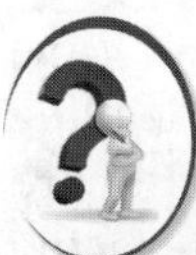

REVIEW QUESTIONS

1. Define expanded role of a nurse. Discuss expanded role of a nurse.
2. Explain role and responsibilities of a graduate nurse.
3. Describe the qualities of a nurse.
4. Explain the trends influencing nursing practice in India.

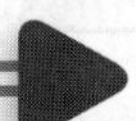 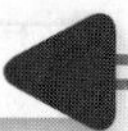

BIBLIOGRAPHY

1. Chitty KK. Professional nursing: Concepts and challenges, 2nd edition. WB Sounders company Philadelphia, Ministry of Health, Ethiopia; 1993.
2. Doheny MO, Cook CB. Stopper MC. The discipline of nursing: an introduction, 4th edition. Stanford CT: Appleton and Lange; 1997.
3. Expanded role of Nurses—Nursing Management [Internet]. Brain Kart. [cited 2023, Apr10]. Available from: https://www.brainkart.com/article/Expanded-Role-of-Nurses_37907/#:~:text=Role%20of%20 Nurses-,An%20expanded%20role%20of%20nursing%20is%20one%20in%20which%20a,cases%20 practice%20with%20greater%20autonomy.&text=Clinical%20Nurse%20specialist.&text=Nurse%20 entrepreneur.&text=Operating%20home%20Nurse
4. Kozier B, ERB G, Blais K, Wilkinson J, Leuven K. Fundamentals of nursing: Concepts, processes and practices, 5th edition. Addi son Weskley Longman, Inc, California; 1998.
5. Mudgal SK. Assess learning needs of nursing students and effectiveness of workshop on knowledge regarding extended and expanded role of nurses. Intl J Nurs Edu. 2018;10(3):109-13.
6. Potter PA, Perry AG, Stockhert PA, Hall AM, Sharma SK. Potter and Perry's fundamentals of Nursing, 2nd edition. New Delhi: Elsevier; 2017.
7. Purtilo R, Cassel C. Ethical Dimensions in the Health Professions, 1st edition. Philadelphia: WB Sounders; 2005.
8. Resnick B. Where is a good nurse when you need one? Advanced Practice Nursing eJournl. 2002;2(4). Available at: Http://Www.Medscape.Com/Viewarticle/442734
9. Royal College of Nursing. Defining Nursing. Http://Www.Rcn.Org.Uk/__data/Assets/Pdf_ file/0003/78564/001983.Pdf. [2003].
10. Tayler C, Carol L, Priscilla L. Fundamentals of nursing the art and science of nursing. care. J.b. Lippincott Company; 1999.

Nursing Education in India

☞ **Learning Objectives**

- Define education and identify its key components.
- Explain the significance of lifelong learning and its role in adapting to the changing demands of the world.
- Describe the concept of nursing education.
- Discuss the milestones for development of nursing education in India.
- Recognize the importance of nursing education in shaping the future of nursing.
- Summarize the different definitions of education provided by various thinkers and understand their perspectives on the transformative power of education.
- Discuss the goals of nursing education.
- Analyze the trends influencing nursing education.

■ INTRODUCTION

Education, in general, is a lifelong process that involves acquiring knowledge, skills, and values through formal and informal methods. It is a fundamental aspect of personal and societal development, enabling individuals to grow intellectually, socially, and professionally. When it comes to nursing education, it encompasses specialized training and preparation for individuals seeking to enter the nursing profession.

Nursing education is a unique branch of education that focuses on equipping individuals with the knowledge, skills, and competencies required to provide safe, competent, and compassionate care to patients across diverse healthcare settings. It blends theoretical knowledge with practical training, ensuring that aspiring nurses are well-prepared to meet the challenges and demands of the nursing profession.

By undergoing nursing education, individuals gain the foundation necessary to enter the nursing profession, pursue specialized areas of practice, and make a positive impact on the health and well-being of those they serve. Nursing education is a vital component of the healthcare system, shaping the future of nursing and ensuring the provision of safe, effective, and patient-centered care.

■ CONCEPT OF EDUCATION

Education encompasses a broad range of subjects and disciplines, including sciences, humanities, social sciences, arts, mathematics, and more. It promotes intellectual growth, fosters creativity, and encourages individuals to explore diverse perspectives and ideas.

Education is not limited to academic pursuits alone. It also includes the development of social, emotional, and moral competencies. Education cultivates values such as empathy, tolerance, respect, and ethical conduct, nurturing well-rounded individuals who can contribute positively to their communities and promote social justice.

Furthermore, education is not confined to a specific age group or stage of life. It begins in early childhood with foundational learning and continues throughout a person's lifetime. Lifelong learning is an integral aspect of education, encouraging individuals to continually seek new knowledge, adapt to changing circumstances, and acquire new skills to meet the evolving demands of the world.

In summary, education is a dynamic process that involves the acquisition of knowledge, skills, values, and attitudes. It prepares individuals for personal fulfillment, professional success, and active participation in society. Education equips individuals with the tools to understand, question, and shape the world around them, fostering personal growth, societal progress, and the advancement of knowledge.

DEFINITIONS OF EDUCATION

Education is a fundamental aspect of human development and societal progress. It equips individuals with the knowledge, skills, and values necessary to navigate the complexities of life, contribute meaningfully to society, and pursue personal fulfillment. Over the years, numerous thinkers, philosophers, and leaders have offered their perspectives on the essence and significance of education. These definitions shed light on the multifaceted nature of education, emphasizing its transformative power, the cultivation of character, and the pursuit of enlightenment.

- "Education is the process of facilitating learning, or the acquisition of knowledge, skills, values, beliefs, and habits. Educational methods include teaching, training, storytelling, discussion, and directed research." *—UNESCO*
- "Education is the passport to the future, for tomorrow belongs to those who prepare for it today." *—Malcolm X*
- "Education is the process of living and not the preparation for future living." *—John Dewey*
- "Education is a shared commitment between dedicated teachers, motivated students, and enthusiastic parents with high expectations." *—Bob Beauprez*
- "Education is the manifestation of perfection already in humans." *—Swami Vivekananda*
- "Education is the most powerful weapon we can use to change the world." *—Dr Sarvepalli Radhakrishnan*
- "Education is the process by which character is formed, strength of mind is increased, and intellect is sharpened, as a result of which one can stand on one's own feet." *—Dr BR Ambedkar*
- "Education is the passport to the future, for tomorrow belongs to those who prepare for it today." *—Dr APJ Abdul Kalam*
- "Education is not the amount of information that is put into your brain and runs riot there, undigested, all your life. We must have life-building, man-making, character-making assimilation of ideas." *—Rabindranath Tagore*
- "By education, I mean an all-round drawing of the best in the child and man, in body, mind, and spirit." *—Mahatma Gandhi*

NURSING EDUCATION

The concept of nursing education evolves to adapt to changes in healthcare, technology, and patient needs. It embraces innovative teaching methods, such as simulation, technology-enhanced learning, and experiential learning opportunities. Nursing education is a dynamic process that prepares individuals to enter the nursing profession and make a positive impact on the health and well-being of individuals, families, and communities.

Definitions of Nursing Education

Here are definitions of nursing education by different authors:

- "Nursing education is the systematic process of preparing individuals to become professional nurses capable of providing comprehensive, safe, and effective care to individuals, families, and communities."
  —*National League for Nursing (NLN)*
- "Nursing education is the process of developing the knowledge, skills, and attitudes necessary to practice nursing competently and ethically in a variety of settings."   —*Judith M Wilkinson*
- "Nursing education is the cultivation of students' abilities to think critically, communicate effectively, and provide safe and compassionate care to patients using evidence-based practice."
  —*Diane M Billings*
- "Nursing education is a dynamic and lifelong process that prepares individuals to practice nursing, engage in ongoing professional development, and adapt to the changing healthcare landscape."
  —*Patricia S Yoder-Wise*
- "Nursing education is a deliberate and structured process that facilitates the development of competent nursing professionals who are prepared to meet the complex healthcare needs of individuals and communities."   —*Joyce J Fitzpatrick*

These definitions reflect the importance of preparing nursing students to deliver safe, effective, and patient-centered care while emphasizing the need for ongoing professional growth and adaptability in the ever-changing healthcare environment.

Goals of Nursing Education

The goals of nursing education encompass a wide range of objectives aimed at preparing individuals to enter the nursing profession and provide high-quality, safe, and compassionate care to patients. These goals include:

- **Develop a strong foundation of knowledge:** Nursing education aims to provide students with a comprehensive understanding of the biological, physical, and social sciences relevant to nursing practice. This includes knowledge of anatomy, physiology, pharmacology, pathophysiology, and other health-related disciplines.
- **Develop clinical competence:** Nursing education aims to provide students with the knowledge, skills, and clinical competence required to deliver safe and effective nursing care. Students learn essential nursing skills, such as patient assessment, medication administration, wound care, and therapeutic interventions, in simulated and real healthcare settings.
- **Foster critical thinking and clinical reasoning:** Nursing education emphasizes the development of critical thinking and clinical reasoning abilities. Students learn to analyze complex situations, make sound judgments, and apply evidence-based practices to provide optimal care for patients. They are taught to evaluate information, consider various perspectives, and solve problems encountered in nursing practice.
- **Cultivate professionalism and ethical practice:** Nursing education instils professionalism and ethical conduct in students. They learn to uphold ethical principles, respect patient autonomy, maintain confidentiality, and advocate for the rights and well-being of patients. Students are taught to adhere to professional standards, demonstrate accountability, and work collaboratively within interdisciplinary healthcare teams.
- **Promote patient-centered care:** Nursing education focuses on the importance of patient-centered care. Students learn to recognize and respect the unique needs, preferences, and values of patients and their families. They are trained to

communicate effectively, develop therapeutic relationships, and engage in shared decision-making to ensure the delivery of care that is responsive to individual patient needs.

- **Foster cultural sensitivity and diversity:** Nursing education promotes cultural competence and sensitivity to diverse populations. Students learn about different cultural, religious, and social backgrounds to deliver culturally appropriate care. They are educated on the importance of addressing health disparities, advocating for equity, and providing inclusive care to individuals from various backgrounds.
- **Promote lifelong learning and professional development:** Nursing education encourages students to embrace lifelong learning and ongoing professional development. They are introduced to the concept of evidence-based practice, research methodologies, and the importance of staying updated with advancements in healthcare. Students are equipped with the skills to critically appraise research findings, integrate new knowledge into practice, and contribute to the advancement of nursing knowledge through research.
- **Prepare for leadership roles:** Nursing education aims to prepare students for leadership positions in healthcare. They develop skills in healthcare management, delegation, and decision-making. Students are encouraged to take on leadership roles, advocate for change, and contribute to quality improvement initiatives within healthcare organizations.
- **Promote evidence-based practice:** Nursing education aims to promote the use of evidence-based practice in nursing care. This includes an understanding of research methodology and the ability to critically evaluate and apply research findings to clinical practice.

- **Develop communication and inter-personal skills:** Nursing education aims to promote the development of communication and interpersonal skills necessary for effective collaboration with patients, families, and healthcare team members.

Overall, the goals of nursing education revolve around equipping students with the knowledge, skills, values, and attitudes necessary to provide competent, patient-centered, and ethical care. It aims to prepare them for the challenges of nursing practice, instil a commitment to lifelong learning, and cultivate leaders who can contribute to the advancement of the nursing profession.

DEVELOPMENT OF NURSING EDUCATION IN INDIA

The development of nursing education in India has undergone significant transformations over the years. It has evolved from a rudimentary form of training to a structured and comprehensive system that prepares nurses to deliver safe and competent care across diverse healthcare settings. The development of nursing education in India can be traced through the following key stages:

- **Late 19th Century:** The British colonial rulers established some of the earliest nursing schools in India to train local women as nurses. The focus was on providing basic nursing skills to serve in hospitals.
- **Early 20th Century:**
  - The Lady Reading Health School (currently known as the Rajkumari Amrit Kaur College of Nursing) was founded in Delhi in 1916, making it one of the oldest nursing schools in India.
  - The Trained Nurses Association of India (TNAI) was established in 1908, playing a crucial role in advocating for nursing education and professional development.

- **1920s–1940s:** Several nursing schools were established across the country, primarily associated with hospitals and missionary organizations.
- **1947:** The Indian Nursing Council (INC) was established as a statutory body under the Indian Nursing Council Act, 1947. It became responsible for setting standards and regulating nursing education in India.
- **1950s–1960s:**
  - The development of nursing education saw a significant shift, with the introduction of formal education and integration of science subjects into nursing curricula.
  - Diploma in General Nursing and Midwifery (GNM) became the standard nursing qualification, providing a three-year training program.
- **1960s–1970s:**
  - The first Bachelor of Science in Nursing (BSc Nursing) program was introduced in India in the 1960s, aimed at preparing nurse graduates with a broader understanding of healthcare.
  - Nurse practitioners and specialized nursing roles began to emerge in areas like psychiatric nursing and community health nursing.
- **1980s–1990s:**
  - Master's programs in nursing (MSc Nursing) were established, offering specialization in various nursing disciplines.
  - Private nursing colleges and institutions started to emerge, contributing to the growth of nursing education.
- **2000s:**
  - The focus on competency-based education gained prominence, emphasizing specific skills and abilities required for nursing practice.
  - The Indian Nursing Council revised nursing curricula to align with international standards, promoting evidence-based practice and research.
- **2010s:**
  - Doctoral programs in nursing (PhD Nursing) were introduced in India, encouraging nursing research and academic advancement.
  - Partnerships and collaborations with international nursing institutions increased, providing opportunities for exchange programs and research collaborations.
- **Recent Years:**
  - Technology-enhanced learning and simulation-based education were integrated into nursing curricula to enhance practical training and critical thinking skills.
  - The emphasis on continuing professional development and lifelong learning became more significant, encouraging nurses to pursue further education and specialization.

It is important to note that the development of nursing education in India is an ongoing process, continuously adapting to the changing healthcare landscape and addressing the healthcare needs of the population. The nursing profession continues to play a vital role in India's healthcare system, and nursing education remains critical in producing skilled and competent nurses to meet the healthcare challenges of the country.

TRENDS INFLUENCING NURSING EDUCATION

Trends in nursing education reflect the evolving needs of the healthcare industry, advancements in technology, and changes in patient demographics. These trends shape the way nursing education programs are designed and delivered. There are several key trends that are influencing nursing education. These trends reflect the changing healthcare landscape, advancements in technology, and evolving patient needs. Here are some of the significant trends influencing nursing education:

- **Emphasis on interprofessional education (IPE):** There is a growing recognition of the importance of collaborative practice in healthcare. Nursing education is integrating interprofessional education, bringing together students from different healthcare disciplines, such as medicine, pharmacy, and social work, to foster teamwork, communication, and a patient-centered approach to care.
- **Integration of technology:** Technology is playing an increasingly prominent role in nursing education. Simulation labs, virtual reality, and other technological tools are being utilized to provide realistic clinical scenarios, enhance critical thinking skills, and improve clinical decision-making. Online learning platforms and mobile applications are also being used to deliver educational content and facilitate remote learning.
- **Shift toward competency-based education:** Nursing education is shifting towards a competency-based approach, focusing on the attainment of specific skills and abilities. This approach ensures that graduates possess the necessary competencies to provide safe and effective care. Competency-based education allows for individualized learning, assessment, and progression based on demonstrated abilities.
- **Emphasis on cultural competence and diversity:** With the increasing diversity of patient populations, nursing education is placing a greater emphasis on cultural competence. Students are being taught to provide culturally sensitive care, recognize and address health disparities, and promote equitable healthcare for all individuals, regardless of their cultural background.
- **Focus on population health and community-based care:** Nursing education is aligning with the shift in healthcare towards a population health approach and community-based care.

Students are being educated on the social determinants of health, health promotion, disease prevention, and the importance of addressing the health needs of communities.
- **Advancements in evidence-based practice:** Nursing education is promoting the integration of evidence-based practice into clinical decision-making. Students are taught to critically appraise research findings, apply evidence-based guidelines and interventions, and contribute to the generation of nursing knowledge through research.
- **Lifelong learning and professional development:** The concept of lifelong learning and continuing professional development is gaining prominence in nursing education. Programs are emphasizing the importance of ongoing learning, encouraging nurses to pursue advanced degrees, certifications, and engage in continuous professional development throughout their careers.
- **Leadership and management skills:** Nursing education is recognizing the need to prepare nurses for leadership and management roles in healthcare. Courses and experiences are being incorporated to develop leadership, organizational, and management skills, enabling nurses to effectively contribute to the administration and management of healthcare organizations.
- **Increased research and evidence-based practice:** Nursing education is placing a greater emphasis on research and evidence-based practice. Students are being taught how to critically appraise research findings, conduct research studies, and apply evidence-based approaches to patient care. This empowers nurses to contribute to the development of nursing knowledge and improve patient outcomes.
- **Global perspective and international experiences:** Nursing education

is increasingly incorporating a global perspective. Programs are offering opportunities for international exchanges, cultural immersion experiences, and collaborations with nursing institutions worldwide. These experiences promote cultural awareness, global health understanding, and prepare nurses to work in diverse healthcare settings.

These trends in nursing education reflect the need to adapt to the changing healthcare environment and equip nursing students with the knowledge, skills, and competencies required to provide high-quality, patient-centered care in a variety of settings. By embracing these trends, nursing education can prepare future nurses to meet the evolving needs of patients and communities.

CHAPTER SUMMARY

1. Education as a lifelong process that involves acquiring knowledge, skills, and values through formal and informal methods.
2. Education is essential for personal and societal development, fostering intellectual, social, and professional growth.
3. Nursing education equips individuals with the knowledge, skills, and competencies needed to provide safe and compassionate care to patients in various healthcare settings.
4. Nursing education combines theoretical knowledge with practical training, preparing aspiring nurses to meet the challenges of the profession.
5. Various definitions of education and nursing education from renowned authors and organizations, highlighting the transformative power and significance of education in shaping individuals and society.
6. The goals of nursing education are outlined, focusing on developing a strong knowledge foundation, clinical competence, critical thinking, professionalism, patient-centered care, cultural sensitivity, and lifelong learning.
7. Current trends influencing nursing education worldwide include interprofessional education, the integration of technology, competency-based learning, cultural competence, population health focus, evidence-based practice, and the importance of leadership and international experiences.

REVIEW QUESTIONS

1. Define education and discuss the significance of nursing education as a lifelong process.
2. Define nursing education and explain the goals of nursing education.
3. Discuss the evolution of nursing education in India.
4. Analyze the trends influencing nursing education.

BIBLIOGRAPHY

1. Bakshi S. History and evolution of nursing education in India. Indian J Palliat Care. 2014;20(1):3-7.
2. Bloomfield JG, Jones A, Jackson D. A new era for nursing education: From challenge comes change. Nurse Educ Pract. 2018;30:79-80.
3. Douglas MK, Rosenkoetter M, Pacquiao DF, Callister LC, Hattar-Pollara M, Lauderdale J, et al. Guidelines for implementing culturally competent nursing care. J Transcult Nurs. 2017;28(4):317-33.
4. Gilmartin MJ. Leadership and management skills in nursing and healthcare: An action research project. J Nurs Manag. 2017;25(1):65-72.
5. Gulliver P, Towell A, March L. Global perspectives in nursing education: The internationalising of nursing curricula. Nurse Educ Today. 2017;50:1-3.
6. Indian Nursing Council (INC). (n.d.). About INC. Retrieved from http://www.indiannursingcouncil.org/about.php.
7. Kulbok PA, Thatcher E, Park E, Meszaros PS. Evolving public health nursing roles: Focus on community participatory health promotion and prevention. The Online J Issues Nurs. 2018;23(3):10.
8. Leary S, Baker P, Reynolds J, Poland F, Fox A. Recognising and managing the deteriorating patient in hospital: A systematic review. Br J Nurs. 2018;27(12):694-700.
9. Melnyk BM, Fineout-Overholt E. Evidence-based Practice in Nursing and Healthcare: A Guide to Best Practice, 4th edition. Wolters Kluwer; 2018.
10. National League for Nursing (NLN). (2020). Nursing Education Perspectives. https://www.nln.org/publications/nursing-education-perspectives.
11. Oermann MH, Gaberson KB. Evaluation and testing in nursing education, 5th edition. Springer Publishing Company; 2018.
12. Patel RR, Mullan PB, Gardner JR. The impact of interprofessional education in healthcare on students' attitudes toward collaboration. J Clin Nurs. 2018;27(1-2):e203-e16.
13. Rajkumari Amrit Kaur College of Nursing. (n.d.). About Us. Retrieved from http://www.rakcon.com/about-us.aspx.
14. Reddy P. Trends in nursing education: A reflection from India. J Nurs Care. 2016;5(6):1-3.
15. Sahu M. Emerging trends in nursing education in India. Int. J Health Sci. 2019;7(3):15-20.

Professional Organizations and Regulatory Bodies

☞ Learning Objectives

- Define the concept of professional organizations in the context of nursing.
- Outline the purpose and significance of professional nursing organizations in advancing the nursing profession and advocating for nurses' interests.
- Identify and describe key international nursing organizations for Nursing and Midwifery.
- Discuss the missions, objectives, and activities of these organizations in promoting global nursing standards, research, education, and policy development.
- List and provide an overview of prominent national nursing organizations within the participant's country or region.
- Define regulatory bodies in nursing and describe the functions and responsibilities of regulatory bodies.

INTRODUCTION

Professional organizations play a vital role in shaping and advancing various fields and professions, including healthcare. These organizations bring together professionals within a specific field, providing them with a platform to collaborate, share knowledge, advocate for their profession, and promote professional development. They serve as a collective voice for the profession, working towards the improvement of standards, ethics, and quality of practice. Professional organizations also provide valuable resources, networking opportunities, and continuing education to their members.

CONCEPT OF PROFESSIONAL ORGANIZATION IN NURSING

The concept of a professional organization in nursing is based on the understanding that nursing is a distinct and specialized profession with unique knowledge, skills, and responsibilities. These organizations provide a platform for nurses to come together, collaborate, and address common issues and challenges they face in their practice.

Professional organizations serve as a unifying force within a profession, fostering collaboration, promoting excellence, and advocating for the best interests of professionals and the communities they serve. They play a crucial role in advancing the profession, ensuring the highest standards of practice, and supporting the professional growth and development of their members.

MEANING OF PROFESSIONAL ORGANIZATION IN NURSING

A professional organization in nursing refers to an association or society that represents and serves the interests of nurses and the nursing profession as a whole. These organizations are dedicated to advancing nursing practice, promoting professional development, and advocating for the well-being of nurses and the quality of patient care.

The meaning of a professional organization in nursing encompasses several key aspects:

- **Representation:** Professional nursing organizations represent the collective voice of nurses. They advocate for the profession at local, national, and international levels, influencing healthcare policies, regulations, and practices that impact nurses and patient care. These organizations provide a unified voice to address concerns and promote the interests of the nursing profession.

- **Professional development:** Professional nursing organizations play a crucial role in promoting ongoing professional development among nurses. They offer educational resources, conferences, seminars, and workshops to enhance nursing knowledge, skills, and competencies. These organizations provide opportunities for networking, mentorship, and career advancement, supporting nurses throughout their professional journey.

- **Standards and ethics:** Nursing organizations establish and uphold professional standards and ethical guidelines that guide nursing practice. They develop codes of ethics that outline the ethical principles and behaviors expected of nurses. These organizations contribute to the development and dissemination of evidence-based practice guidelines, ensuring that nurses deliver safe, competent, and ethical care.

- **Collaboration and networking:** Professional nursing organizations foster collaboration and networking among nurses. They provide platforms for nurses to connect with peers, share best practices, and engage in interprofessional collaboration. Through these interactions, nurses can exchange knowledge, ideas, and experiences, promoting professional growth and innovation in nursing practice.

- **Advocacy:** Nursing organizations advocate for the well-being of nurses and the profession as a whole. They address issues such as nurse staffing, workplace safety, nurse-patient ratios, and the recognition of nursing as a critical profession. These organizations work towards creating supportive work environments, improving working conditions, and ensuring that nurses have a voice in decision-making processes.

In summary, professional organizations in nursing are dedicated to advancing the nursing profession, supporting the professional development of nurses, promoting standards of practice and ethics, and advocating for the well-being of nurses and the quality of patient care. They serve as a collective force that brings nurses together, empowering them to contribute to the growth and advancement of the nursing profession.

PROFESSIONAL NURSING ORGANIZATIONS

There are many professional nursing organizations worldwide that cater to the unique needs and interests of nurses in specific countries or regions. Here are some notable professional organizations in the field of nursing:

International Professional Organizations

The International Council of Nurses

The International Council of Nurses (ICN) is a federation of national nursing associations that represents nurses worldwide. It was founded in 1899 and is headquartered in Geneva, Switzerland. The ICN is the global voice of nursing and works to promote and advance nursing education, practice, and policies to improve healthcare outcomes.

The ICN organizes the International Council of Nurses Congress, which is held every four years, bringing together nurses from around the world to share research findings, innovative practices, and discuss issues of global importance to nursing and health care.

The ICN also collaborates with other international organizations, such as the World Health Organization (WHO), to promote nursing's role in achieving global health goals and addressing health disparities.

Vision of the International Council of Nurses

The vision of the International Council of Nurses (ICN) is to work towards a healthy world through the advancement of nursing and healthcare. The ICN envisions a future where the nursing profession plays a central role in promoting and achieving health for all individuals, families, and communities.

The ICN's vision encompasses the following key elements:

- **Universal access to quality healthcare:** The ICN envisions a world where every individual has equitable access to quality healthcare services. This includes ensuring that nursing care is accessible and available to all, regardless of their socio-economic status, geographical location, or cultural background. The vision emphasizes the importance of healthcare systems that prioritize primary healthcare, prevention, health promotion, and the provision of comprehensive, holistic care.
- **Empowered and respected nursing profession:** The ICN aims to empower and elevate the nursing profession to its full potential. The vision recognizes the critical role that nurses play in healthcare delivery, advocating for the rights of nurses, and promoting their professional growth and development. It emphasizes the need for nursing to be recognized and valued as a key profession, with nurses having the authority, resources, and support to provide safe, evidence-based, and person-centered care.
- **Collaborative and interprofessional practice:** The ICN envisions a future where healthcare is delivered through collaborative and interprofessional practice. The vision recognizes the importance of teamwork, communication, and partnerships among healthcare professionals to provide coordinated and integrated care. It highlights the value of interprofessional collaboration in improving health outcomes, enhancing patient safety, and optimizing healthcare delivery.
- **Leadership and advocacy:** The ICN's vision includes fostering nursing leadership and advocacy at all levels of healthcare. The vision emphasizes the need for nurses to be actively involved in shaping healthcare policies, contributing to decision-making processes, and advocating for the health needs and rights of individuals and populations. It envisions nurses as leaders in healthcare organizations, policy development, and the advancement of evidence-based practice.
- **Ethical and culturally sensitive care:** The ICN's vision encompasses the provision of ethical, culturally sensitive, and compassionate care. The vision recognizes the importance of respecting individuals' autonomy, rights, and cultural beliefs in healthcare delivery. It emphasizes the need for nursing care that is rooted in ethical principles, human rights, and social justice, promoting dignity, equality, and inclusivity for all.

The vision of the ICN serves as a guiding principle for its work, advocacy efforts, and collaborations with national nursing associations, governments, and international organizations. It drives the ICN's commitment to advancing nursing practice, improving healthcare outcomes, and working towards a healthier world for all.

Functions of the International Council of Nurses

The International Council of Nurses (ICN) serves several key functions to support and advance the nursing profession worldwide. These functions include:

- **Representation:** The ICN represents nurses and nursing associations at the global level. It serves as a unified voice for the nursing profession, advocating for its interests, concerns, and contributions in international forums, conferences, and policy-making processes. The ICN ensures that nursing perspectives are included in global health discussions and decisions.

- **Advocacy:** The ICN advocates for the rights, interests, and welfare of nurses globally. It works to ensure that the unique perspectives and contributions of nurses are recognized and incorporated into healthcare policies, legislation, and decision-making processes. The ICN promotes nursing as a vital profession and seeks to address issues related to working conditions, professional development, and nursing leadership.

- **Leadership and professional development:** The ICN supports the development of nursing leadership and promotes the professional growth of nurses. It provides opportunities for nurses to enhance their knowledge, skills, and competencies through educational programs, conferences, workshops, and networking events. The ICN fosters leadership development at all levels, from frontline nurses to nursing administrators and policymakers.

- **Standards and guidelines:** The ICN plays a crucial role in developing and promoting evidence-based standards, guidelines, and best practices for nursing education, practice, and regulation. It collaborates with nursing experts and organizations to establish guidelines that ensure safe, effective, and ethical nursing care. The ICN also contributes to the development of global nursing curricula, competency frameworks, and ethical codes.

- **Knowledge sharing and capacity building:** The ICN facilitates the exchange of knowledge, best practices, and experiences among nurses globally. It promotes the dissemination of evidence-based research, guidelines, and innovations in nursing through publications, conferences, workshops, and online platforms. The ICN also supports capacity building by offering educational programs, training opportunities, and professional development resources for nurses and nursing associations.

- **Collaboration and networking:** The ICN serves as a global platform for collaboration, networking, and knowledge exchange among nurses and nursing associations worldwide. It fosters partnerships and alliances with other international healthcare organizations, governments, and stakeholders to address global health challenges, promote nursing leadership, and influence health policy.

- **Global health advocacy:** The ICN actively participates in global health initiatives and advocates for the central role of nursing in achieving global health goals. It collaborates with international organizations like the World Health Organization (WHO) to ensure that nursing perspectives are considered in global health strategies, programs, and policies. The ICN works towards addressing health disparities, promoting health equity, and advancing the health of populations worldwide.

- **Research and evidence-based practice:** The ICN supports nursing research and the use of evidence-based practice to enhance healthcare outcomes. It promotes research funding, provides research grants, and encourages the integration of research findings into nursing education and practice. The ICN advocates for the importance of research in informing nursing policies and improving the delivery of quality care.

- **Ethics and professional conduct:** The ICN promotes ethical standards and professional conduct among nurses globally. It develops ethical codes and guidelines that guide nurses' behavior, ensuring the provision of compassionate, culturally sensitive, and patient-centered care. The ICN supports initiatives to strengthen nurses' awareness of ethical principles and their application in practice.

These functions collectively contribute to the ICN's mission of advancing nursing and improving health outcomes globally. By providing a unified voice for nurses worldwide, the ICN empowers the profession and supports its growth, recognition, and impact on healthcare systems and the well-being of individuals and communities.

The International Confederation of Midwives

The International Confederation of Midwives (ICM) is a global organization that represents midwives and promotes the profession of midwifery worldwide. Established in 1954, the ICM is a federation of national midwifery associations and represents midwives from over 140 countries. The ICM works to strengthen the role of midwives in maternal and new born health and advocates for the rights of women and new born to receive quality midwifery care.

The International Confederation of Midwives plays a vital role in advocating for midwives, promoting quality midwifery care, and strengthening the profession worldwide. Through its activities, the ICM works towards ensuring that women and new born receive safe, respectful, and evidence-based care during pregnancy, childbirth, and the postpartum period.

Vision of the International Confederation of Midwives

The vision of the International Confederation of Midwives (ICM) is to strive for a world where every childbearing person has access to a midwife's care for a safe and fulfilling birth experience. The ICM envisions a future where midwives are recognized as autonomous and respected professionals, working in partnership with women and their families to ensure the best possible outcomes for maternal and newborn health.

The ICM's vision encompasses the following key elements:

- **Universal access to midwifery care:** The ICM envisions a world where all individuals, regardless of their geographical location or socio-economic background, have equitable access to midwifery care throughout their reproductive journey. This includes access to prenatal care, skilled attendance during childbirth, postnatal care, and comprehensive sexual and reproductive healthcare services.

- **Safe and fulfilling birth experiences:** The ICM aims to promote and facilitate safe and fulfilling birth experiences for women and their families. This vision emphasizes the importance of respectful, woman-centered care that supports the physical, emotional, and cultural needs of childbearing individuals. The ICM advocates for evidence-based practices, informed decision-making, and continuity of care to enhance the overall birth experience.

- **Recognition and autonomy of midwives:** The ICM envisions a future where midwives are recognized as essential healthcare professionals and valued members of the healthcare team. This includes acknowledging midwives' expertise, skills, and unique role in providing primary healthcare to women and newborns. The vision encompasses the empowerment of midwives to practice autonomously and contribute to policy-making, shaping healthcare systems, and advocating for the needs and rights of childbearing individuals.

- **Collaboration and partnerships:** The ICM recognizes the importance of collaboration and partnerships to achieve its vision. This involves fostering strong collaborations with governments, international organizations, healthcare providers, and communities to strengthen midwifery services, advocate for policy changes, and improve maternal and newborn health outcomes. The vision embraces a multidisciplinary approach, recognizing the value of collaboration among healthcare professionals to ensure comprehensive and integrated care for women and newborns.

- **Equity and social justice:** The ICM's vision encompasses a commitment to equity and social justice in maternal and newborn healthcare. This involves addressing disparities and inequalities in access to quality care, advocating for the rights of marginalized populations, and striving for equitable health outcomes for all individuals. The vision emphasizes the importance of culturally sensitive care and a human rights-based approach to midwifery practice.

The vision of the ICM serves as a guiding principle for its activities and initiatives, shaping its advocacy efforts, policy development, and capacity-building programs to improve the lives of childbearing individuals and promote the profession of midwifery worldwide.

Functions of the International Confederation of Midwives

The International Confederation of Midwives (ICM) performs several important functions to support and advance the profession of midwifery globally. These functions include:

- Representation and Advocacy for midwives at the global level.
- Promotion and development of Professional Standards and Education in midwifery.
- Facilitation of knowledge sharing and best practices among midwives worldwide.
- Capacity building and leadership development for midwives.
- Support for research and evidence-based practice in midwifery.
- Collaboration with global partners and stakeholders to advance maternal and new born health.

These functions collectively contribute to the ICM's mission of promoting and advancing the profession of midwifery globally, advocating for the rights of women and new born to receive quality midwifery care, and improving maternal and new born health outcomes.

The International Federation of Perioperative Nurses

The formation of the federation was initiated in 1997, and it was launched officially in July 1999. The IFPN is a "federation of national perioperative nurses' associations or an equivalent nurses group affiliated to the official nurse's organization of the member country, and which are in compliance with its constitution and have been formally admitted to membership".

The International Federation of Perioperative Nurses (IFPN) is a global organization dedicated to actively promoting perioperative nursing. The IFPN serves as a platform for perioperative nurses from different countries to collaborate, share knowledge, and promote excellence in perioperative nursing practice. The IFPN mission is "to support perioperative nurses working towards improving patient care globally; by promoting a safe surgical experience for patients, through evidence-based best researched practice standards and education, together with member organizations and other relevant collaborators".

Functions of the International Federation of Perioperative Nurses

The International Federation of Perioperative Nurses (IFPN) functions to promote and advance the specialty of perioperative nursing on a global scale. While specific functions may vary, here are some common areas of focus for organizations like the IFPN:

- **Professional development:** The IFPN aims to support the professional development of perioperative nurses by providing educational resources, organizing conferences and workshops, and facilitating networking opportunities. This helps perioperative nurses enhance their knowledge and skills, stay updated with the latest developments in perioperative care, and promote best practices in their respective settings.
- **Standards and guidelines:** The IFPN contributes to the development and

dissemination of standards, guidelines, and evidence-based practices in perioperative nursing. These resources provide a framework for perioperative nurses to deliver safe and quality care to patients undergoing surgical procedures. The IFPN may collaborate with national nursing organizations and other professional bodies to develop and endorse these standards.

- **Advocacy and representation:** The IFPN serves as an advocate for perioperative nurses and the perioperative nursing profession at a global level. It may engage in activities aimed at raising awareness about the importance of perioperative nursing, advocating for the rights and interests of perioperative nurses, and promoting the role of perioperative nursing in healthcare systems.
- **Research and innovation:** The IFPN promotes research in perioperative nursing and encourages evidence-based practice. It may support research initiatives, facilitate collaboration among researchers, and disseminate research findings to improve perioperative care outcomes. The organization may also foster innovation in perioperative nursing, exploring new technologies, techniques, and approaches that enhance patient safety and surgical outcomes.
- **Collaboration and partnerships:** The IFPN collaborates with national and international nursing organizations, surgical associations, and other healthcare stakeholders to strengthen perioperative nursing globally. This includes sharing knowledge and best practices, collaborating on projects and initiatives, and advocating for the recognition and inclusion of perioperative nursing in healthcare policies and frameworks.

In summary, the IFPN works toward improving patient care by promoting, preserving, and advancing the role of perioperative nurses in member organizations.

It is engaged actively in providing educational opportunities and support to perioperative nurses and assisting with humanitarian perioperative nursing projects. The organization seeks collaborative partnerships with recognized international nurse and health care organizations to achieve its mission.

Indian Professional Nursing Organizations

The Trained Nurses Association of India

The Trained Nurses Association of India (TNAI) is a professional organization representing nurses in India. Established in 1908, TNAI has a long-standing history of promoting the nursing profession and advocating for the rights and welfare of nurses across the country. It serves as a platform for nurses to come together, collaborate, and contribute to the advancement of nursing practice, education, and research. TNAI plays a crucial role in promoting the interests and welfare of nurses, as well as advancing the nursing profession in the country.

Functions of the Trained Nurses Association of India

Here are some key aspects and functions of the Trained Nurses Association of India:

- Representing and advocating for the interests and welfare of nurses in India.
- Promoting professional development through educational programs, conferences, and workshops.
- Establishing and disseminating nursing standards and best practices.
- Engaging in policy discussions and initiatives related to nursing and healthcare in India.
- Facilitating collaboration and networking among nurses across the country.
- Supporting continuing education and research activities for nurses.
- Publishing journals, newsletters, and other publications to share knowledge and information.

- Providing a platform for nurses to showcase their work and contribute to the nursing profession.
- Addressing issues related to working conditions, remuneration, and career progression for nurses.
- Promoting the value and recognition of nursing in Indian society.
- Fostering unity and camaraderie among nurses through professional activities and initiatives.

Overall, the Trained Nurses Association of India (TNAI) plays a vital role in advancing the nursing profession in India. It strives to uphold the professional integrity and well-being of nurses, enhance the quality of patient care, and contribute to the overall development of the healthcare system in the country.

The Student Nurses' Association of India

Under the aegis of TNAI, the Student Nurses' Association of India (SNAI) is an affiliated association of student nurses. The fundamental motivation for the founding of SNAI was to protect the dignity and foster a sense of belonging among students with professional ethics.

SNAI was founded in 1929 in Madras during the TNAI Annual Conference. The first Honorary Organizing Secretary of SNAI was Miss L Rina Jeans, Nursing Superintendent at Government General Hospital in Madras. The General Hospital in Madras became home to the first SNA unit. Delhi hosted the first SNA Annual Conference in November 1932. In 1951, the first one day SNA Conference took place, and in 1961, Nagpur hosted the inaugural biennial SNA Conference.

Objectives

- To foster a sense of teamwork among students in pursuit of a common objective;
- To assist students in upholding the dignity of the profession.
- To aid students in developing a sense of professional ethics.

- To promote students' adoption of a positive outlook on the nursing profession
- To promote the students' overall growth by helping them acquire leadership qualities and strong communication abilities.
- To inspire students to take part in and compete in a range of events at regional, state, and international conferences.

Activities of SNA

To accomplish the goals of the association, the SNAI members are given a variety of tasks at different levels. At the unit, state, and national levels, the professional, educational, social, cultural, and recreational activities are set up to strengthen their curriculum and co-curricular components. One of the crucial activities that offers a venue for the members to discuss and find answers for the many issues faced by the students is the organization of conferences and meetings at all levels. Here are some common activities carries out by SNAI:

- **Educational workshops and seminars:** SNA organizes workshops and seminars to enhance the knowledge and skills of student nurses. These sessions may cover various topics such as clinical skills, evidence-based practice, nursing ethics, and professional development.
- **Conferences and conventions:** SNA may hold conferences or conventions where student nurses can attend lectures, presentations, and panel discussions by nursing professionals. These events provide opportunities for networking, learning about new research and innovations, and gaining insights into current trends in the nursing field.
- **Community outreach programs:** SNA often engages in community outreach programs to serve the community and raise awareness about health-related issues. This can involve organizing health camps, participating in health fairs, conducting health education sessions, or volunteering at local healthcare facilities.
- **Professional development programs:** SNA may offer programs and resources to

support the professional development of student nurses. This can include resume-building workshops, interview preparation sessions, career counseling, and mentorship programs where experienced nurses guide and advise student nurses.

- **Health promotion initiatives:** SNA may initiate health promotion campaigns targeting specific health concerns in the community. This can involve organizing awareness campaigns, conducting health screenings, promoting healthy lifestyles, and disseminating information about preventive healthcare measures.
- **Collaboration with nursing organizations:** SNA often collaborates with larger nursing organizations, such as state or national nursing associations, to advocate for the rights and interests of student nurses. This can involve participating in advocacy efforts, attending meetings or conferences, and staying updated on policy developments related to nursing education.
- **Research and publications:** SNA may encourage student nurses to engage in research activities and publish their findings. This can include conducting research projects, presenting research posters or papers at conferences, and contributing to nursing journals or publications.
- **Social and networking events:** SNA organizes social events, such as mixers, fundraisers, or social gatherings, to foster a sense of community among student nurses. These events provide opportunities for networking, building friendships, and creating a support system within the nursing student community.

In addition, there are numerous other activities in the shape of article writing, poetry writing, flower arrangement, cooking, sewing, interior decoration and gardening, etc., are also encouraged. The personality contest Mr. SNA and Miss SNA was introduced for the first time in the SNA Platinum Jubilee and XXI Biennial conference.

These activities aim to support the educational and professional growth of student nurses, enhance their skills and knowledge, promote their well-being, and prepare them for successful careers in nursing.

The Christian Nurses' League

The Christian Nurses' League (CNL) is an organization affiliated with the Christian Medical Association of India (CMAI). It is a professional and faith-based association specifically for nurses who identify as Christians in India. The CNL aims to bring together Christian nurses, promote Christian values in nursing practice, and support the professional and spiritual growth of its members.

Functions

The Christian Nurses' League of the Christian Medical Association of India carries out several activities and functions, including:

- **Spiritual support:** The CNL provides spiritual support and encouragement to Christian nurses through prayer meetings, Bible studies, retreats, and fellowship gatherings. It aims to nurture the faith and spiritual well-being of its members.
- **Professional development:** The CNL organizes conferences, seminars, and workshops focused on enhancing the professional knowledge and skills of Christian nurses. These events address topics such as evidence-based nursing practice, ethical considerations in nursing, and leadership development.
- **Networking and collaboration:** The CNL facilitates networking among Christian nurses across India, allowing them to connect, share experiences, and collaborate on projects or initiatives that promote Christian values in healthcare and nursing practice.
- **Advocacy and ethical guidelines:** The CNL advocates for the integration of Christian values in healthcare policies and practices. It promotes ethical nursing standards and guidelines based on Christian principles

and facilitates discussions on ethical dilemmas and challenges faced by Christian nurses.

- **Service and outreach:** The CNL encourages Christian nurses to actively engage in community service and outreach programs. This may involve volunteering in medical camps, participating in health education initiatives, or providing nursing care to underserved populations.
- **Support and counseling:** The CNL offers support and counseling services to Christian nurses, addressing their professional and personal concerns. This may include guidance on career advancement, work-related challenges, or personal well-being.
- **Research and publication:** The CNL encourages research and scholarly activities among its members. It may publish journals, articles, or newsletters to disseminate knowledge, share best practices, and promote research in the field of Christian nursing.

The Christian Nurses' League of the Christian Medical Association of India serves as a platform for Christian nurses to unite, grow spiritually, and contribute to the development of nursing practice and healthcare in India. It strives to uphold Christian values and ethics while providing professional support and fostering holistic care.

The Indian Society of Psychiatric Nurses

The Indian Society of Psychiatric Nurses (ISPN) is a professional organization dedicated to advancing the field of psychiatric nursing in India. It is a national association that brings together psychiatric nurses from various settings and provides a platform for professional development, research, advocacy, and collaboration in the field of mental health nursing.

Functions of ISPN

The Indian Society of Psychiatric Nurses (ISPN) carries out several activities and functions, including:

- Organizing conferences, workshops, seminars, and continuing education programs for professional development
- Promoting research in psychiatric nursing and disseminating research findings
- Advocating for recognition and importance of psychiatric nursing in healthcare systems
- Influencing policies related to mental health, nursing education, and workforce development
- Contributing to the development of standards and guidelines for psychiatric nursing practice
- Facilitating networking and collaboration among psychiatric nurses and other healthcare professionals
- Conducting public awareness campaigns and community outreach programs to reduce mental health stigma
- Providing support, mentorship, and guidance to students pursuing psychiatric nursing education
- Promoting interdisciplinary teamwork and partnerships for enhanced mental health care delivery.

REGULATORY BODY

A regulatory body, also known as a regulatory agency or regulatory authority, is an organization established by the government or a relevant authority to regulate and oversee specific industries or sectors. Its primary purpose is to ensure compliance with laws, regulations, and standards related to the operation, conduct, and safety of those industries.

Regulatory bodies are responsible for creating and enforcing rules and regulations that govern various aspects of industry operations, such as safety standards, consumer protection, quality control, environmental protection, financial regulations, and fair competition. They have the authority to issue licenses, permits, certifications, and approvals, as well as to conduct inspections to ensure compliance.

Regulatory bodies play a crucial role in maintaining order, protecting public interests, and ensuring the smooth functioning of particular sector by promoting fair practices, preventing abuse or fraud, and safeguarding the welfare of society, employees, and the environment.

REGULATORY BODIES IN NURSING

Regulatory bodies in nursing are organizations or agencies that are responsible for regulating and overseeing the nursing profession. These bodies establish and enforce rules, regulations, and standards to ensure the competence, professionalism, and ethical conduct of nurses. They play a vital role in safeguarding the public and maintaining the quality of nursing practice.

Concept

The concept of regulatory bodies in nursing is rooted in the recognition that nursing is a regulated profession, and maintaining high standards of practice is essential to protect the public and ensure quality care. These bodies act as guardians of the nursing profession, fostering professionalism, accountability, and ethical conduct among nurses while advocating for patient safety and well-being.

Purposes

Their primary purpose is to ensure the safety, quality, and ethical practice of nursing, while protecting the interests of the public. Other purposes of regulatory bodies in nursing can be summarized as follows:

- **Public protection:** The primary objective of regulatory bodies in nursing is to safeguard the public's health and well-being. By setting and enforcing standards of practice, they aim to ensure that nurses provide safe and quality care to patients.
- **Licensure and registration:** Regulatory bodies grant nursing licenses or registrations to individuals who meet the required educational and competency standards. They ensure that only qualified individuals can practice nursing and protect the public from unqualified practitioners.
- **Standards and practice guidelines:** These bodies develop and maintain standards of practice for nursing, including clinical, ethical, and professional guidelines. They set expectations for nurses regarding their scope of practice, clinical skills, ethical responsibilities, and professional conduct.
- **Education and accreditation:** Regulatory bodies often have a role in accrediting and approving nursing education programs. They establish the educational requirements and ensure that nursing schools provide a quality education that prepares students for safe and competent practice.
- **Continuing competence:** Regulatory bodies promote ongoing professional development and competence among nurses. They may require nurses to participate in continuing education programs and maintain evidence of their ongoing learning to ensure they stay updated and competent in their practice.
- **Complaints and disciplinary actions:** Regulatory bodies investigate complaints against nurses and take disciplinary actions when necessary. This could include suspending or revoking licenses, imposing fines, or implementing remedial measures to protect the public and maintain professional standards.
- **Public protection:** The primary focus of regulatory bodies in nursing is to protect the public by ensuring that nurses provide safe, competent, and ethical care. They establish and enforce regulations that promote patient safety, prevent misconduct, and address any risks or concerns related to nursing practice.

By establishing and enforcing these regulations and standards, regulatory bodies in nursing contribute to the overall quality, professionalism, and accountability of the nursing profession. They serve as a regulatory authority to maintain public trust in nursing and ensure that healthcare recipients receive safe and effective nursing care.

NATIONAL REGULATORY BODIES IN NURSING

Indian Nursing Council

The Indian Nursing Council (INC) is the regulatory body for nursing education and practice in India. It is an autonomous body under the Government of India, established under the Indian Nursing Council Act, 1947. The council was constituted in 1949. The INC plays a crucial role in setting and maintaining standards of nursing education, training, and practice in the country.

The Indian Nursing Council works in collaboration with state nursing councils, nursing associations, and other stakeholders to regulate and develop the nursing profession in India. It plays a vital role in maintaining the quality of nursing education, ensuring competent nursing professionals, and safeguarding the interests of the public.

Objectives

The main objectives of the Indian Nursing Council include:

- **Regulation of nursing education:** The INC establishes and regulates the educational standards and requirements for nursing programs in India. It sets guidelines for curriculum, infrastructure, faculty quali-fications, and student intake in nursing institutions across the country.
- **Recognition and approval of nursing institutions:** The INC is responsible for granting recognition and approval to nursing institutions, including schools of nursing, colleges of nursing, and nursing training centers. Institutions must meet the prescribed standards and criteria to be recognized by the INC.
- **Curriculum development:** The INC develops and updates the curriculum for nursing education, ensuring that it aligns with contemporary healthcare needs and best practices. The curriculum covers theoretical knowledge, clinical training, and practical skills required for nursing practice.
- **Registration and licensing:** The INC maintains a central register of qualified nurses, midwives, auxiliary nurse-midwives, and health visitors in India. It sets the criteria and guidelines for registration and licensing, ensuring that only qualified and competent professionals are allowed to practice nursing.
- **Promotion of research and continuing education:** The INC promotes and supports nursing research and continuing education activities in India. It encourages nurses to engage in research, evidence-based practice, and lifelong learning to enhance their knowledge and skills.
- **Standards of nursing practice**: The INC sets and maintains standards of nursing practice, including ethical and professional guidelines. These standards serve as a reference for nurses to ensure safe and quality care delivery and uphold professional ethics.

Functions

The Indian Nursing Council (INC) performs several important functions in the regulation and development of nursing education and practice in India. Here are the key functions of the Indian Nursing Council:

- Regulating nursing education and training standards in India.
- Recognizing and approving nursing institutions and programs.
- Developing and updating the curriculum for nursing education.
- Maintaining a central register of qualified nurses, midwives, auxiliary nurse-midwives, and health visitors.
- Setting criteria and guidelines for registration and licensing of nursing professionals.
- Promoting and supporting nursing research and continuing education.

- Establishing and enforcing standards of nursing practice.
- Collaborating with state nursing councils and nursing associations to regulate and develop the nursing profession.
- Providing guidance and support to nursing institutions, educators, and professionals.
- Ensuring compliance with the Indian Nursing Council Act and related regulations.
- Addressing complaints and disciplinary actions related to nursing practice.
- Advocating for the interests and welfare of the nursing profession in India.

The Organizational Structure of the Indian Nursing Council

The organizational structure of the INC consists of various levels and entities responsible for the governance, decision-making, and implementation of its functions. Here is an overview of the organizational structure of the INC:

- **General body:** The General Body is the highest decision-making authority of the INC. It comprises members representing the central government, state governments, nursing institutions, nursing associations, and other stakeholders. The General Body approves policies, regulations, and major decisions related to nursing education and practice.
- **Executive committee:** The Executive Committee is responsible for the day-to-day functioning of the INC. It is composed of elected members from the General Body, including the President, Vice-President, Secretary, Treasurer, and other office bearers. The Executive Committee oversees the implementation of policies, manages financial matters, and guides the activities of the INC.
- **President:** The President of the INC is the highest-ranking official and represents the organization. They provide leadership, preside over meetings, and ensure the effective functioning of the council.
- **Vice-President:** The Vice-President supports the President and assumes their responsibilities in their absence. They assist in decision-making, coordination, and overall management of the INC's activities.
- **Secretary:** The Secretary of the INC is responsible for the administrative affairs of the organization. They coordinate with various stakeholders, manage records and correspondence, and ensure compliance with regulations and procedures.
- **Treasurer:** The Treasurer oversees the financial matters of the INC. They manage budgets, financial reporting, and financial planning to ensure the proper utilization of resources.
- **Sections and committees:** The INC has various sections and committees to focus on specific areas of nursing education and practice. These may include the Education Section, Examination Section, Accreditation Committee, Research Committee, and others. Each section or committee is responsible for specific functions, such as curriculum development, accreditation of institutions, examination administration, research promotion, and professional development.
- **Regional centers:** The INC has established regional centers in different parts of the country to facilitate its functions at the regional level. These centers assist in implementing the policies and guidelines of the INC and provide support to nursing institutions and professionals in their respective regions.
- **State nursing councils:** The state nursing councils work in collaboration with the INC at the state level. They are responsible for implementing nursing education and practice regulations within their respective states and ensuring compliance with the guidelines set by the INC.

The organizational structure of the INC is designed to ensure effective governance, representation, and coordination in regulating and developing nursing education and practice in India. It allows for decision-making, implementation, and oversight of various functions related to nursing education, registration, standards, and research.

State Nursing Councils in India

State Nursing Councils in India are regulatory bodies that operate at the state level and are responsible for the regulation and supervision of nursing education and practice within their respective states. These councils work in collaboration with the INC, which is the national regulatory body for nursing education and practice in India. Here are some key points regarding State Nursing Councils in India:

Structure

Each state in India has its own State Nursing Council, which operates under the provisions of the Indian Nursing Council Act, 1947. The council consists of members appointed or elected from various stakeholders, including nursing professionals, nursing institutions, and government representatives.

Functions

State Nursing Councils perform several important functions, including:

- Maintaining a register of qualified nurses, midwives, auxiliary nurse-midwives, and health visitors within the state.
- Granting registration and licensing to nursing professionals who meet the required qualifications and criteria.
- Granting recognition and approval to nursing institutions and programs within the state.
- Monitoring and assessing the quality of nursing education, curriculum, faculty, and infrastructure.
- Establishing and enforcing standards and guidelines for nursing education and practice at the state level.
- Conducting inspections and assessments of nursing institutions to ensure compliance with standards.
- Conducting examination of nursing students (General Nursing and Midwifery and Auxiliary Nurse Midwife) with standards.
- Promoting and facilitating continuing education programs for nursing professionals.
- Handling complaints and conducting investigations into allegations of professional misconduct.
- Taking appropriate disciplinary actions against nursing professionals when necessary.
- Collaborating with the Indian Nursing Council and adhering to the guidelines and regulations set by the INC.
- Providing guidance and support to nursing institutions, educators, and professionals within the state.
- Representing the state's nursing profession and advocating for its interests and welfare.
- Contributing to policy development and decision-making related to nursing education and practice at the state level.
- Ensuring the delivery of safe, competent, and ethical nursing care to the public within their jurisdiction.

State nursing councils play a crucial role in ensuring the quality and regulation of nursing education and practice at the state level in India. They work to protect the interests of the public, maintain professional standards, and uphold the ethics and integrity of the nursing profession.

National Examination Board and Universities in Nursing

In India, there are several examination boards and universities that are involved in nursing education, licensure, and certification. Here are some examples:

Universities

- **All India Institute of Medical Sciences (AIIMS):** AIIMS is a premier medical institution in India that offers undergraduate and postgraduate nursing programs. It is recognized for its quality education and research in the field of nursing.

- **Rajiv Gandhi University of Health Sciences (RGUHS):** RGUHS is a health sciences university in Karnataka that offers various nursing programs, including Bachelor of Nursing (BSc Nursing), Master of Nursing (MSc Nursing), and Doctor of Philosophy (PhD) in Nursing.
- **Rajasthan University of Health Sciences (RUHS):** RUHS is a health sciences university in Rajasthan that offers various nursing programs, including Bachelor of Nursing (BSc Nursing), Master of Nursing (MSc Nursing), and Doctor of Philosophy (PhD) in Nursing.
- **Tamil Nadu Dr MGR Medical University:** This university in Tamil Nadu offers nursing programs at the undergraduate and postgraduate levels. It focuses on promoting excellence in nursing education and research.
- **West Bengal University of Health Sciences:** This university in West Bengal offers nursing programs and conducts examinations for nursing students in the state. It aims to ensure the quality of nursing education and practice in the region.
- **Maharashtra University of Health Sciences:** This university in Maharashtra offers nursing programs and conducts examinations for nursing students in the state. It strives to promote quality nursing education and research.

These are just a few examples, and there are several other universities and examination boards across India that offer nursing education and regulate the nursing profession. It's important to check with the respective universities and nursing councils for the most accurate and up-to-date information on nursing education, examinations, and licensure in India.

CHAPTER SUMMARY

1. Professional organizations play a crucial role in shaping and advancing various fields and professions, including healthcare. In nursing, professional organizations represent the collective voice of nurses, advocate for the profession, and promote standards of practice and ethics.
2. The ICN advocates for universal access to quality healthcare, empowered and respected nursing profession, collaborative practice, leadership and advocacy, and ethical and culturally sensitive care.
3. The ICM promotes universal access to midwifery care, safe and fulfilling birth experiences, recognition and autonomy of midwives, collaboration and partnerships, and equity and social justice.
4. The International Federation of Perioperative Nurses (IFPN) promotes perioperative nursing and provides a platform for collaboration and knowledge sharing among perioperative nurses globally.
5. The Trained Nurses Association of India established in 1908, TNAI represents nurses in India and promotes the nursing profession's advancement.
6. The Student Nurses' Association of India is an affiliated association of student nurses under TNAI.
7. The Christian Nurses' League is a faith-based association affiliated with the Christian Medical Association of India (CMAI).
8. The Indian Society of Psychiatric Nurses is a professional organization dedicated to advancing psychiatric nursing in India.
9. National regulatory bodies in nursing such as Indian Nursing Council, State Nursing Councils and universities in India work together to ensure the safety, quality, and ethical practice of nursing, protect the interests of the public, and maintain the standards of the nursing profession.

REVIEW QUESTIONS

1. What do you mean by professional organization in nursing and discuss about International Nursing Council.
2. Describe the purposes of regulatory bodies in nursing.
3. Explain the functions of Trained Nurses Association of India (TNAI).
4. Enumerate the functions of Indian Nursing Council.

BIBLIOGRAPHY

1. [Internet]. [cited 2023, May 20]. Available from: http://samples.jbpub.com/9781284104899/9781284104981_CH05_Pass03.pdf.
2. [Internet]. [cited 2023, May 20]. Available from: https://ca.indeed.com/career-advice/career-development/nursing-organizations.
3. [Internet]. [cited 2023, May 20]. Available from: https://www.indiannursingcouncil.org/government-of-india-who-international-council-of-nurses-icn-other-stakeholders-guidelines-reports-policies.
4. Catton H. International council of nurses: putting nurses at the centre of the world's policymaking has benefits for us all. Int Nurs Rev. 2019;66(3):299-301.
5. Esmet. All State Nursing Council of India for nurses [Internet]. [cited 2023, May 20]. Available from: https://www.nurseszone.in/nurseszone/all-state-nursing-council-of-india-for-nurses/121.html.
6. http://Www.Indiaedunews.Net/Today/Regulatory_bodies_to_implement_strict_antiRagging_measures_7796/ Regulatory bodies to implement strict anti-ragging measures, 25th March, 2009.
7. International Council of Nurses (ICN) [Internet]. [cited 2023, May 20]. Available from: https://www.icn.ch/.
8. Matthews J. Role of professional organizations in advocating for the nursing profession. The Online J Issues Nurs. 2012;17(1):13.
9. Merton RK. (1958). The functions of the professional association. Am J Nurs. 1958;58(1):50-4.
10. Midwives IC. The International Confederation of Midwives Supports Midwives [Internet]. [cited 2023, May 20]. Available from: https://www.internationalmidwives.org/.
11. Ralph C. Regulation and empowerment of nursing. Int Nurs Rev. 2002;40(2):58-60.
12. Role of regulatory bodies [Internet]. Scribd; [cited 2023, May 20]. Available from: https://www.scribd.com/document/132197878/3-1-Rol-of-Regulatory-Bodies#.
13. Serving on a nursing regulatory agency: Lessons learned from a board member [Internet]. [cited 2023, May 20]. Available from: https://www.aonl.org/news/voice/jan-2021/Serving-on-a-Nursing-Regulatory-Agency.
14. Sue CD, Patricia KL. Fundamentals of nursing standards and practice, 7th edition. Published by Delmar Publishers, pp. 216-17.
15. Woodville L. Historical background on international confederation of midwives. Bulletin of the American College of Nurse-Midwives. 1971;16(2):37-8.

Career Planning

Learning Objectives

♦ Understand the concept of a career and identify the characteristics of a career.
♦ Define career planning in nursing as a deliberate and systematic process.
♦ Recognize the importance of career planning in nursing.
♦ Explore the steps of career planning in nursing.
♦ Compare and contrast career planning and career development.
♦ Describe the career opportunities in nursing in India, including roles in hospital services, educational institutions, and community settings.
♦ Evaluate the significance of career advancement and continuous learning in nursing.

INTRODUCTION

A career is a journey that encompasses the professional choices and achievements an individual makes throughout their working life. It involves a series of employment opportunities, experiences, and personal development that shape a person's professional path. Choosing a career is a significant decision as it can have a profound impact on one's life, satisfaction, and personal fulfillment. A well-chosen career provides opportunities for growth, learning, and progression, allowing individuals to pursue their passions and make a meaningful contribution to their chosen field.

A career in nursing is a rewarding and noble profession that revolves around providing care, support, and advocacy for individuals, families, and communities. Nurses play a vital role in the healthcare system, serving as a bridge between patients and other healthcare professionals. They are responsible for promoting health, preventing illness, and treating patients across various healthcare settings.

MEANING OF CAREER

The word "career" originates from the Latin word "carrus," which means "wheeled vehicle" or "chariot." In ancient Rome, a "carrus" referred to a four-wheeled vehicle used for transportation. Over time, the term "carrus" evolved to "carriera" in medieval Latin, which referred to a racecourse or a path for racing chariots.

The concept of a career evolved to represent the idea of a person's chosen path or vocation, encompassing their employment choices, achievements, and advancement in their chosen field. Today, the word "career" is commonly used to refer to an individual's professional journey and the sequence of jobs, roles, and accomplishments they undertake throughout their working life.

The term "career" refers to the course of professional progression and development that an individual undertakes throughout their working life. It encompasses the sequence of jobs, positions, and roles that a person engages in, often spanning different organizations, industries, or sectors.

A career is not merely a series of jobs or occupations but represents a long-term journey of learning, growth, and achievement. It involves the pursuit of professional goals, the development of skills and expertise, and the accumulation of experience and knowledge in a particular field or industry.

DEFINITIONS

Here are definitions of the term "career" by different authors:

- "A career is a series of professional activities and choices linked together and stretched out over time."

    —*Peiperl M and Baruch Y (2017)*

- "Career is a sequence of employment-related positions, roles, activities, and experiences encountered by an individual throughout his or her lifetime."

    —*Hall and Associates (2002)*

- "A career is a series of connected employment opportunities, occupations, or positions within a particular field pursued by an individual throughout their working life."   —*Savickas (2002)*

- "Career represents the life roles individuals adopt in their work, which encompass their occupation, employment, and profession."

    —*Schein (1978)*

- "A career involves a series of work-related activities and experiences that individuals engage in, including learning, advancement, and development, within a particular occupational field."

    —*Lent, Brown, and Hackett (1994)*

CHARACTERISTICS OF A CAREER

A career is typically characterized by the following aspects **(Fig. 5.1)**:

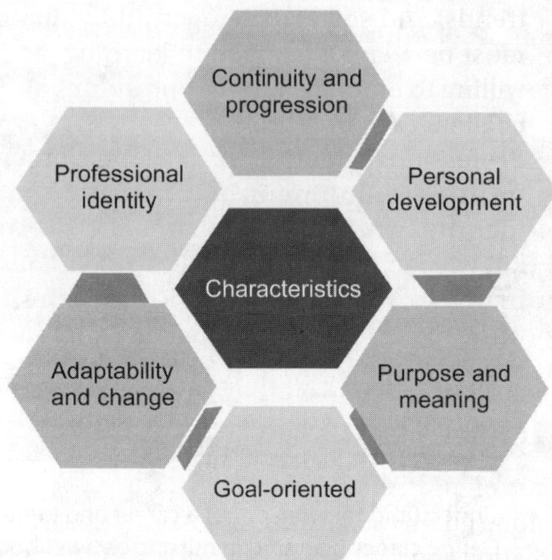

Fig. 5.1: Characteristics of a career.

- **Continuity and progression:** A career is a continuous process of building upon previous experiences and accomplishments. It involves moving forward, advancing to higher levels of responsibility, and achieving professional milestones.

- **Personal development:** A career provides opportunities for personal growth and development. Through education, training, and practical experience, individuals acquire new skills, expand their knowledge, and enhance their capabilities.

- **Purpose and meaning:** A career is often associated with a sense of purpose and fulfillment. It allows individuals to pursue their passions, align their work with their values, and make a meaningful contribution in their chosen field.

- **Goal-oriented:** A career involves setting and pursuing specific goals and objectives. These goals may include achieving certain positions, acquiring new qualifications, gaining recognition, or making a positive impact in a particular domain.

- **Adaptability and change:** Careers are influenced by external factors such as technological advancements, economic trends, and societal changes. Individuals must be adaptable, open to learning, and willing to embrace new opportunities and challenges as they arise.

- **Professional identity:** A career contributes to the development of a professional identity, which encompasses the skills, knowledge, and expertise that individuals bring to their work. It reflects their unique strengths, values, and areas of specialization.

CAREER PLANNING

Career planning refers to the process of setting goals, making informed decisions, and creating a roadmap to guide your professional development and progression. It involves assessing your skills, interests, values, and goals, exploring career options, and developing strategies to achieve your desired career outcomes.

Career planning is a dynamic and ongoing process. It requires continuous self-reflection, exploration, and adaptation to navigate the ever-changing job market and professional landscape. Stay proactive, seek growth opportunities, and be willing to adjust your plans to achieve your career aspirations.

CAREER PLANNING IN NURSING

Career planning in nursing is a vital process that allows nurses to set goals, make informed decisions, and create a roadmap for their professional development and advancement within the nursing profession. It involves assessing one's skills, interests, and values, exploring various nursing specialties, and strategically planning steps to achieve desired career outcomes.

By engaging in career planning, nurses can align their career goals with their personal interests, values, and strengths. It enables them to make informed decisions about their professional development, such as pursuing advanced degrees, acquiring certifications, or transitioning to leadership roles. Career planning in nursing empowers nurses to take charge of their professional growth, adapt to the changing healthcare landscape, and make meaningful contributions to patient care and the nursing profession as a whole.

Definition

- Career planning in nursing refers to the deliberate and systematic process that nurses undertake to set and achieve their professional goals within the nursing profession.
- Career planning in nursing empowers nurses to take an active role in their professional development, make deliberate choices about their career trajectory, and maximize their potential for success and satisfaction in the nursing profession.

Importance of Career Planning in Nursing

- Provides direction and focus for nurses in their professional development.
- Helps nurses align their career goals with their personal interests and values.
- Enables nurses to make informed decisions about educational pursuits and specialization.
- Facilitates the acquisition of skills and knowledge necessary for career advancement.
- Assists in identifying opportunities for professional growth and development.
- Allows nurses to anticipate and prepare for changes in the healthcare industry.
- Enhances job satisfaction and fulfillment by pursuing a career path aligned with personal aspirations.
- Promotes lifelong learning and continuous improvement in nursing practice.
- Provides a framework for nurses to set and achieve career milestones and objectives.
- Enhances employability and opens doors to new opportunities within the nursing field.
- Supports effective career transitions, such as moving from clinical practice to leadership roles.
- Provides a sense of purpose and motivation in the nursing profession.

- Enables nurses to make a positive impact on patient care and healthcare outcomes.
- Facilitates networking and building professional connections within the nursing community.
- Helps nurses navigate the complexities of the nursing profession and make informed choices.

Steps of Career Planning in Nursing

Career planning in nursing involves several steps to guide nurses in setting and achieving their professional goals. Here are the key steps in the career planning process for nurses:

- **Self-assessment:** Reflect on your skills, interests, values, and goals. Identify your strengths, areas for improvement, and what motivates you in the nursing profession. Consider your preferred patient population, clinical settings, and areas of specialization.
- **Explore nursing specialties:** Research and gather information about various nursing specialties. Learn about the required qualifications, job responsibilities, work environments, and potential growth opportunities in different specialties. Consider shadowing or speaking with nurses working in those areas to gain firsthand insights.
- **Set career goals:** Based on your self-assessment and exploration, set specific and achievable career goals in nursing. Define short-term and long-term goals that align with your aspirations. Ensure your goals are realistic and measurable.
- **Identify education and training requirements:** Determine the educational and training requirements for your desired nursing specialty. Research the academic programs, certifications, or additional training needed to advance in your chosen field. Consider the level of education required, such as pursuing a bachelor of science in nursing (BSN) or advanced degrees.
- **Develop a career plan:** Create a detailed career plan that outlines the steps and timeline for achieving your career goals. Include specific milestones, such as completing educational programs, gaining clinical experience, or obtaining certifications. Break down larger goals into smaller, actionable steps.
- **Gain clinical experience:** Seek opportunities to gain practical experience in your desired nursing specialty. Consider internships, clinical rotations, or entry-level positions in healthcare settings relevant to your career goals. Obtain hands-on experience to develop and refine your clinical skills.
- **Pursue continuing education and professional development:** Nursing is a field that requires ongoing learning and professional development. Stay updated on current nursing practices, research, and advancements. Seek out opportunities for continuing education, specialized certifications, and attending conferences or workshops.
- **Network and seek mentorship:** Build a network of nursing professionals by connecting with colleagues, joining professional nursing organizations, and attending networking events. Seek mentorship from experienced nurses or nurse leaders who can provide guidance, support, and valuable insights into your career path.
- **Review and adjust:** Regularly review your career plan, reassess your goals, and make adjustments as needed. Stay informed about industry trends, changes in healthcare policies, and emerging opportunities within nursing. Be open to new possibilities and be willing to adapt your plan as circumstances evolve.
- **Seek career guidance:** Consider seeking guidance from nursing career counselors or mentors who can provide valuable advice and help you navigate your career options. They can offer support, insights, and expertise to guide you in making informed career decisions.

Remember that career planning is an ongoing process. Regularly evaluate your progress, update your goals, and adapt your plan as you gain experience and new opportunities arise. Stay motivated, remain proactive in your professional development, and continuously strive for growth and advancement in your nursing career.

CAREER DEVELOPMENT IN NURSING

Career development in nursing refers to the process of continuous growth, learning, and advancement within the nursing profession. It involves deliberate actions and strategies to enhance knowledge, skills, and experiences, with the aim of achieving professional goals and maximizing one's potential as a nurse.

The goal of career development in nursing is to enhance clinical competence, expand professional opportunities, and achieve career satisfaction and fulfillment. It recognizes the importance of staying current with advancements in nursing practice, research, and technology, as well as adapting to the changing healthcare landscape.

Through career development, nurses can pursue leadership roles, advance their careers, and contribute to the improvement of patient care and outcomes. It emphasizes the continuous pursuit of knowledge, skills, and professional growth, with the aim of delivering high-quality care, assuming greater responsibilities, and making a meaningful impact in the nursing profession.

DIFFERENCES BETWEEN CAREER PLANNING AND CAREER DEVELOPMENT

Career planning and career development are related but distinct concepts. Career planning provides the initial structure and direction, while career development ensures continuous growth and adaptation to achieve long-term career success. Here are the key differences between career planning and career development **(Table 5.1)**:

STAGES OF CAREER PLANNING AND DEVELOPMENT

Exploration (Usually Age Range: 21–25 Years)

The exploration stage occurs before securing permanent employment. During this stage, individuals may be completing their undergraduate or graduate degrees. It is a critical phase that shapes their professional aspirations. As the idea of a long-term career becomes more tangible, individuals start narrowing down their options and focusing on a few professions of interest.

Several factors influence career choices, including personal background, upbringing, communication from parents, feedback from teachers, and education. When embarking on a job search, individuals in the exploration stage typically engage in the following activities:

- **Discovering interests:** Identifying their passions, motivations, and careers that align with their personality.
- **Developing basic skills:** Taking relevant courses and successfully passing state or national exams if required, such as medical licensing exams.
- **Creating expectations:** Considering the desired lifestyle, salary range, future family plans, and work-life balance preferences.

Establishment (Usually Age Range: 25–35 Years Old)

The establishment stage refers to the period when you begin your job search, apply for positions, and secure your first long-term job. Typically, you will accept an entry-level or mid-level position with relatively limited responsibilities.

This stage is characterized by learning, career development, and finding your place in the professional world. The realities of your job replace the expectations you had during the exploration stage. It is common to experience uncertainty and anxiety as you enter the workforce for the first time

Table 5.1: Difference between career planning vs career development.

Based on	Career planning	Career development
Definition	Career planning refers to the process of setting goals, making decisions, and creating a roadmap to guide one's professional development and advancement	Career development refers to the ongoing process of managing and advancing one's career over time through continuous learning, skill development, and growth
Focus	It primarily focuses on the initial stages of identifying career goals, exploring options, and creating a plan to achieve those goals	Focuses on the ongoing process of acquiring new skills, knowledge, and experiences to enhance one's professional growth and advance in their career
Timeframe	It typically occurs at specific points in an individual's career, such as when entering a new field, seeking a promotion, or making a career change	It is a continuous and lifelong process that evolves throughout an individual's career, encompassing ongoing learning, skill enhancement, and adaptation to changing job requirements
Scope	It involves activities such as self-assessment, exploring career options, setting goals, and creating a career plan	It encompasses a broader range of activities, including acquiring education and training, gaining experience, seeking advancement opportunities, networking, and ongoing professional development
Orientation	It is more future-oriented, focusing on setting goals and creating a strategic plan to achieve those goals	Is both present and future-oriented, emphasizing continuous growth, learning, and adaptation to advance and excel in one's career.
Process vs outcome	It is more focused on the process of setting goals and creating a plan, with the outcome being a well-defined career path and direction	It emphasizes the ongoing process of acquiring new skills, experiences, and opportunities, with the outcome being professional growth, advancement, and increased job satisfaction.

and encounter new situations and people. However, this stage also brings excitement as you embark on a new phase in your life and look ahead to the future.

The primary objectives during the establishment stage include:

- Learning the responsibilities of your new job.
- Gaining acceptance from your colleagues and peers.
- Developing and improving your skills.

Mid-career (Usually Age Range: 35–45 Years Old)

The mid-career stage can be characterized by two possibilities: maintaining career stability and advancement within the same profession, or transitioning into a new profession or field. Many professionals at this stage reach their peak levels of productivity and possess a specific skill set related to their role. These years demonstrate your dedication to your work and help solidify your position. By remaining committed to your current job, you have the potential to gain more responsibility, along with the accompanying rewards and recognition.

During this stage, it is natural to expect progress in your career, such as a promotion or salary increase. If such advancements do not occur, you may consider reassessing your role. In the mid-career stage, it is common to reevaluate your goals, interests, and skills. Like many professionals at this point, you may face a decision between pursuing greater success within your current role or transitioning to a new position or even an entirely different career.

Furthermore, achieving work-life balance often becomes a concern during this stage.

Balancing professional success with family commitments and outside activities can present challenges that require careful navigation.

Late-career (Usually Age Range: 45–55 Years Old)

Assuming you have progressed successfully through the mid-career stage, the late-career stage presents an opportunity for a less demanding work environment. Rather than acquiring new skills or knowledge, individuals in this stage can focus on sharing their expertise, mentoring others, and identifying and training a potential successor.

While there may be fewer opportunities for advancement during this stage, you can find fulfillment in tasks such as mentoring younger employees. Job changes are less likely, as your reputation and good standing provide a sense of security in your current position.

During the late-career stage, you can start envisioning what your life will be like after retirement. You may begin to allocate less time to work and dedicate more time to activities and pursuits that bring you enjoyment outside of the workplace.

Decline (Usually Age Range: 55–65 Years Old)

After completing a fulfilling career and spending several decades in the workforce, many individuals reach a point where they are ready to retire.

Upon retirement, you may choose to embrace the opportunity to take a break from work and allocate more time to activities such as spending quality time with family and friends, traveling, and pursuing past hobbies or developing new interests. Additionally, you can utilize your skills and knowledge by engaging in volunteer work.

Depending on your financial circumstances, desired lifestyle, and energy levels, you might also consider alternative ways to generate income, such as:

- Working part-time.
- Offering consulting services on a freelance basis.
- Exploring new full-time employment opportunities.

■ NURSING AS A CAREER

Nursing is a rewarding and respected profession that involves providing compassionate and holistic care to individuals, families, and communities. Nurses play a crucial role in the healthcare system, working collaboratively with other healthcare professionals to promote and restore health, prevent illnesses, and support patients in their healing journey. Here are some key aspects of nursing as a career:

- **Patient care:** Nurses are at the forefront of patient care, delivering direct care to individuals of all ages and backgrounds. They assess patient needs, administer medications, perform treatments, and provide emotional support, ensuring the well-being and comfort of patients.
- **Diverse specialties:** Nursing offers a wide range of specialties and areas of practice, allowing nurses to pursue their interests and passions. These specialties include critical care, pediatrics, maternity, mental health, geriatrics, community health, and more. Nurses can choose to specialize in a particular area or explore various fields throughout their career.
- **Lifelong learning:** Nursing is a profession that requires continuous learning and professional development. Nurses stay up-to-date with advancements in healthcare, research, and technology. They participate in ongoing education, attend conferences, obtain certifications, and engage in evidence-based practice to provide the highest quality care to patients.
- **Teamwork and collaboration:** Nurses collaborate with interdisciplinary teams, including doctors, therapists, pharmacists, and other healthcare professionals. Effective communication, teamwork, and coordination are essential in providing

comprehensive and coordinated care to patients.

- **Career advancement:** Nursing offers various opportunities for career advancement and growth. Nurses can pursue higher education, such as earning advanced degrees (e.g., Master of Science in Nursing or Doctor of Nursing Practice), becoming nurse educators, researchers, or advanced practice nurses (e.g., nurse practitioners, nurse anesthetists, nurse midwives). Leadership roles in nursing management and administration are also available.
- **Impactful and meaningful work:** Nursing provides an opportunity to make a positive impact on individuals and communities. Nurses have the privilege of helping patients during challenging times, advocating for their needs, and improving health outcomes. The personal satisfaction that comes from providing care and making a difference in someone's life is one of the most rewarding aspects of a nursing career.
- **Job stability and demand:** Nursing is a profession with high job stability and demand. With an aging population and evolving healthcare needs, the demand for qualified nurses continues to grow. Nurses have diverse employment options, including hospitals, clinics, long-term care facilities, schools, research institutions, and government agencies.

Overall, nursing is a dynamic and fulfilling career path that offers opportunities for personal and professional growth, the ability to positively impact lives, and the satisfaction of being part of a vital profession dedicated to caring for others.

CAREER OPPORTUNITIES IN NURSING IN INDIA

In India, nursing offers a range of career opportunities across various healthcare sectors. Here are some of the career opportunities available in nursing in India:

In Hospital Services

- **Staff nurse/nursing officer:** This is the entry-level position for registered nurses in India. Staff nurses work in hospitals, clinics, nursing homes, and other healthcare settings, providing direct patient care, administering medications, and assisting with medical procedures.
- **Nursing supervisor/in-charge/senior nursing officer:** Nursing supervisors are responsible for overseeing the nursing staff, ensuring quality patient care, managing nursing schedules, and coordinating with other healthcare professionals. They play a crucial role in maintaining smooth operations within healthcare facilities.
- **Nurse educator:** Nurse educators work in nursing schools and colleges, teaching and mentoring nursing students. They develop curriculum, deliver lectures, supervise clinical training, and assess student performance. Nurse educators contribute to the development of competent nursing professionals.
- **Nurse administrator/manager:** Nurse administrators or managers are responsible for managing nursing departments or units within healthcare organizations. They oversee budgets, staffing, quality improvement initiatives, and ensure compliance with regulatory standards. Nurse administrators play a vital role in the effective functioning of healthcare facilities.
- **Nurse practitioner:** In recent years, the role of nurse practitioners (NPs) has been evolving in India. NPs are advanced practice registered nurses who can provide comprehensive healthcare services, including diagnosing and treating common illnesses, prescribing medications, and offering health promotion and disease prevention services.
- **Clinical nurse specialist:** Clinical nurse specialists (CNS) are specialized nurses who focus on a specific area of healthcare, such as critical care, oncology, or mental

health. They provide expert clinical care, develop and implement care protocols, and serve as resources for both patients and nursing staff.

- **Nurse researcher:** Nurse researchers contribute to the advancement of nursing knowledge and practice through research studies. They design and conduct research, collect and analyze data, and disseminate findings to improve patient care and healthcare policies.

In Educational Institutions

- **Nursing college administrator/principal:** Nursing colleges require strong leadership to oversee the entire institution. As an administrator or principal, you would be responsible for strategic planning, financial management, faculty recruitment and development, student affairs, and maintaining the overall academic environment of the nursing college.
- **Nursing faculty:** Nursing colleges require qualified and experienced nursing faculty members who can teach various nursing subjects and mentor students. As a nursing faculty member, you would be responsible for developing and delivering lectures, designing curriculum, evaluating student performance, and guiding students in their clinical training.
- **Nursing tutor/clinical instructor:** Nursing colleges often hire nursing tutors or clinical instructors who work closely with students in clinical settings. They provide hands-on training, supervise clinical experiences, and ensure that students develop practical skills and competencies required in nursing practice.
- **Nursing researcher:** Nursing colleges in India encourage research and evidence-based practice. As a nursing researcher, you would have the opportunity to conduct research studies, contribute to nursing knowledge, and address healthcare challenges specific to the Indian context.

This role involves designing research projects, collecting and analyzing data, and disseminating research findings through publications and presentations.

- **Nursing administrator:** Nursing colleges require efficient administrators who can manage the day-to-day operations, oversee academic programs, handle administrative tasks, and ensure compliance with regulatory standards. Nursing administrators play a crucial role in maintaining the quality and reputation of the nursing college.
- **Nursing curriculum developer:** As the field of nursing evolves, nursing colleges need professionals who can develop and update nursing curricula to meet the changing healthcare needs and industry standards. Nursing curriculum developers work closely with faculty members, industry experts, and regulatory bodies to design relevant and comprehensive nursing programs.
- **Nursing education consultant:** Nursing colleges may seek the expertise of nursing education consultants who can provide guidance and support in curriculum development, program accreditation, faculty development, and overall improvement of nursing education standards.
- **Nursing quality improvement coordinator:** Nursing colleges emphasize quality improvement initiatives to enhance the educational experience and outcomes for students. Nursing quality improvement coordinators assess the effectiveness of teaching methodologies, develop strategies for continuous improvement, and ensure that the nursing college meets the required standards of excellence.

In Community Settings

- **Public health nurse:** Public health nurses work in community settings, focusing on preventive healthcare and promoting public health. They conduct health screenings, immunizations, health education programs, and collaborate with community organizations to address health concerns.

- **Lady health visitor (LHV) or female health supervisor:** LHVs play a crucial role in providing primary healthcare services, promoting community health, and overseeing the work of Auxiliary Nurse Midwives (ANMs) and other healthcare workers.
- **Auxiliary nurse midwife or multi-purpose health worker:** The role of an ANM or Multi-purpose health worker (female)/health worker (male) is a vital position in the healthcare system, particularly in India. ANMs play a crucial role in providing primary healthcare services and promoting maternal and child health.
- **Occupational health nurse:** Occupational health nurses work in industrial or corporate settings, ensuring the health and safety of employees. They provide health assessments, monitor workplace hazards, develop health promotion programs, and facilitate employee wellness initiatives.

In Ministry

- **Nursing advisor of the Government of India (GOI):** The position of Nursing Advisor of the GOI is a significant role that involves providing expert guidance, advice, and support in matters related to nursing and healthcare policy. The Nursing Advisor serves as a key official within the government's healthcare department and plays a crucial role in shaping nursing education, practice, and policy initiatives.
- **The Assistant Director General of Nursing Services (ADGNS):** The Assistant Director General of Nursing Services (ADGNS) is a high-level administrative position within the healthcare system, particularly in India. The ADGNS serves as a key official responsible for overseeing and managing nursing services at the national level.

These are some of the career opportunities available in nursing in India. The demand for qualified and skilled nurses is high, and the healthcare industry continues to grow, offering numerous avenues for career advancement, specialization, and professional development.

CHAPTER SUMMARY

1. A career is a journey that encompasses an individual's professional choices and achievements throughout their working life. It involves a series of employment opportunities, experiences, and personal development that shape one's professional path.
2. A career in nursing is a rewarding profession centered around providing care, support, and advocacy for individuals, families, and communities.
3. Career planning is the process of setting goals, making informed decisions, and creating a roadmap for professional development.
4. Career planning in nursing empowers nurses to align their goals with their interests, values, and strengths. It helps nurses make informed decisions about education, specialization, and career transitions.
5. Career development in nursing focuses on continuous growth, learning, and advancement within the profession. It involves acquiring new skills, knowledge, and experiences to enhance clinical competence and expand opportunities.
6. Career planning and career development differ in their focus, timeframe, scope, and orientation.
7. The stages of career planning and development include exploration, establishment, mid-career, and late career. Each stage involves specific objectives and challenges for individuals in their professional journey.

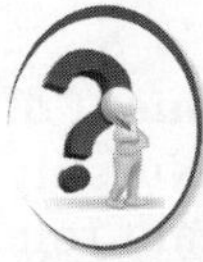

REVIEW QUESTIONS

1. Define career and explain characteristics of a career.
2. Explain steps of career planning in nursing and differentiate between career planning and career development.
3. Discuss nursing as a career and enumerate career opportunities in nursing in India.
4. What do you mean by career development. Describe stages of career development.
5. Discuss the importance of career planning in nursing.

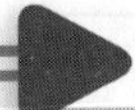 **BIBLIOGRAPHY** 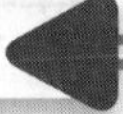

1. Arthur MB, Hall DT, Lawrence BS (Eds). Handbook of career theory. Cambridge: Cambridge University Press; 1989.
2. Career planning [Internet]. [cited 2023, May 21]. Available from: https://www.cna-aiic.ca/en/nursing/career-development/career-planning.
3. Clements J, Parrinello K. Climbing higher. Nurs Manage. 1998;29(12):41-5.
4. Donner GJ, Wheeler MM. Building and sustaining a career culture. Can Nurse. 2005;101(8):30-1.
5. Edu TL. Career Planning and Development [Internet]. Leverage Edu; 2021 [cited 2023, May 21]. Available from: https://leverageedu.com/blog/career-planning-and-development/
6. Hall LM, Waddell J, Donner G, Wheeler MM. Outcomes of a career planning and development program for registered nurses. Nurs Econ. 2004;22(5):231–8,227.
7. Jong N, Wisse B, Heesink JA, van der Zee KI. Personality traits and career role enactment: Career Role Preferences as a mediator. Front Psychol. 2019;10. doi:10.3389/fpsyg.2019.01720.
8. Nelson JM, Cook PF. Evaluation of a career ladder program in an ambulatory care environment. Nurs Econ. 2008;26(6), 353-60.
9. Pool I, Poell R, ten Cate O. Nurses' and managers' perceptions of continuing professional development for older and younger nurses: A focus group study. Int J Nurs Stud. 2013;50(1):34-43.
10. Shermont H, Krepcio D, Murphy J. Career mapping: Developing nurse leaders, reinvigorating careers. J Nurs Adm. 2009;39(10):432-7.
11. Shirey M. Building an extraordinary career in nursing: promise, momentum, and harvest. J Contin Educ Nurs. 2009;40(9):394-400.
12. Sonmez B, Yildirim A. What are the career planning and development practices for nurses in hospitals? Is there a difference between private and public hospitals? J Clin Nurs. 2009;18(24):3461-71.
13. Waddell J, Bauer M. Career planning and development for students: Building a career in a professional practice discipline. Can J Program Eval. 2005;4(2)4-13
14. Walsh K, Weeks LC. PACE: A unique career development program. J Nurs Adm. 1995;25(1):10-1.
15. Wesarat P-O, Sharif M, Majid A. A review of organizational and individual career management: A dual perspective. Int J Hum Resour. 2014;4:101.
16. Yan Y, Li L, Tang J, Zhang T, Zhai Y. Influencing factors and strategy to the career planning of operating room nurses. Nurs Open. 2021;8(5):2637-44.

Code of Ethics and Professional Conduct

Learning Objectives

- Define the concept of ethics in nursing and its significance in guiding ethical decision-making and providing quality care to patients.
- Identify the key ethical principles in nursing.
- Differentiate between ethics and moral values, understanding their relationship and how they influence nurses' behavior and decision-making.
- Analyze the importance of ethical competence in nursing practice.
- Evaluate the ethical considerations and implications arising from advances in medical technology, changes in healthcare policies, and cultural diversity in nursing practice.
- Describe the ethical responsibilities and obligations outlined in the Code of Ethics by the International Council of Nurses (ICN) and its significance in guiding professional conduct for nurses worldwide.
- Illustrate the concept of moral values and their role in shaping an individual's behavior, decision-making, and sense of right and wrong.
- Examine the ethical principles and guidelines outlined in the Code of Ethics by the Indian Nursing Council (INC) and their implications for nursing practice in India.

INTRODUCTION

Ethics in nursing is an essential aspect of healthcare that guides nurses in making ethical decisions and providing quality care to patients. Nurses are faced with numerous moral dilemmas and challenging situations on a daily basis, where they must navigate complex ethical issues. These ethical considerations are rooted in a set of values and principles that govern their professional conduct.

In today's rapidly evolving healthcare landscape, ethical dilemmas have become more intricate and multifaceted. Advances in medical technology, changes in healthcare policies, and cultural diversity present new ethical challenges for nurses. Moreover, the increasing complexity of healthcare decisions and the need for interprofessional collaboration further highlight the significance of ethical competence in nursing practice.

MEANING OF ETHICS

The term "ethics" finds its origin in the ancient Greek word "Ethikos," which signifies a connection to an individual's character. "Ethikos" is derived from the root word "ethos." The Greek word "ethos," which means "character" or "custom."

Ethics refers to the branch of philosophy that deals with moral principles, values, and codes of conduct that guide human behavior and decision-making. It explores questions of what is morally right or wrong, good or bad, and how individuals should behave in various situations. Ethics provides a framework for evaluating actions and determining the moral implications and consequences of one's choices. In the context of nursing, ethics plays a crucial role in guiding nurses' actions and ensuring the provision of ethical and compassionate care to patients.

DEFINITIONS OF ETHICS

- According to Aristotle, ethics is the study of character and how individuals can live virtuous lives by cultivating good habits and virtues.
- Immanuel Kant defines ethics as the pursuit of moral principles and universal laws that guide human actions, emphasizing the importance of moral duty and rationality.
- John Stuart Mill views ethics as the pursuit of maximizing happiness and well-being for the greatest number of people, known as utilitarianism.
- **American Nurses Association (ANA):** The ANA defines ethics in nursing as the principles and values that guide the profession of nursing, including the moral responsibility to provide safe, competent, and ethical care to individuals, families, and communities.
- **International Council of Nurses (ICN):** The ICN defines ethics in nursing as the ethical principles and values that guide nurses in their professional practice, emphasizing the importance of respecting human rights, dignity, and the autonomy of patients.

MORAL VALUE

Moral values refer to the fundamental principles or beliefs that guide an individual's behavior and decision-making, shaping their sense of right and wrong. These values are deeply ingrained and are often influenced by cultural, societal, and personal factors. Moral values provide a framework for individuals to evaluate their actions and choices, determining what is considered morally acceptable.

Difference Between Ethics and Moral Value

Ethics and moral values are related concepts, but they have distinct differences **(Table 6.1)**:

In summary, ethics provides a broader framework of principles and rules that guide behavior within a specific context, while moral values represent an individual's personal beliefs and principles about what is morally right or wrong. Ethics is more universal and objective, while moral values are subjective and can vary between individuals.

CODE OF ETHICS

The Code of Ethics in nursing is a set of principles and guidelines that outline the professional standards and ethical responsibilities of nurses. It serves as a foundation for ethical decision-making and guides nurses in providing safe, compassionate, and competent care to individuals, families, and communities.

The history of nursing ethics dates back to the early days of the nursing profession. Florence Nightingale, often considered the founder of modern nursing, emphasized the importance of ethical practice in nursing. She recognized the need for nurses to uphold high moral standards and maintain a commitment to patient welfare.

Over the years, nursing ethics has evolved and become more formalized. In the mid-20th century, nursing organizations started developing codes of ethics to provide a clear framework for professional conduct. These codes addressed various ethical issues and established guidelines for ethical decision-making in nursing practice.

Ethical Principles for Nurses

Ethical principles in nursing provide a framework for nurses to make morally sound decisions and guide their professional conduct. Here are some key ethical principles in nursing:

- **Respect for human dignity:** Nurses respect the inherent dignity, worth and uniqueness of every person.

Table 6.1: Difference between ethics and moral value.

Content	Ethics	Moral values
Definition	Ethics refers to a set of principles or rules that govern behavior within a particular context or profession, guiding individuals on what is considered right or wrong	Moral values are personal beliefs and principles that individuals hold about what is morally right or wrong
Scope	Ethics is broader in scope and encompasses a system of principles that can be applied in various situations or professions. It provides a framework for making ethical decisions within a specific context	Moral values are more individualistic and subjective, representing personal beliefs and values that guide an individual's behavior and decision-making
Universality	Ethics is often considered to be more universal and objective, applicable to all individuals within a particular context or profession. It provides a shared set of principles or guidelines that guide the behavior of individuals within that context	Moral values, however, can vary between individuals and may be influenced by personal beliefs, cultural norms, and individual experiences
Context	Ethics is often associated with professional contexts, such as business ethics, medical ethics, or legal ethics. It provides guidelines and standards for professionals within those fields	Moral values extend beyond specific contexts and are applicable to personal behavior and decision-making in various aspects of life

- **Autonomy:** Nurses promote the right of individuals to make decisions about their own health care.
- **Beneficence:** Nurses act in ways that benefit patients and other people who are receiving nursing care.
- **Non-maleficence:** Nurses avoid causing harm to patients and other people who are receiving nursing care.
- **Justice:** Nurses ensure that all people have access to health care that is fair and equitable.
- **Fidelity:** Nurses are faithful to their patients and to the profession of nursing.
- **Confidentiality:** Nurses protect the privacy and confidentiality of patients and other people who are receiving nursing care.
- **Accountability:** Nurses are accountable for their actions and for the quality of care they provide.
- **Integrity:** Upholding high moral and ethical standards, being accountable for one's actions, and acting consistently with professional values and ethical principles.

These ethical principles serve as guiding principles for nurses to navigate complex ethical dilemmas, promote patient-centered care, and maintain professional integrity in their practice. They help ensure that nursing care is delivered with compassion, respect, and ethical decision-making.

CODE OF ETHICS BY INTERNATIONAL COUNCIL OF NURSES

The Code of Ethics developed by the International Council of Nurses (ICN) is a widely recognized and respected ethical framework for the nursing profession. The ICN, a global organization representing millions of nurses worldwide, first adopted its Code of Ethics in 1953. The code has since been revised and updated to reflect the evolving ethical landscape of nursing practice.

The Code of Ethics by the International Council of Nurses (ICN) consists of several key elements that guide ethical practice in nursing. These elements encompass various principles and standards that nurses should uphold in their professional roles. Here are the core elements of the ICN Code of Ethics:

- **Nurses and people or patients requiring care:** This element emphasizes the importance of nurses' commitment to respecting the dignity, rights, and cultural beliefs of individuals, families, and communities. Nurses strive to build trusting relationships, promote health, and provide compassionate care that meets the unique needs of each person.

- Nurses have a fundamental professional obligation to individuals, families, communities, or populations in need of nursing care, referred to as "patients" or "people requiring care."

- Nurses foster an environment where the human rights, values, customs, religious beliefs, and spiritual beliefs of individuals, families, and communities are respected and promoted by all.

- Nurses ensure that individuals receive accurate, sufficient, and timely information in a culturally appropriate manner to make informed decisions regarding their care and treatment.

- Nurses maintain the confidentiality of personal information and uphold the privacy, confidentiality, and interests of patients in the lawful collection, use, access, transmission, storage, and disclosure of this information.

- Nurses respect the privacy and confidentiality of colleagues and individuals in their care, upholding the integrity of the nursing profession in personal interactions and across all forms of media, including social media.

- Nurses share with society the responsibility to take initiative and support actions that address the health and social needs of all individuals.

- Nurses advocate for equity and social justice in the allocation of resources, access to healthcare, and other social and economic services.

- Nurses embody professional values such as respect, justice, responsiveness, compassion, empathy, trustworthiness, and integrity.

- Nurses provide care that is evidence-informed and centered around the individual, recognizing and incorporat-ing the values and principles of primary health care and health promotion.

- Nurses encourage a culture of safety in healthcare and raise concerns regarding the safety of individuals and healthcare services.

- Nurses support and protect the right to self-determination of all patients and other healthcare professionals.

- Nurses ensure that the use of technology and scientific advancements aligns with the safety, dignity, and rights of individuals. In the case of devices such as robots, nurses ensure that care remains centered around the individual and that such devices support, rather than replace, human relationships.

- **Nurses and practice:** This element highlights the professional responsibilities and accountabilities of nurses. It emphasizes the need for nurses to maintain competence, engage in lifelong learning, and deliver safe, evidence-based practice. Nurses are encouraged to advocate for health equity, address health disparities, and contribute to improving healthcare systems.

- Nurses hold personal responsibility and are accountable for their nursing practice, as well as for maintaining competence through ongoing learning. They actively engage in continuous professional development and lifelong learning.

- Nurses ensure that they are fit to practice in order to maintain their ability to provide care without compromise.

- Nurses practice within the boundaries of their individual competence and exercise judgment when accepting and delegating responsibilities.

- Nurses prioritize their own dignity, well-being, and health. They understand that positive practice environments, characterized by professional recognition, education, support structures, adequate resources, effective management practices, and occupational health and safety, are essential for achieving these goals.

- Nurses consistently maintain standards of personal conduct that reflect positively on the nursing profession, enhance its image, and inspire public confidence. They recognize and establish appropriate personal boundaries in their professional role.
- Nurses willingly share their knowledge and provide feedback, mentorship, and guidance to support the professional development of nursing students, novice nurses, other nurses, and healthcare providers.
- Nurses cultivate and sustain a practice culture that promotes ethical behavior and encourages open dialogue.
- Nurses have the right to conscientiously object to participating in specific medical procedures or research studies, but they must ensure that individuals still receive the necessary care.
- Nurses respect an individual's right to provide or withdraw informed consent when accessing their genetic information, including activities related to genetic and genomic-based research. They protect the use, privacy, and confidentiality of genetic information and human genome materials. They also advocate for equitable access to genomic technologies.
- Nurses foster and maintain collaborative and respectful relationships with colleagues and other members of the healthcare team. They recognize and respect their knowledge, skills, and perspectives.
- Nurses take appropriate action to protect individuals, families, and communities when their health is at risk due to the actions of a coworker, another person, a policy, a practice, or the misuse of technology.
- Nurses actively contribute to promoting patient safety. They uphold ethical conduct when errors or near misses occur, speak up when patient safety is threatened, and collaborate with others to reduce the potential for errors.

- **Nurses and the profession:** This element focuses on promoting and maintaining the integrity and reputation of the nursing profession. Nurses are expected to uphold ethical standards, demonstrate professional conduct, and contribute to the development and advancement of nursing knowledge. They collaborate with colleagues, mentor others, and engage in professional organizations and activities.
  - Nurses play a central role in establishing and implementing acceptable standards for clinical nursing practice, management, research, and education.
  - Nurses actively contribute to the development of a solid foundation of research-based knowledge that supports practice informed by evidence.
  - Nurses actively contribute to the development and maintenance of a set of professional values.
  - Nurses, through their professional organizations, actively participate in creating a positive practice environment that supports individual nursing practice, ensures the provision of safe and high-quality care, and upholds safe, fair, and equitable working conditions for nurses.
  - Nurses contribute to fostering positive and ethical organizational environments while challenging unethical practices and settings.
  - Nurses actively engage in the generation, dissemination, and utilization of research.
  - Nurses are prepared for and respond to emergencies, disasters, conflicts, epidemics, and situations involving limited resources.

- **Nurses and the global health:** Nurses play a crucial role in global health, contributing to the well-being and healthcare of individuals, families, communities, and populations worldwide. The International Council of

Nurses (ICN) recognizes the significance of nurses' involvement in global health and emphasizes their responsibilities and contributions in this domain.

- Nurses acknowledge the importance of healthcare access as a fundamental human right, emphasizing the need for universal health coverage.
- Nurses uphold the dignity, autonomy, and inherent worth of every individual and actively oppose all forms of exploitation, including human trafficking and child labor.
- Nurses play a leading role or contribute to the development of health policies.
- Nurses support and actively work towards achieving the Sustainable Development Goals established by the United Nations.
- Nurses recognize the critical impact of social determinants of health and actively contribute to, and advocate for, policies and programs aimed at addressing them.
- Nurses collaborate with others and take action to preserve, sustain, and protect the natural environment, acknowledging its implications for health. They advocate for initiatives that reduce environmentally harmful practices to promote health and well-being.
- Nurses collaborate with other healthcare professionals and the public to uphold principles of justice, promoting human rights, equity, fairness, and the overall well-being of individuals and the planet.

CODE OF ETHICS BY INDIAN NURSING COUNCIL

The Indian Nursing Council is the regulatory body for nursing education and practice in India. They have established a code of ethics that sets the standards and guidelines for ethical conduct and professional behavior expected from nurses in India.

Here are the core elements of the ICN Code of Ethics:

- **The nurse respects the uniqueness of individual in provision of care**
  Nurse:
  - Deliver care to individuals regardless of factors such as caste, creed, religion, culture, ethnicity, gender, socio-economic and political status, personal characteristics, or any other criteria.
  - Tailor the care they provide to consider the individual's beliefs, values, and cultural sensitivities.
  - Acknowledge the role of the individual within their family and community and encourage the involvement of significant others in their care.
  - Establish and foster trusting relationships with individuals.
  - Acknowledge the individuality of each person's response to interventions and adjust their approach accordingly.
- **The nurse respects the rights of individuals as partner in care and help in making informed choices**
  Nurse:
  - Acknowledge and respect the individual's autonomy in making decisions about their own care by providing them with sufficient and accurate information, enabling them to make informed choices.
  - Show respect for the decisions made by individuals regarding their own care.
  - Nurses safeguard the public by preventing the spread of misinformation and misinterpretations.
  - Advocate for the implementation of specific measures to safeguard and support vulnerable individuals or groups.
- **The nurse respects individual's right to privacy, maintains confidentiality, and shares information judiciously**
  Nurse:
  - Acknowledge and uphold the individual's right to privacy regarding their personal information.

- Ensure the confidentiality of privileged information, except in situations where there is a threat to life, and exercise discretion when sharing information.
- Obtain informed consent and maintain anonymity when collecting information for quality assurance, academic, or legal purposes.
- Restrict access to personal records, both written and computerized, only to authorized individuals.

- **Nurse maintains competence in order to render quality nursing care**
  Nurse
  - The provision of nursing care should be exclusively carried out by registered nurses.
  - Make efforts to uphold the standards of care and ensure the delivery of high-quality nursing services.
  - Recognize the importance of continuous education and actively seek opportunities for self-improvement and professional growth.
  - Appreciate the significance of research in advancing the nursing profession and engage in nursing research while adhering to ethical principles.

- **The nurse is obliged to practice within the framework of ethical, professional and legal boundaries**
  Nurse
  - Abide by the code of ethics and code of professional conduct for nurses in India, which have been established by the Indian Nursing Council.
  - Ensure they are knowledgeable about the applicable laws and practices that align with the legal requirements of the state.

- **Nurse is obliged to work harmoniously with members of the health team**
  Nurse
  - Recognizes and values the collaborative efforts involved in providing care.

  - Actively engages in cooperation, coordination, and collaboration with other healthcare team members to effectively meet the needs of individuals.

- **Nurse commits to reciprocate the trust invested in nursing profession by society**
  Nurse
  - Exhibits proper manners and behavior in all interactions.
  - Displays professional characteristics and qualities in all interactions.

PROFESSIONAL CONDUCT

Professional conduct refers to the behavior, actions, and attitudes exhibited by individuals in a specific profession. It encompasses the ethical principles, standards, and norms that guide professionals in their interactions with colleagues, clients, and the broader community. Professional conduct is essential for maintaining trust, integrity, and credibility within a profession and ensuring the delivery of high-quality services or products. It involves adhering to professional codes of ethics, demonstrating professionalism in one's work, respecting boundaries, communicating effectively, maintaining confidentiality, upholding professional standards, and continuously striving for personal and professional growth.

CONCEPT OF PROFESSIONAL CONDUCT IN NURSING

Professional conduct in nursing refers to the ethical behavior, attitudes, and standards of practice that guide nurses in their interactions with patients, colleagues, and the healthcare system as a whole. It encompasses the values and principles that uphold the integrity of the nursing profession and ensure the delivery of safe, compassionate, and competent care.

By adhering to the principles of professional conduct, nurses uphold the trust and confidence placed in them by patients and society. They contribute to the advancement of nursing practice and play a vital role in providing safe and compassionate care to individuals, families, and communities.

Code of Professional Conduct for Nurses in India

- **Professional responsibility and accountability**
  Nurse
  - Values and embraces personal worth and fosters its development
  - Upholds personal conduct that reflects positively on the nursing profession
  - Performs responsibilities within the established professional boundaries
  - Assumes accountability for adhering to the practice standards set by the Indian Nursing Council
  - Takes responsibility for individual decisions and actions
  - Demonstrates compassion
  - Takes responsibility for continuous improvement of current practices
  - Provides individuals with sufficient information to make informed choices
  - Engages in health-promoting behaviors
- **Nursing Practice**
  Nurse
  - Delivers care in accordance with established practice standards
  - Treats all individuals and families with dignity while addressing their physical, psychological, emotional, social, and spiritual needs
  - Respects individuals and families within the context of their traditional and cultural practices, promoting healthy behaviors and discouraging harmful practices
  - Provides truthful and realistic information in all situations to facilitate autonomous decision-making by individuals and families

- Encourages the active participation of individuals and their significant others in their care
- Ensures the practice of safe care
- Seeks consultation, coordination, collaboration, and appropriate follow-up when individuals' care needs exceed the nurse's level of competence.
- **Communication and Interpersonal Relationships**
  Nurse
  - Develops and maintains positive and effective relationships with individuals, families, and communities
  - Respects the dignity of team members and fosters positive interpersonal relationships with them
  - Recognizes and supports the professional roles of team members
  - Collaborates with other healthcare professionals to address the needs of individuals, families, and communities.
- **Valuing Human Being**
  Nurse
  - Implements necessary measures to safeguard individuals from unethical practices that may cause harm
  - Makes conscientious decisions based on relevant information, prioritizing the best interests of individuals
  - Empowers and advocates for individuals to express their own views regarding matters concerning their health and well-being
  - Respects and supports the choices made by individuals, honoring their autonomy and preferences.
- **Management**
  Nurse
  - Ensures appropriate and efficient utilization of available resources
  - Contributes to the supervision and education of students and other healthcare providers

- Exercises judgment in accepting and delegating responsibilities based on individual competence
- Cultivates a supportive work environment to achieve institutional goals
- Communicates effectively using appropriate channels of communication
- Engages in performance appraisal processes
- Participates in the evaluation of nursing services
- Contributes to policy decisions, promoting equity and accessibility of services
- Collaborates with individuals to identify their needs and advocates for resource allocation to policymakers and funding agencies

- **Professional Advancement**
  Nurse
  - Safeguards human rights while actively seeking knowledge advancement
  - Contributes to the enhancement of nursing practice
  - Participates in the establishment and delivery of high-quality care
  - Takes personal responsibility for continuous learning and skill development
  - Contributes to the body of professional knowledge through research involvement and collaboration.

CHAPTER SUMMARY

1. Ethics in nursing is an essential aspect of healthcare that guides nurses in making ethical decisions and providing quality care to patients.
2. In today's rapidly evolving healthcare landscape, ethical dilemmas have become more intricate and multifaceted.
3. Advances in medical technology, changes in healthcare policies, and cultural diversity present new ethical challenges for nurses.
4. The term "ethics" finds its origin in the ancient Greek word "Ethikos," which signifies a connection to an individual's character. "Ethikos" is derived from the root word "ethos," which means "character" or "custom."
5. Ethics refers to the branch of philosophy that deals with moral principles, values, and codes of conduct that guide human behavior and decision-making.
6. Moral values refer to the fundamental principles or beliefs that guide an individual's behavior and decision-making, shaping their sense of right and wrong.
7. Ethics and moral values are related concepts but have distinct differences.
8. The Code of Ethics in nursing is a set of principles and guidelines that outline the professional standards and ethical responsibilities of nurses.
9. Ethical principles in nursing provide a framework for nurses to make morally sound decisions and guide their professional conduct.
10. Some key ethical principles in nursing include respect for human dignity, autonomy, beneficence, non-maleficence, justice, fidelity, confidentiality, accountability, and integrity.
11. Codes of ethics emphasize the importance of respecting individuals' rights, providing compassionate care, maintaining competence, and collaborating with other healthcare professionals.
12. Professional conduct in nursing refers to the ethical behavior, attitudes, and standards of practice that guide nurses in their interactions with patients, colleagues, and the healthcare system.

REVIEW QUESTIONS

1. Define ethics in nursing and explain its significance in guiding ethical decision-making and providing quality care to patients.
2. Identify and discuss the key ethical principles in nursing.
3. Differentiate between ethics and moral values in the context of nursing.
4. Evaluate the factors affecting ethical considerations and implications.
5. Describe the ethical responsibilities and obligations outlined in the Code of Ethics by the International Council of Nurses (ICN).
6. Illustrate the concept of moral values and differentiate it from ethics.

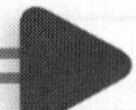 ## BIBLIOGRAPHY 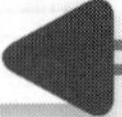

1. American Nurses Association. (2015). Code of Ethics for Nurses with Interpretive Statements. Retrieved from: https://www.nursingworld.org/coe-view-only.
2. Beauchamp TL, Childress JF. Principles of Biomedical Ethics. Oxford University Press; 2019.
3. Borhani F, Alhani F, Mohammadi E, Abbaszadeh A. Lived experience of Iranian Nurses. Ethical codes in nursing. Iran J Public Health. 2017;46(9):1271-7.
4. Burkhardt MA, Nathaniel AK. Ethics and issues in contemporary nursing. Cengage Learning; 2014.
5. Canty L, Gardner MD. Ethical Competence in Nursing Practice: Competencies, Skills, Decision-Making. Springer Publishing Company; 2014.
6. Delgado C. Ethical decision making: Codes of ethics and beyond. J Soc Work Values and Ethics. 2014;11(1):6-13.
7. Dierckx de Casterlé B, Izumi S, Godfrey NS, Denhaerynck K, Nurses MD. Nurses' responses to ethical dilemmas in nursing practice: Meta-analysis. J Adv Nurs. 2016;72(6):1209-24.
8. Epstein B, Turner M, Chmielinski K, Pazdernik V. Moral distress, compassion fatigue, and perceptions about medication errors in certified critical care nurses. Dimens Crit Care Nurs. 2017;36(3):159-65.
9. Gaur R, Mudgal SK. Ethical Issues and Ethical Dilemma. In: Sharma SK (Ed). Professionalism, Professional Values and Ethics in Nursing. New Delhi: Jaypee Brothers Medical Publishers; 2023.
10. International Council of Nurses. (2012). ICN Code of Ethics for Nurses. Retrieved from:https://www.icn.ch/sites/default/files/inline-files/2012_ICN_Codeofethicsfornurses_%20eng.pdf.
11. Johnstone M-J. Bioethics: A Nursing Perspective. Elsevier Australia; 2020.
12. Lamiani G, Borghi L, Argentero P, Vegni E. The impact of workload and moral distress on the intention to quit the job in emergency and critical care nurses. Journal of Emergency Nursing, 2017;43(2):141-50.
13. Mudgal SK, Gaur R. Ethics and Bioethics. In: Sharma SK (Ed). Professionalism, Professional Values and Ethics in Nursing. New Delhi: Jaypee Brothers Medical Publishers; 2023.
14. Papathanassoglou ED, Karanikola MN, Kalafati M. Ethical challenges in nursing practice: An overview. Health Sci J. 2018;12(3):1-4.
15. Park M, Kjervik D, Crandell J, Oermann MH. The relationship of ethics education to moral sensitivity and moral reasoning skills of nursing students. Nurs Ethics. 2012;19(5):568-80.
16. Pavlish C, Brown-Saltzman K, Hersh M. Shaping moral distress: An analysis of healthcare providers' narratives. J Clin Ethics. 2011;22(2):124-34.
17. Singer PA, Viens AM. The Cambridge Textbook of Bioethics. Cambridge University Press; 2020.
18. Valizadeh L, Zamanzadeh V, Lotfi M, Johansson H, Griffiths P. Training nurses and creating a supportive work environment are essential to sustaining moral distress. Int Nurs Rev. 2018;65(4):512-20.
19. Yıldırım N, Şenyuva E, Aşiret GD, İncir Ş, Kızılcık AY. The effect of ethics education on the moral sensitivity of nursing students. Nurs Ethics. 2018;25(2):191-200.

2 Section

Foundations of Nursing Practice: Ethical, Legal, and Developmental Considerations

Section Outline

Issues in Nursing

Learning Objectives

♦ Identify and analyze common ethical issues in nursing practice.
♦ Apply ethical principles and frameworks to navigate complex ethical dilemmas.
♦ Demonstrate an understanding of the importance of maintaining professional boundaries and cultural competence in providing patient-centered care.
♦ Define legal issues in nursing and identify the sources from which legal issues arises.
♦ Classify the types of law relevant to nursing.
♦ Describe intentional and unintentional torts in nursing.
♦ Articulate the importance of law in nursing practice.
♦ Analyze the legal responsibilities of nurses and their role in health care.
♦ Identify other critical issues faced by the nursing profession.
♦ Discuss the challenges posed by technological advancements in health care.

INTRODUCTION

Nursing is a critical profession that plays a vital role in the healthcare system. Nurses are responsible for providing direct patient care, promoting health, and advocating for the well-being of individuals, families, and communities. However, like any profession, nursing faces several challenges and issues that impact the delivery of quality care and the overall well-being of both nurses and patients.

ETHICAL ISSUES

Nursing is a noble profession that requires not only technical skills but also a strong ethical foundation. Nurses are entrusted with the responsibility of providing compassionate care, upholding patient rights, and making complex decisions in challenging situations. However, they often encounter ethical issues that can pose significant moral dilemmas and require careful consideration and resolution.

DEFINITIONS

- **American Nurses Association (ANA):** The ANA defines ethical issues in nursing as "situations in which nurses must make decisions that involve conflicting values."
- **International Council of Nurses (ICN):** The ICN defines ethical issues in nursing as "situations in which nurses must make decisions that involve the rights, responsibilities, and well-being of patients, families, and communities."
- **Beauchamp and Childress:** Beauchamp and Childress are two philosophers who have written extensively on ethics. They define ethical issues as "situations in which there is a conflict between two or more moral principles."

COMMON ETHICAL ISSUES IN NURSING

Ethical issues are an integral part of nursing practice and involve complex dilemmas that require careful consideration and decision-making. Nurses often find themselves facing various ethical challenges as they strive to provide patient-centered care while upholding professional standards and maintaining the highest ethical principles. Let's delve into some common ethical issues in nursing practice in more detail (**Fig. 7.1**):

Patient Autonomy

Respecting patient autonomy is a fundamental ethical principle in nursing. It means recognizing and honoring an individual's right to make decisions about their own healthcare. However, situations may arise where a patient's autonomous decision conflicts with medical recommendations or poses risks to their well-being. Nurses must navigate these dilemmas by ensuring patients are provided with adequate information, promoting informed consent, and collaborating with patients to find a balance between respecting autonomy and promoting patient safety.

In nursing, patient autonomy presents several ethical considerations and challenges:

- **Informed consent:** Nurses have a responsibility to provide patients with accurate and understandable information about their medical condition, available treatment options, risks, benefits, and alternatives. Informed consent is a process that ensures patients have the necessary information to make autonomous decisions about their care. Nurses must actively engage in this process, answer questions, address concerns, and ensure that patients have the capacity to understand the information provided.

- **Shared decision-making:** Collaborative decision-making involves active participation and shared responsibility between the healthcare team and the patient. It recognizes that patients are experts in their own lives and should have a voice in determining their treatment plans. Nurses play a vital role in facilitating

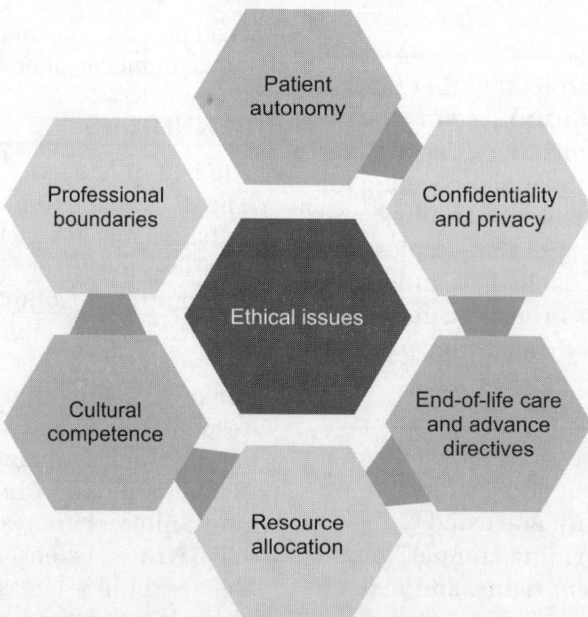

Fig. 7.1: Ethical issues in nursing.

discussions, providing information, and ensuring that patients are involved in decision-making processes. This approach enhances patient autonomy and promotes patient-centered care.

- **Respect for patient values and preferences:** Nurses must respect the diverse values, beliefs, and cultural backgrounds of their patients. This includes recognizing and acknowledging the individuality of each patient and their right to make choices that align with their personal values and goals. Nurses should avoid imposing their own values and biases on patients and strive to provide culturally sensitive and appropriate care.
- **Challenging situations:** Ethical dilemmas can arise when patients' autonomous decisions conflict with medical recommendations or pose potential risks to their well-being. For example, a patient may refuse a life-saving treatment or request a treatment that healthcare professionals deem unnecessary or ineffective. In such situations, nurses must balance the principles of patient autonomy with their duty to promote the patient's best interests and ensure patient safety. Ethical decision-making frameworks, collaboration with the healthcare team, and seeking ethical consultation can help navigate these challenging situations.
- **Vulnerable populations:** Certain patient populations, such as children, individuals with cognitive impairments, or those with mental health conditions, may have limitations in exercising full autonomy. In these cases, nurses have a responsibility to advocate for the patient's best interests and act as their surrogate decision-makers when necessary. Balancing patient autonomy with the duty to protect vulnerable individuals requires careful ethical considerations and adherence to legal frameworks.

Respecting patient autonomy in nursing practice requires a commitment to open communication, providing information, fostering trust, and promoting patient empowerment. Nurses must advocate for patients' rights, facilitate shared decision-making, and ensure that patients' values and preferences are at the forefront of their care. By upholding patient autonomy, nurses contribute to patient-centered care and the ethical practice of nursing.

Confidentiality and Privacy

Maintaining patient confidentiality and privacy is crucial to establish trust and protect patients' rights. Nurses have a legal and ethical duty to safeguard patient information and only disclose it with appropriate consent or as required by law. However, ethical challenges can arise when there is a potential conflict between patient confidentiality and the need to protect the patient or others from harm. Nurses must navigate these situations by understanding the limits of confidentiality, following organizational policies, and seeking guidance from ethical committees or supervisors.

Here is a closer look at confidentiality and privacy as ethical issues in nursing:

- **Trust and therapeutic relationship:** Confidentiality is a fundamental aspect of building trust and establishing a therapeutic relationship between nurses and patients. Patients must feel confident that their personal information, medical history, and conversations with healthcare providers will be kept confidential. Respecting confidentiality helps foster open and honest communication, enabling patients to share sensitive information without fear of judgment or unauthorized disclosure.
- **Legal and ethical obligations:** Nurses are bound by legal and ethical standards that require them to protect patient privacy. Laws, such as the Health Insurance Portability and Accountability Act (HIPAA) in the United States, establish guidelines for maintaining patient confidentiality and safeguarding electronic health records. Violations of patient confidentiality can

lead to legal consequences and erode trust in healthcare providers.

- **Informed consent and autonomy:** Confidentiality is closely tied to informed consent and patient autonomy. Before obtaining a patient's informed consent, nurses must provide clear and comprehensive information about the intended procedures, potential risks and benefits, and available alternatives. Patients can make autonomous decisions when they have access to accurate information and trust that their personal details will be kept confidential.

- **Sharing information with the healthcare team:** While nurses have a duty to maintain confidentiality, they also need to collaborate and share relevant patient information with the healthcare team to provide comprehensive care. Ethical challenges may arise in determining what information should be shared, ensuring that it is done on a need-to-know basis, and balancing the patient's privacy rights with the necessity of communication for coordinated care.

- **Balancing confidentiality and duty to protect:** Nurses may encounter situations where confidentiality conflicts with their duty to protect patients or others from harm. Ethical dilemmas may arise when a patient's condition raises concerns about their safety or the safety of others. Nurses must carefully navigate these situations, seeking guidance from ethical frameworks, institutional policies, and legal obligations to strike a balance between respecting confidentiality and ensuring the welfare of individuals involved.

- **Digital privacy and technology:** With the increasing use of electronic health records, telehealth, and other digital platforms, nurses must be vigilant in protecting patient privacy in the digital realm. This includes maintaining secure passwords, encrypting data, and being cautious when sharing patient information through electronic means to prevent unauthorized access or breaches.

Nurses must undergo regular training and education to understand the importance of confidentiality and privacy, stay updated with legal requirements, and adhere to institutional policies and guidelines. Respecting patient confidentiality and privacy not only upholds ethical standards but also contributes to building trust, promoting patient autonomy, and ensuring the overall well-being of patients in the healthcare setting.

End-of-Life Care and Advance Directives

End-of-life care presents complex ethical dilemmas for nurses. Patients may have varying preferences regarding life-sustaining treatments, resuscitation, or palliative care. Nurses must respect the patient's autonomy by ensuring their wishes are known and honored. However, conflicts may arise when patients' choices conflict with healthcare providers' or family members' beliefs or when the patient's decision-making capacity is impaired. Ethical decision-making involves careful discussions, exploring the patient's values and goals, and collaborating with the healthcare team and family to provide compassionate and appropriate end-of-life care.

Let's explore the ethical considerations related to end-of-life care and advance directives:

- **Autonomy and respect for patient wishes:** End-of-life care and advance directives are deeply rooted in the principle of patient autonomy. It recognizes that individuals have the right to make decisions about their healthcare, even when they are no longer able to communicate those decisions. Nurses have an ethical obligation to respect and honor patients' advance directives, such as living wills or do-not-resuscitate (DNR) orders, which outline their preferences regarding medical interventions and end-of-life care.

- **Informed decision-making:** Nurses play a crucial role in providing patients and their families with accurate and comprehensive information about end-of-life options, including the benefits, risks, and possible outcomes. Informed decision-making involves discussing prognosis, explaining treatment alternatives, and addressing any concerns or misconceptions. Nurses must ensure that patients and their families have the necessary knowledge to make informed choices about their care.

- **Shared decision-making:** End-of-life care decisions are often complex and emotionally charged. Nurses have a responsibility to facilitate shared decision-making, involving patients, families, and the healthcare team in the process. This collaborative approach helps ensure that patient preferences are respected, family concerns are addressed, and decisions are made collectively with the patient's best interests in mind.

- **Palliative care and pain management:** Ethical considerations arise when balancing the goals of curative treatment with the need for palliative care and pain management. Nurses must advocate for patients' comfort, dignity, and quality of life, even when curative options are limited. Providing appropriate pain relief, managing symptoms, and addressing psychological, emotional, and spiritual needs are integral parts of end-of-life care.

- **Cultural and religious considerations:** End-of-life care is influenced by cultural and religious beliefs, which may vary greatly among individuals and communities. Nurses must approach end-of-life care with cultural sensitivity, respecting patients' cultural and religious practices, values, and preferences. Ethical dilemmas may arise when cultural or religious beliefs conflict with medical recommendations. Nurses must engage in open and respectful communication, seek cultural guidance, and collaborate with the healthcare team to find a balance that respects patients'

autonomy while providing compassionate care.

- **Family dynamics and conflict resolution:** Family dynamics can significantly impact end-of-life decision-making. Conflicts may arise when family members hold differing opinions about treatment options or advance directives. Nurses must navigate these challenging situations by promoting effective communication, providing emotional support, and engaging in ethical discussions to help families reach a consensus that aligns with the patient's wishes and best interests.

- **Withdrawal of life-sustaining treatment:** Withdrawing life-sustaining treatment, such as ventilators or feeding tubes, raises ethical questions. Nurses must ensure that decisions to withdraw or withhold treatment are made in accordance with the patient's wishes, advance directives, and ethical guidelines. Open communication, documentation, and collaboration with the healthcare team are essential to ensure transparency and accountability in these decisions.

Nurses should continually engage in ethical reflection, seek support from ethics committees or clinical supervisors, and stay updated on legal and ethical guidelines regarding end-of-life care and advance directives. By navigating these ethical issues with compassion and sensitivity, nurses can provide holistic care that respects patient autonomy and preserves dignity during the end-of-life journey.

Resource Allocation

In healthcare settings with limited resources, nurses may face ethical challenges related to the fair distribution of resources among patients. This includes medications, treatments, or healthcare interventions. Nurses must make decisions based on factors such as medical urgency, potential benefits, and equitable distribution. Ethical considerations such as the principles of justice, minimizing bias or discrimination, and ensuring transparency are essential. Nurses should work collaboratively with the healthcare team, following established protocols and guidelines, to make fair decisions regarding resource allocation.

Here are the key ethical considerations related to resource allocation in nursing:

- **Justice and fairness:** Resource allocation requires nurses to consider the principles of justice and fairness. They must strive to distribute resources equitably, ensuring that all patients have access to the necessary care, regardless of their socioeconomic status, age, gender, or other factors. This principle aims to prevent discrimination and promote equal opportunities for healthcare.

- **Utilitarianism and maximizing benefits:** Utilitarian ethical theories argue for resource allocation decisions that maximize overall benefits and outcomes for the greatest number of patients. Nurses may need to assess the potential benefits and expected outcomes of different treatment options and allocate resources accordingly. This approach focuses on the overall welfare of the population and aims to achieve the best possible outcomes for the majority.

- **Proportionality and need:** Nurses must consider the severity of patients' conditions and allocate resources based on the principle of proportionality. This means directing resources to those with the greatest need or those who stand to benefit the most from the intervention. Prioritizing patients based on the urgency and severity of their condition helps ensure that resources are used effectively and efficiently.

- **Transparency and accountability:** It is crucial to maintain transparency in the decision-making process and communicate clearly with patients, families, and healthcare providers. Nurses should explain the reasons behind resource allocation decisions, outline the criteria used, and provide opportunities for discussion and appeals. Transparency fosters trust, promotes understanding, and allows stakeholders to participate in the decision-making process.

- **Ethical dilemmas and difficult choices:** Resource allocation often involves making difficult choices between patients with similar needs or allocating scarce resources to one patient at the expense of another. Nurses may face ethical dilemmas when balancing the principles of equity, utility, and individual patient needs. Ethical decision-making frameworks, ethical consultation, and collaboration with multidisciplinary teams can help navigate these challenging situations.

- **Advocacy and ethical responsibility:** Nurses have an ethical responsibility to advocate for their patients and ensure they receive appropriate care. They must be proactive in identifying and addressing issues related to resource allocation that may affect patient outcomes. Nurses can collaborate with healthcare administrators, policymakers, and ethics committees to develop policies and guidelines that promote fair resource allocation and minimize ethical challenges.

- **Ongoing education and reflection:** Given the dynamic nature of healthcare and the constant evolution of resource availability, nurses should engage in continuous education and reflection on ethical issues related to resource allocation. Staying informed about current guidelines, participating in discussions and ethical case reviews, and seeking ethical guidance contribute to ethical decision-making in resource allocation.

By approaching resource allocation with ethical principles and a patient-centered perspective, nurses can strive to ensure fairness, maximize benefits, and advocate for equitable access to healthcare resources. Effective communication, transparency, and collaboration among healthcare professionals and stakeholders are essential in addressing the ethical complexities of resource allocation in nursing.

Cultural Competence

Nursing is practiced in diverse cultural contexts, and nurses encounter patients from various cultural backgrounds. Providing culturally competent care involves respecting and understanding patients' values, beliefs, and healthcare practices. However, ethical challenges may arise due to cultural clashes, differing views on healthcare interventions, or conflicts between patients' cultural practices and evidence-based care. Nurses must strive for cultural sensitivity, open communication, and finding common ground while ensuring the delivery of safe and appropriate care that respects patients' autonomy and cultural identity.

Here's a closer look at cultural competence as an ethical issue in nursing:

- **Respect for cultural diversity:** Cultural competence embodies the ethical principle of respect for persons and the recognition of the inherent worth and dignity of every individual. Nurses have an ethical obligation to respect and value the cultural beliefs, practices, and values of their patients. They should strive to provide care that is sensitive to cultural diversity and avoids imposing their own cultural biases on patients.
- **Health equity and eliminating disparities:** Cultural competence is closely linked to the ethical principle of justice, which emphasizes the fair distribution of healthcare resources and the elimination of health disparities. Nurses must recognize that cultural factors can influence health outcomes and access to care. By understanding and addressing these factors, they can work towards promoting health equity and reducing disparities among diverse populations.
- **Effective communication:** Effective communication is a cornerstone of cultural competence. Nurses must be able to communicate with patients from different cultural backgrounds in a way that respects their language preferences, health literacy levels, and communication styles. This includes being mindful of nonverbal cues, using appropriate interpreters when necessary, and engaging in active listening to ensure accurate understanding.
- **Individualized care:** Cultural competence recognizes that individuals within the same cultural group may have unique beliefs, values, and preferences. Nurses must provide individualized care that takes into account each patient's cultural context, personal experiences, and needs. This involves engaging in a collaborative and culturally sensitive approach to care, incorporating the patient's input and involving their family or community as appropriate.
- **Overcoming stereotypes and biases:** Nurses must be aware of their own biases and stereotypes that may affect the delivery of culturally competent care. Self-reflection and ongoing education are essential in identifying and addressing these biases. Nurses should continuously strive to challenge stereotypes, examine their own cultural assumptions, and work towards providing care that is free from discrimination or prejudice.
- **Cultural safety:** Cultural safety goes beyond cultural competence and emphasizes creating a safe and respectful healthcare environment for individuals from diverse cultures. Nurses must ensure that their practice settings are culturally safe, where patients feel empowered to express their cultural identity and voice concerns without fear of judgment or discrimination. This includes addressing systemic barriers, power imbalances, and promoting inclusive and welcoming care environments.
- **Continuous learning and development:** Cultural competence is a lifelong learning process. Nurses should actively seek opportunities for education and training to enhance their cultural knowledge,

awareness, and skills. By staying informed about diverse cultural practices, beliefs, and healthcare disparities, nurses can continually improve their ability to provide culturally competent care.

By embracing cultural competence as an ethical imperative, nurses can promote respectful, patient-centered care, and contribute to the overall well-being and satisfaction of patients from diverse cultural backgrounds. It fosters trust, improves health outcomes, and upholds the ethical principles of respect, justice, and equity in nursing practice.

PROFESSIONAL BOUNDARIES

Maintaining professional boundaries is essential for ensuring patient safety, trust, and professional integrity. Nurses must establish appropriate boundaries to prevent any exploitation, emotional harm, or breach of professional standards. Ethical challenges may arise when nurses face situations that blur the boundaries, such as engaging in dual relationships with patients, crossing emotional boundaries, or becoming personally involved. Nurses must receive adequate education on professional boundaries, regularly reflect on their own practices, and seek supervision or consultation when faced with challenging situations.

Here is an in-depth look at professional boundaries as an ethical issue in nursing:

- **Power imbalance:** Nurses hold a position of power and authority within the healthcare setting, while patients are often in vulnerable positions due to their health conditions. Professional boundaries help mitigate the inherent power imbalance between healthcare professionals and patients, ensuring that care is delivered in a respectful and ethical manner. Nurses must recognize the power they hold and use it responsibly, prioritizing the best interests and autonomy of the patient.
- **Patient safety:** Maintaining professional boundaries is essential for protecting the safety and well-being of patients.

Boundaries help prevent situations of exploitation, abuse, or manipulation. By adhering to appropriate professional conduct, nurses create a safe environment where patients feel comfortable sharing sensitive information and seeking care without fear of their boundaries being violated.

- **Confidentiality and privacy:** Professional boundaries include maintaining patient confidentiality and privacy. Nurses have an ethical obligation to respect and protect patient information. They must refrain from sharing patient details or engaging in discussions about patients outside the necessary professional context. Respecting confidentiality helps build trust, maintains patient autonomy, and upholds the ethical principle of privacy.
- **Dual relationships:** Dual relationships occur when nurses engage in personal, social, or financial relationships with patients or their families outside the professional context. Nurses must avoid such relationships as they can compromise objectivity, impartiality, and the nurse-patient therapeutic relationship. Dual relationships can blur boundaries and lead to conflicts of interest or exploitation.
- **Emotional boundaries:** Nurses often build close relationships with their patients as they provide emotional support and compassionate care. However, it is crucial to maintain emotional boundaries to ensure professional objectivity and prevent emotional dependency. Nurses must navigate the fine line between empathy and professional detachment, ensuring they do not become personally involved beyond the scope of their professional responsibilities.
- **Social media and digital boundaries:** With the rise of social media, nurses must be mindful of the potential risks related to maintaining professional boundaries in the online realm. Nurses must avoid engaging in unprofessional or boundary-crossing behavior on social media platforms and refrain from sharing patient information

or engaging in inappropriate discussions. Maintaining digital boundaries protects patient privacy and maintains professional integrity.

- **Self-awareness and reflection:** Nurses must engage in self-reflection and continuously evaluate their own behaviors and interactions to ensure they maintain appropriate professional boundaries. This includes recognizing personal biases, cultural differences, and power dynamics that may influence their relationships with patients. Nurses should seek feedback, engage in supervision or mentorship, and participate in ongoing professional development to enhance their self-awareness and ethical practice.

Ethical nursing practice requires nurses to establish and maintain professional boundaries, ensuring that their relationships with patients are grounded in trust, respect, and patient-centered care. By adhering to professional boundaries, nurses protect patient safety, maintain confidentiality, and contribute to the ethical integrity of the nursing profession.

◼ DO NOT RESUSCITATE

Do Not Resuscitate (DNR), orders are an important aspect of end-of-life care and an ethical issue that nurses often encounter. A DNR order is a medical directive that instructs healthcare providers not to perform cardiopulmonary resuscitation (CPR) if a patient's heart stops or they stop breathing. It is a decision made by a competent patient or their designated healthcare proxy, reflecting their wishes regarding resuscitative efforts.

When it comes to DNR orders, several ethical considerations come into play:

- **Patient autonomy:** DNR orders are grounded in the principle of patient autonomy, respecting an individual's right to make decisions about their own healthcare. It allows patients to have control over the extent of medical interventions they receive and aligns with their personal values and goals of care.

- **Informed consent:** Nurses have a crucial role in facilitating discussions about DNR orders, ensuring that patients and their families understand the implications, risks, and potential outcomes of CPR. Informed consent involves providing comprehensive information, answering questions, and clarifying any misconceptions to enable patients to make well-informed decisions.

- **Shared decision-making:** The decision to have a DNR order should be a collaborative process involving the patient, their family, and the healthcare team. Nurses play a critical role in facilitating these discussions, ensuring that patients' preferences and values are heard and respected. Shared decision-making fosters a patient-centered approach and ethical practice.

- **Emotional impact:** DNR discussions can be emotionally challenging for patients, families, and nurses themselves. It requires sensitivity, empathy, and effective communication to address fears, provide emotional support, and guide individuals through the decision-making process. Nurses should create a supportive environment that allows open dialogue and respects the emotional needs of everyone involved.

- **Ethical dilemmas:** Ethical dilemmas may arise when there is a disagreement between patients, families, and healthcare providers regarding the appropriateness of a DNR order. Conflicts can occur if family members have differing opinions or if cultural or religious beliefs influence the decision-making process. In such cases, nurses must facilitate open discussions, consider all perspectives, and seek ethical consultation to find a resolution that upholds patient autonomy and ensures the provision of compassionate care.

- **Documentation and communication:** Accurate documentation of the DNR order is essential to ensure its implementation and communication to the entire healthcare team. Nurses are responsible for properly documenting the DNR order, updating the patient's medical records, and ensuring that all relevant team members are aware of the patient's wishes.

Nurses must navigate these ethical considerations surrounding DNR orders with sensitivity, respect, and adherence to professional and legal standards. Open communication, collaborative decision-making, and ongoing support for patients and their families are essential in promoting ethical care at the end of life. Additionally, nurses should stay updated with legal requirements and institutional policies regarding DNR orders to ensure compliance and provide optimal end-of-life care to patients.

Overall, in addressing these ethical issues, nurses can rely on ethical frameworks, such as the principles of autonomy, beneficence, nonmaleficence, and justice, to guide their decision-making. Collaboration with the healthcare team, seeking ethical consultation or guidance from ethical committees or supervisors, and engaging in continuous education and reflective practices are essential in navigating these complex ethical dilemmas.

By recognizing and addressing these ethical issues, nurses can contribute to improved patient outcomes, enhanced trust in healthcare, and the promotion of ethical practice within the nursing profession.

LEGAL ISSUES IN NURSING

Legal issues in nursing encompass a wide range of topics related to the legal framework that governs nursing practice. Nurses are expected to adhere to laws and regulations to ensure patient safety, protect their professional integrity, and avoid legal consequences.

DEFINITIONS

- **Barbara K Redman** defines legal issues in nursing as "those situations in which a nurse may be held liable for harm to a patient." She goes on to say that "legal issues can arise from a variety of sources, including the nurse's actions, omissions, or decisions."
- Linda J Nelson defines legal issues in nursing as "any situation that could result in a lawsuit against a nurse." She includes in this definition "situations where a nurse has provided substandard care, violated a patient's rights, or engaged in unprofessional conduct."
- Margaret A Barnsteiner defines legal issues in nursing as "the intersection of law and nursing practice." She says that "legal issues can arise from any aspect of nursing practice, including patient care, education, research, and administration."

CONCEPT OF LAW

The word "law" has a rich linguistic history and has evolved over time. Its derivation can be traced back to different origins:

- **Proto-Indo-European Root:** The English word "law" is believed to have originated from the Proto-Indo-European root "*legh-", which means "to lay" or "to put." This root gave rise to various related words in different Indo-European languages.
- **Old English:** In Old English, the word "law" was spelled "lagu" or "laʒu" and referred to a rule or custom. It was derived from the Old Norse word "lag," meaning "law" or "layer." This term likely entered Old English through Viking invasions and settlements.
- **Germanic influence:** The Germanic languages, including Old English, have a shared linguistic heritage. The German word for "law" is "Gesetz," which also shares a common root with the English word.

DEFINITIONS

- **John Locke:** "Law is a rule of civil conduct prescribed by the supreme power in a state, commanding what is right and prohibiting what is wrong."
- **Thomas Aquinas:** "Law is nothing else than an ordinance of reason for the common good, made by him who has care of the community, and promulgated."
- **John Austin:** "Law is the aggregate of rules set by men as politically superior or sovereign to men as politically subject."

- **Oliver Wendell Holmes Jr:** "The prophecies of what the courts will do in fact, and nothing more pretentious, are what I mean by the law."

SOURCES OF LAW IN NURSING

In nursing, various sources of law provide the legal framework that governs the profession. These sources of law establish the rights and responsibilities of nurses, outline the standards of practice, and regulate the delivery of healthcare. Here are the primary sources of law in nursing:

- **Statutory law:** Statutory law consists of laws passed by legislative bodies at the federal, state, or local levels. In nursing, statutory law includes statutes and regulations specifically related to healthcare and nursing practice. Examples include the Nurse Practice Act, which defines the scope of practice for nurses in a particular jurisdiction, and healthcare regulations issued by government agencies such as the Centers for Medicare and Medicaid Services (CMS).
- **Common law:** Common law is based on legal precedents established through court decisions. In nursing, common law evolves over time as courts interpret and apply laws to specific cases. Court decisions related to nursing practice, malpractice claims, and patient rights contribute to the body of common law in nursing.
- **Administrative law:** Administrative law comprises rules, regulations, and decisions issued by administrative agencies, such as state boards of nursing and professional regulatory bodies. These agencies are responsible for implementing and enforcing statutes related to nursing practice. Administrative law plays a crucial role in setting standards of practice, licensing requirements, and disciplinary actions for nurses.
- **Constitutional law:** Constitutional law refers to the body of laws derived from a country's constitution or constitutional principles. Constitutional provisions may impact nursing practice by defining the rights of individuals, including patients, healthcare providers, and healthcare organizations. Constitutional law protects individual rights, such as privacy, due process, and freedom from discrimination, which have implications for nursing practice.
- **Case law:** Case law, also known as judicial precedent, is the body of law established through court decisions in specific legal cases. These decisions interpret and apply statutory and common law to the specific circumstances of the case. Case law contributes to the development of legal principles and can influence nursing practice and legal interpretations of ethical issues.

TYPES OF LAW

There are various types of law that exist within legal systems. Here are two of the most common types of law in nursing:

1. **Criminal Law:** Criminal law deals with offenses committed against society as a whole. It encompasses crimes such as murder, theft, assault, and fraud. Criminal law sets out the legal framework for investigating, prosecuting, and punishing individuals who violate these laws.
2. **Civil Law:** Civil law governs the relationships between individuals or entities and deals with noncriminal matters. It covers areas such as contracts, property, torts (personal injuries and civil wrongs), family law, and employment law. Disputes in civil law are typically resolved through lawsuits and can result in monetary compensation or specific performance of a legal obligation.

TORTS

In the context of nursing, torts can be categorized as intentional or unintentional based on the nature of the harm caused to the patient and the intent of the nurse. Here's an explanation of intentional and unintentional torts in nursing:

Intentional Torts

Intentional torts occur when a nurse deliberately performs an action that results in harm to a patient. These torts involve the intent to cause harm or the intent to engage in conduct that is substantially certain to cause harm. Examples of intentional torts in nursing include:

- **Assault:** Intentionally causing apprehension of harmful or offensive contact with a patient, such as threatening physical harm. For example, a nurse who threatens to harm a patient has committed assault.
- **Battery:** Intentional and unauthorized physical contact or touching of a patient without their consent, even if it is not necessarily harmful. For example, a nurse who forcefully restrains a patient without their consent has committed battery.
- **False imprisonment:** Intentionally confining or restraining a patient without legal justification or without their consent. For example, a nurse who locks a patient in a room without their consent has committed false imprisonment.
- **Invasion of privacy:** Deliberately violating a patient's right to privacy or confidentiality by disclosing private information without consent. For example, a nurse who reads a patient's medical records without their consent has committed invasion of privacy.
- **Defamation:** Defamation occurs when false statements are made about an individual that harm their reputation. It can be either slander (spoken defamation) or libel (written or printed defamation). Nurses must be cautious in discussing patient information to avoid making false statements that could damage a patient's reputation.

Intentional torts are considered willful acts and may result in both civil liability (requiring the nurse to compensate the injured party) and potential criminal charges, depending on the jurisdiction and severity of the actions.

Unintentional Torts

Unintentional torts, also known as negligence, occur when a nurse fails to provide the expected standard of care, resulting in harm to a patient. These torts involve actions or omissions that are considered to be below the standard of care expected of a reasonably competent nurse. Examples of unintentional torts in nursing include:

- **Negligence:** Failing to provide adequate care or exercising a lack of reasonable care that leads to harm, such as medication errors, failure to monitor or assess patients adequately, or not following established protocols.
- **Malpractice:** Professional negligence that occurs when a nurse's actions or omissions deviate from the accepted standards of practice, resulting in harm to the patient. For example, a doctor who fails to diagnose a patient's cancer has committed malpractice.

Unintentional torts are typically addressed through civil litigation, and the injured party must establish the elements of duty, breach of duty, causation, and damages to prove negligence or malpractice. Nurses can be held liable for damages caused by their negligent actions or omissions.

It is important for nurses to understand the distinction between intentional and unintentional torts to ensure they provide safe and ethical care. Nurses should strive to act in the best interests of their patients, avoid intentional harm, and practice within the accepted standards of care to minimize the risk of tort claims, whether intentional or unintentional.

IMPORTANCE OF LAW IN NURSING

Law plays a crucial role in nursing and healthcare in several ways. Here are some of the key reasons why law is important in the nursing profession:

- Ensures patient safety and quality care.
- Defines the scope of nursing practice and professional responsibilities.

- Upholds ethical standards and principles.
- Establishes legal accountability for nurses.
- Guides the process of obtaining informed consent from patients.
- Regulates documentation and recordkeeping for accurate and comprehensive patient information.
- Protects patient privacy and confidentiality.
- Aligns with professional standards and guidelines.
- Provides legal protection for nurses and patients.
- Promotes trust and respect between healthcare providers and patients.
- Facilitates communication, continuity of care, and collaboration in healthcare settings.
- Supports evidence-based practice and continuous improvements in healthcare.

LEGAL RESPONSIBILITIES AND ROLE OF A NURSE

Nurses have important legal responsibilities and play a crucial role in healthcare. These responsibilities and roles are guided by various laws, regulations, and professional standards. Here are some key aspects of the legal responsibilities and role of a nurse:

- **Providing safe and competent care:** Nurses have a legal duty to provide safe, competent, and ethical care to their patients. This includes performing assessments, administering medications, implementing treatments, and monitoring patient progress while adhering to the accepted standards of practice.
- **Maintaining patient confidentiality and privacy:** Nurses are obligated to protect patient confidentiality and privacy. They must follow laws and regulations, such as HIPAA, to ensure that patient information remains confidential and is only shared with authorized individuals for appropriate purposes.
- **Documenting patient care:** Accurate and timely documentation of patient care is a legal responsibility of nurses. Documentation serves as a record of the care provided, facilitates communication among healthcare professionals, and may be used in legal proceedings or audits.
- **Obtaining informed consent:** Nurses have a responsibility to ensure that patients or their authorized representatives provide informed consent before any treatment or procedure. This involves explaining the nature, risks, benefits, and alternatives of the proposed intervention so that patients can make informed decisions about their healthcare.
- **Recognizing and reporting adverse events:** Nurses are responsible for promptly recognizing and reporting adverse events, errors, or incidents that may harm patients. This includes documenting and reporting incidents to appropriate individuals or departments within the healthcare organization to initiate appropriate action and ensure patient safety.
- **Advocating for patient rights:** Nurses are advocates for their patients, promoting and protecting their rights. They should ensure that patients' voices are heard, their concerns are addressed, and their autonomy is respected. Nurses may also advocate for patients at the organizational or policy level to improve healthcare delivery and patient outcomes.
- **Continuing education and professional development:** Nurses have a legal and ethical obligation to engage in lifelong learning, keeping their knowledge and skills up to date. They should participate in continuing education programs, maintain professional certifications, and stay informed about new research, evidence-based practices, and legal updates relevant to their practice.
- **Recognizing and reporting abuse or neglect:** Nurses have a legal obligation to recognize and report any signs of abuse, neglect, or exploitation of vulnerable individuals, such as children, elderly patients, or individuals with disabilities. Reporting such incidents protects the

welfare of the patients and fulfills legal requirements.

- **Adhering to professional standards and codes of ethics:** Nurses must abide by the standards of practice and codes of ethics established by their professional nursing organizations. These standards provide guidance on professional conduct, ethical principles, and accountability in nursing practice.

It is essential for nurses to be knowledgeable about the laws and regulations that govern their practice and to maintain their competence in providing safe, ethical, and patient-centered care. Regularly consulting legal resources, staying updated on professional guidelines, and seeking guidance when faced with legal or ethical dilemmas are important steps for nurses to fulfill their legal responsibilities and ensure high-quality care.

OTHER ISSUES IN NURSING

Apart from ethical and legal issues, the nursing profession faces numerous challenges and issues that impact nurses, patients, and the overall healthcare system. These issues range from workforce shortages and high levels of stress to the need for continuous professional development. The following sections will delve into specific challenges faced by nurses, including:

- **Nurse shortage:** One of the major issues in nursing is the ongoing nursing shortage. Many countries around the world are experiencing a shortage of qualified nurses, which can have detrimental effects on patient care. The demand for nursing services is increasing due to an aging population, a rise in chronic diseases, and advances in medical technology. However, the supply of nurses is not keeping pace with this demand, leading to understaffed healthcare facilities, increased workloads for nurses, and compromised patient safety.
- **Workforce fatigue:** Workplace stress and burnout are significant problems in the nursing profession. Nurses often work long hours, handle high patient caseloads, and face challenging situations regularly. This can lead to physical and emotional exhaustion, resulting in decreased job satisfaction and an increased risk of medical errors. The consequences of nurse burnout not only affect the well-being of nurses but also impact patient outcomes and the overall quality of healthcare.
- **Inadequate staffing:** Nurses also face issue related to inadequate staffing levels. Insufficient staffing can strain nurses' ability to provide optimal care, leading to compromised patient safety and increased stress levels among healthcare providers.
- **Violence against nurses:** Nurses are at an increased risk of violence, both verbal and physical, from patients, families, and visitors. A study by the American Nurses Association found that nearly one in four nurses have been physically assaulted at work. Additionally, unsafe working conditions, such as exposure to infectious diseases, pose risks to nurses' physical and mental health.
- **Lack of professional development:** Another important issue in nursing is the need for continuous professional development and education. The field of healthcare is constantly evolving, with new treatments, technologies, and best practices emerging regularly. Nurses must stay updated with the latest knowledge and skills to provide evidence-based care. However, accessing quality education and training opportunities can be challenging, particularly for nurses working in remote or underserved areas.
- **Lack of professional autonomy:** The issue of professional autonomy and nursing leadership is also relevant in the nursing profession. Nurses are highly skilled professionals who possess valuable expertise and insights into patient care. However, in some healthcare settings,

nurses may face limited decision-making authority and opportunities for leadership roles. Enhancing nurses' autonomy and empowering them to contribute to decision-making processes can positively impact patient care outcomes and the overall effectiveness of healthcare teams.

- **Low pay:** Nurses are often underpaid for the work they do. The median annual salary for registered nurses in the India is Rs. 96,000/- approximately in private sectors and 8,40,000/- in government sector the median annual salary for other healthcare professionals, such as physicians and pharmacists.
- **Technological advancements:** Rapid advancements in healthcare technology have transformed the nursing profession. While technology can enhance efficiency and patient outcomes, it also presents challenges. Nurses need to adapt to and master new technologies, such as electronic health records, telemedicine, and digital monitoring systems. Integrating technology effectively while maintaining a human-centered approach to care delivery is a significant concern.
- **Diversity and cultural competence:** Healthcare is provided to diverse populations with unique cultural, linguistic, and social backgrounds. Nurses must be culturally competent to deliver patient-centered care effectively. However, disparities in access to healthcare and cultural biases can hinder the provision of equitable care. Increasing diversity within the nursing workforce and enhancing cultural competence training are essential to address these challenges.
- **Interprofessional collaboration:** Effective teamwork and collaboration among healthcare professionals are crucial for providing comprehensive and coordinated patient care. Nurses play an integral role in interprofessional collaboration, but challenges such as hierarchies, communication barriers, and role ambiguity can hinder optimal collaboration.
- **Nursing education and training:** There is ongoing discussion about the need to enhance nursing education and training programs to prepare nurses for the evolving healthcare landscape. This includes incorporating advanced technologies, promoting critical thinking skills, and providing opportunities for lifelong learning.

Recognizing and addressing the issues in nursing is crucial for fostering a sustainable and thriving nursing workforce and delivering high-quality patient care. By prioritizing strategies to address workforce shortages, mitigate burnout, enhance ethical decision-making, expand scope of practice, and promote continuous education, stakeholders can collectively work towards building a healthier and more resilient nursing profession.

CHAPTER SUMMARY

1. Ethical issues are an integral part of nursing practice and involve complex dilemmas that require careful consideration and decision-making.
2. Some common ethical issues in nursing include patient autonomy, confidentiality and privacy, end-of-life care and advance directives, resource allocation, and cultural competence.
3. Addressing ethical issues with compassion, sensitivity, and adherence to ethical principles, nurses can provide patient-centered care and contribute to the ethical practice of nursing.

4. Legal issues in nursing encompass a wide range of topics related to the legal framework that governs nursing practice.
5. Nurses are expected to adhere to laws and regulations to ensure patient safety, protect their professional integrity, and avoid legal consequences.
6. Various sources of law, including statutory law, common law, administrative law, constitutional law, and case law, provide the legal framework for nursing practice.
7. Torts, which can be intentional or unintentional, play a significant role in nursing legal issues.
8. Nurses have important legal responsibilities, including providing safe and competent care, maintaining patient confidentiality, documenting patient care, obtaining informed consent, reporting adverse events, advocating for patient rights, continuing education, recognizing and reporting abuse or neglect, and adhering to professional standards and codes of ethics.
9. The other issues in nursing, such as nurse shortage, workforce fatigue, inadequate staffing, violence against nurses, lack of professional development, lack of professional autonomy, low pay, technological advancements, and diversity and cultural competence.

REVIEW QUESTIONS

1. Define issues in nursing. Explain common ethical issues in nursing.
2. Define legal issues in nursing and differentiate between intentional and unintentional tort.
3. Discuss legal responsibilities of a nurse.
4. Describe issues in nursing.
5. Define law and explain importance of law in nursing.

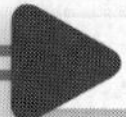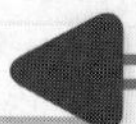

BIBLIOGRAPHY

1. American Nurses Association (ANA). (2015). Code of ethics for nurses with interpretive statements. Silver Spring, MD: ANA.
2. Foss NJ, Ellefsen B. Ethical issues in nursing: A guide to ethical decision-making. London, UK: SAGE Publications; 2016.
3. Gaur R, Mudgal SK. Ethical Issues and Ethical Dilemma, In: Sharma SK (Ed). Professionalism, Professional Values and Ethics in Nursing. New Delhi: Jaypee Brothers Medical Publishers; 2023.
4. Guido GW. Legal and ethical issues in nursing, 7th edition. Pearson; 2017.
5. Jormsri P, Kunaviktikul W, Ketefian S, Chaowalit A. Moral distress: Its prevalence, nature, and impact among professional nurses in Thailand. Nurs Ethics. 2016;23(4):469-81.
6. Kuhlthau KC, Milstead JA. Ethical issues in nursing: A decision-making approach. Sudbury, MA: Jones & Bartlett Learning; 2017.
7. Masters K. Role Development in Professional Nursing Practice, 5th edition. Burlington, MA: Jones & Bartlett Learning; 2020.
8. McGonigl D, Mastrian KG. Nursing Informatics and the Foundation of Knowledge, 4th edition. Burlington, MA: Jones & Bartlett Learning; 2017.
9. Meleis AI. Ethical issues in nursing: Caring in the age of complexity. Philadelphia, PA: FA Davis Company; 2016.

10. Moyer A, Gaba MM, Dellefield ME. The ethical nurse: Integrating ethical issues into clinical practice. MEDSURG Nursing, 2016;25(4):251-4.
11. Mudgal SK, Gaur R. Ethics and Bioethics. In: Sharma SK (Ed). Professionalism, Professional Values and Ethics in Nursing. New Delhi: Jaypee Brothers Medical Publishers; 2023.
12. National Council of State Boards of Nursing (NCSBN): Nurse Practice Act, rules and regulations, 2016. https://www.ncsbn.org/nurse-practice-act.htm.
13. Numminen O, Repo H, Leino-Kilpi H, Suhonen R. Ethical issues in nursing management: The role of codes of ethics. Nurs Ethics. 2015;22(4):432-42.
14. Papathanassoglou EDE, Karanikola MNK, Kalafati M. Exploration of the ethical dimension of nursing care and its integration into undergraduate nursing education. Nurse Educ Today. 2016;41:100-5.
15. Pozgar GD. Legal and ethical issues for health professionals, 4th edition. Burlington, MA, Jones & Bartlett; 2016.
16. Tanner CA. Ethical issues in nursing: Critical thinking and decision-making. Burlington, MA: Jones & Bartlett Learning; 2017.
17. Westrick SJ, Jacob N. Disclosure of errors and apology: law and ethics, J Nurse Pract. 2016;12(2):120.

Health and Illness

Learning Objectives

◆ Define the concept of health and its multidimensional nature.
◆ Compare and contrast various definitions of health provided by organizations.
◆ Explain how the concept of health has evolved over time and has been influenced by cultural, societal, and scientific factors.
◆ Describe the determinants of health and their impact on an individual's well-being.
◆ Differentiate between acute and chronic illnesses.
◆ Analyze the variables influencing illness.
◆ Evaluate the concepts of wellness and well-being.
◆ Illustrate the importance of a holistic approach to healthcare.
◆ Describe the impact of illness on the patient and family.
◆ Discuss the nurse's role in health and illness.

INTRODUCTION

Health is a concept that encompasses the overall well-being of individuals and is essential for a fulfilling and productive life. It goes beyond the absence of disease or infirmity and encompasses physical, mental, and social dimensions. The concept of health is multifaceted and has evolved over time, shaped by cultural, societal, and scientific influences. Understanding the concept of health is crucial for individuals, healthcare professionals, policymakers, and societies as they strive to promote and maintain optimal well-being.

Health is not a static state but a dynamic and evolving concept. It can vary from person to person and can be influenced by various factors, including genetics, lifestyle choices, socioeconomic status, access to healthcare, and environmental conditions. Additionally, health is influenced by broader societal factors, such as education, employment opportunities, and social and economic inequalities.

DEFINITIONS

- The World Health Organization (WHO) defines health as "a state of complete physical, mental, and social well-being and not merely the absence of disease or infirmity."
- The American Medical Association (AMA) defines health as "a state of optimal physical, mental, and social well-being."
- The Centers for Disease Control and Prevention (CDC) defines health as "a state of well-being in which every individual realizes his or her potential for physical, mental, and social well-being and can cope with the normal stresses of life."

CONCEPT OF HEALTH

Health refers to a state of complete physical, mental, and social well-being, not merely the absence of disease or infirmity. It encompasses the overall well-being and functioning of an individual in multiple dimensions. The World Health Organization (WHO) defines health as "a state of complete physical, mental, and social well-being and not merely the absence of disease or infirmity." This definition included three basic dimensions, i.e., physical, mental, and social well-being.

- **Physical health:** Physical health refers to the condition of the body and its ability to perform daily activities without limitations. It involves factors such as good nutrition, regular exercise, adequate sleep, and the absence of physical illnesses or injuries.
- **Mental and emotional well-being:** Mental and emotional well-being encompasses the psychological and emotional aspects of health. It includes having a positive sense of self, managing stress effectively, maintaining good mental health, and having the ability to cope with life's challenges.
- **Social well-being:** Social well-being refers to the quality of an individual's relationships, social interactions, and support systems. It involves having meaningful connections with others, feeling a sense of belonging, and being able to participate in social activities.

However, many other aspects of health need to be considered, viz., spiritual, emotional, vocational, and political dimensions of health. Health is a state of being that people define in relation to their own values, personality, and lifestyle. Each person has a personal concept of health. Pender and colleagues (2015) define health as "the actualization of inherent and acquired human potential through goal-directed behavior, competent self-care, and satisfying relationships with others while adjustments are made as needed to maintain structural integrity and harmony with the environment."

Individuals' views of health vary among different cultural orientations. Pender (1996) explains that "all people free of disease are not equally healthy." Views of health have broadened to include not only physical well-being, but also mental, social, and spiritual well-being and a focus on health at the family and community levels.

DIMENSIONS OF HEALTH

Health is a multidimensional concept that encompasses various dimensions or domains. These dimensions represent different aspects of an individual's overall well-being. While different models and frameworks may propose slightly different dimensions, here are some commonly recognized dimensions of health:

- **Physical health:** This dimension focuses on the body's physical well-being, including factors such as body composition, fitness, mobility, and the absence of illness or disease. It involves maintaining good nutrition, engaging in regular exercise, and receiving appropriate healthcare.
- **Mental health:** Mental health encompasses emotional well-being, cognitive functioning, and psychological resilience. It involves having a positive sense of self, managing stress effectively, experiencing positive emotions, and coping with challenges and adversity.
- **Emotional health:** Emotional health relates to the ability to understand and manage one's emotions in a healthy way. It involves recognizing and expressing emotions, building resilience, and having healthy relationships with oneself and others.
- **Social health:** Social health emphasizes the quality of an individual's relationships, social support networks, and social interactions. It involves effective communication, the ability to establish and maintain meaningful connections, and a sense of belonging and inclusion within communities.
- **Spiritual health:** Spiritual health refers to finding meaning, purpose, and connection

to something greater than oneself. It involves exploring personal values, beliefs, and principles, as well as fostering a sense of inner peace, harmony, and connection with the world.

- **Intellectual health:** Intellectual health focuses on cognitive abilities, intellectual stimulation, and ongoing learning. It involves engaging in activities that promote mental stimulation, critical thinking, creativity, and lifelong learning.
- **Occupational health:** Occupational health relates to one's satisfaction and well-being in the workplace. It involves finding fulfillment, purpose, and a healthy work-life balance, as well as experiencing a sense of productivity, satisfaction, and growth in one's chosen occupation.
- **Environmental health:** Environmental health involves the impact of the physical environment on an individual's well-being. It includes factors such as access to clean air and water, safe and healthy living conditions, and a sustainable and supportive environment.

It is important to note that these dimensions are interconnected and mutually influence each other. Achieving overall well-being involves addressing and nurturing each dimension, recognizing that they are all essential components of a healthy and fulfilling life.

DETERMINANTS OF HEALTH

Determinants of health are factors that influence an individual's health status and well-being. These determinants can be categorized into several broad categories (Fig. 8.1):

- **Individual characteristics:** These include factors such as age, sex, genetics, and personal behaviors. Age can affect health outcomes, as certain health conditions may be more prevalent in specific age groups. Sex can also play a role, as biological differences can influence susceptibility to certain diseases. Genetic factors can contribute to the risk of certain conditions, while personal behaviors like diet, exercise, substance use, and adherence to medical recommendations can significantly impact health.
- **Social and economic factors:** Socio-economic factors play a crucial role in

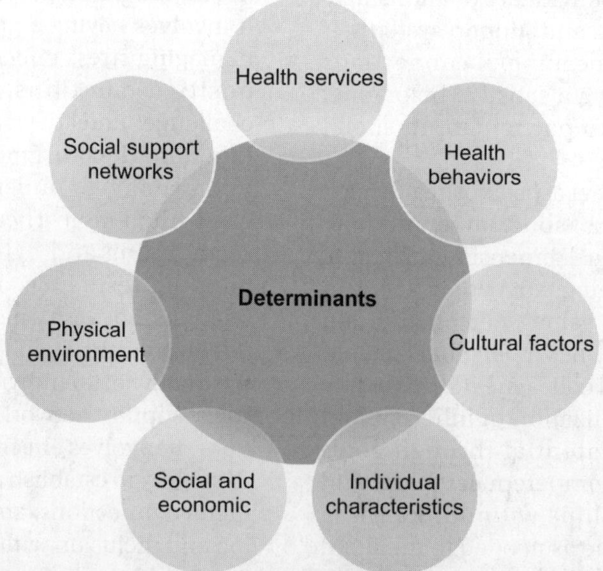

Fig. 8.1: Determinants of health.

health outcomes. Education, income, and occupation influence access to resources, opportunities, and healthcare services. People with higher levels of education and income tend to have better health outcomes and greater access to healthcare. Employment conditions, including job security, workplace safety, and income inequality, can also affect health.

- **Physical environment:** The physical environment encompasses both natural and built surroundings. Factors such as air and water quality, housing conditions, availability of green spaces, access to healthy food options, and exposure to environmental hazards can significantly impact health. Living in a safe and supportive neighborhood with access to parks and recreational areas promotes physical activity and overall well-being.

- **Social support networks:** Social support networks, including family, friends, and community, can have a significant influence on health. Strong social connections and positive relationships provide emotional support, reduce stress, and promote healthy behaviors. Conversely, social isolation and lack of support can contribute to adverse health outcomes.

- **Health services:** Access to quality healthcare services is a crucial determinant of health. Factors such as availability, affordability, and accessibility of healthcare facilities, as well as the quality of healthcare providers and services, can impact health outcomes. Accessible and affordable healthcare services are vital for prevention, early detection, and effective management of health conditions.

- **Health behaviors:** Individual lifestyle choices and behaviors have a significant impact on health. Behaviors such as tobacco and alcohol use, physical activity levels, dietary choices, and adherence to preventive measures (e.g., vaccinations, regular screenings) can influence the risk of developing various health conditions.

- **Cultural factors:** Cultural beliefs, values, norms, and practices can influence health behaviors, help-seeking behaviors, and attitudes towards health and illness. Understanding and respecting diverse cultural perspectives is essential for providing culturally competent and inclusive healthcare.

These determinants interact with each other and can have cumulative effects on health outcomes. Addressing these determinants and promoting health equity is essential for improving population health and reducing health disparities. Policies and interventions that focus on addressing these determinants can contribute to creating healthier environments and improving overall well-being.

CONCEPT OF WELLNESS AND WELL-BEING

The concepts of wellness and well-being are closely related and revolve around achieving a state of optimal health and overall satisfaction in various aspects of life. While they share similarities, they have slightly different focuses:

Wellness

Wellness refers to a holistic approach to health that encompasses multiple dimensions of well-being. It goes beyond the absence of illness and incorporates various aspects of a person's life, including physical, mental, emotional, social, and spiritual dimensions. Wellness emphasizes the pursuit of a balanced and fulfilling life by making conscious choices and taking proactive steps to enhance overall health and well-being.

Well-being

Well-being is a broader concept that encompasses the state of being healthy, happy, and prosperous in all aspects of life. It goes beyond the absence of illness and focuses on the individual's subjective experience of their quality of life. Well-being is influenced by various factors, including physical health, mental and emotional well-being, social relationships, work-life balance, financial security, and a sense of purpose and fulfillment.

Well-being takes into account individual perceptions, subjective feelings, and life satisfaction. It recognizes that well-being is multifaceted and can vary from person to person based on their unique circumstances, values, and goals. Achieving well-being involves balancing different aspects of life, nurturing positive relationships, pursuing personal growth, and finding fulfillment in various domains, including work, relationships, leisure activities, and personal development.

In summary, wellness and well-being focus on achieving a state of optimal health, satisfaction, and fulfillment in various dimensions of life. While wellness emphasizes a holistic approach to health, encompassing multiple dimensions, well-being encompasses broader aspects of overall satisfaction and quality of life. Both concepts encourage individuals to take proactive steps, make healthy choices, and foster a balanced and fulfilling life.

CONCEPT OF ILLNESS

Illness is a broader concept than disease. It refers to the overall impact of a health condition on a person's physical, emotional, social, intellectual, developmental, and spiritual functioning. Disease, on the other hand, is a specific medical condition that can cause illness. For example, two people with cancer may experience the disease very differently. One person may be able to continue their normal activities while receiving treatment, while the other person may experience significant physical and emotional side effects that impact their ability to function.

Nurses need to be aware of both disease and illness. They need to understand the medical aspects of a health condition, but they also need to be able to assess the impact of the condition on the patient's overall well-being. This allows nurses to provide comprehensive care that addresses the physical, emotional, and social needs of their patients.

DEFINITIONS

- **Adolf Meyer (1951):** "Illness is not just a matter of disease, but of the whole person in his environment."
- **George Engel (1977):** "Illness is a biopsychosocial process that involves the interaction of biological, psychological, and social factors."
- **Arthur Kleinman (1988):** "Illness is a culturally constituted experience that is shaped by the patient's beliefs, values, and social context."

These definitions highlight the complex nature of illness. It is not simply a biological problem, but a social, psychological, and cultural one as well. This understanding of illness is important for healthcare providers, as it allows them to provide more comprehensive and effective care for their patients.

ACUTE AND CHRONIC ILLNESS

Acute and chronic illnesses are two distinct categories of health conditions that differ in their duration, onset, and progression. Here is an overview of acute and chronic illnesses (**Table 8.1**):

Acute Illness

- Acute illnesses are characterized by their sudden onset and relatively short duration.
- They are often caused by infections, injuries, or other acute factors.
- Acute illnesses typically have a clear beginning, a defined course, and an eventual resolution.
- Examples of acute illnesses include the flu, common cold, acute appendicitis, and acute injuries like a sprained ankle.
- Treatment for acute illnesses often focuses on relieving symptoms, promoting healing, and managing any complications that may arise.

Table 8.1: Differences between acute and chronic illnesses.

Feature	*Acute illness*	*Chronic illness*
Onset	Sudden	Slow and gradual
Duration	Short-term (days to weeks)	Long-term (months to years)
Treatment	Usually resolves on its own with rest, fluids, and medication; in some cases, surgery may be necessary	Requires ongoing treatment, such as medication, lifestyle changes, or surgery
Prognosis	Usually good, with most people making a full recovery	Varies depending on the specific condition; some chronic illnesses can be managed well with treatment, while others can be more serious and may lead to disability or death

Chronic Illness

- Chronic illnesses, on the other hand, are long-term health conditions that persist over an extended period, typically lasting for months to years or even a lifetime.
- They often develop gradually and may not have a specific endpoint or cure.
- Chronic illnesses can result from various factors, including genetic predispositions, lifestyle choices, environmental factors, or underlying medical conditions.
- Examples of chronic illnesses include diabetes, hypertension, asthma, arthritis, chronic kidney disease, and mental health conditions like depression and anxiety disorders.
- Managing chronic illnesses involves ongoing medical care, long-term treatment plans, lifestyle modifications, and regular monitoring of symptoms and health status.

VARIABLES INFLUENCING ILLNESS

Several factors can influence the occurrence and development of illness in individuals. These factors can be categorized into four main groups:

Biological Factors

- **Genetics:** Inherited genetic traits and predispositions can make individuals more susceptible to certain illnesses.
- **Age:** Different age groups may be more prone to specific health conditions or have varying immune responses.
- **Sex:** Biological differences between males and females can influence susceptibility to certain diseases or conditions.

Environmental Factors

- **Physical environment:** Exposure to pollutants, toxins, radiation, or hazardous substances in the environment can contribute to the development of illnesses.
- **Socioeconomic environment:** Socioeconomic conditions, such as poverty, inadequate housing, or lack of access to clean water and sanitation, can increase the risk of certain diseases.
- **Occupational hazards:** Exposure to occupational hazards, such as chemicals, physical strain, or infectious agents, can lead to work-related illnesses.

Lifestyle Factors

- **Diet and nutrition:** Poor nutrition, imbalanced diets, and excessive intake of unhealthy foods can contribute to various health conditions, including obesity, cardiovascular diseases, and diabetes.
- **Physical activity:** Lack of regular physical activity and sedentary lifestyles can increase the risk of obesity, heart disease, and other chronic conditions.
- **Substance abuse:** The use of tobacco, alcohol, drugs, or other substances can have detrimental effects on health and increase the risk of addiction, mental health disorders, and physical illnesses.

Socioeconomic and Psychosocial Factors

- **Socioeconomic status:** Lower socio-economic status can lead to limited access to healthcare, inadequate nutrition, and increased stress, which can impact overall health.
- **Education and literacy:** Limited education and health literacy levels can affect individuals' ability to understand and engage in preventive measures and make informed healthcare decisions.
- **Social support:** Strong social support networks and positive relationships can have a protective effect on health, while social isolation and lack of support may contribute to poor health outcomes.
- **Stress:** Chronic stress, such as from work, financial difficulties, or interpersonal conflicts, can weaken the immune system and increase vulnerability to illness.

It is important to note that these factors often interact and influence each other. Additionally, individual circumstances and contexts may contribute to the impact of these factors on an individual's health and the development of illness. By recognizing and addressing these factors, healthcare providers, policymakers, and individuals themselves can work towards promoting healthier environments, lifestyles, and well-being.

STAGES OF ILLNESS

Edward A Suchman, a sociologist, developed a model of illness behavior. Suchman's model has been influential in understanding how individuals experience and respond to illness. It has been used to develop interventions to improve patient adherence to treatment regimens and to reduce health disparities. Here are the five stages:

1. **Symptom experience:** The symptom experience can be quite variable, from a mild discomfort to a severe pain or other disruption. The individual's interpretation of the symptom is also influenced by their past experiences, cultural beliefs, and social expectations. For example, someone who has a family history of heart disease may be more likely to interpret chest pain as a sign of a heart attack, while someone who has never experienced chest pain before may be more likely to ignore it.

2. **Labeling:** Once the individual has experienced a symptom, they must decide whether it is a sign of illness. This labeling process is influenced by a number of factors, including the individual's knowledge about health and illness, their past experiences, and their cultural beliefs. For example, someone who has recently been exposed to a contagious illness may be more likely to label a mild fever as a sign of illness, while someone who has never been sick before may be more likely to ignore it.

3. **Decision to seek care:** Once the individual has labeled the symptom as a sign of illness, they must decide whether to seek medical attention. This decision is influenced by a number of factors, including the severity of the symptom, the individual's beliefs about the cause of the symptom, and their access to healthcare. For example, someone who experiences a severe headache that is not relieved by over-the-counter pain medication is more likely to seek medical attention than someone who experiences a mild headache that goes away on its own.

4. **Patient role assumption:** If the individual decides to seek medical attention, they will likely assume the sick role. The sick role is a socially defined role that allows the individual to receive medical care and be excused from their usual responsibilities. The sick role has a number of expectations, including the following:

- The individual is not responsible for their illness.
- The individual should seek help from a competent professional.
- The individual should cooperate with the treatment plan.
- The individual should try to get well as quickly as possible.

5. **Recovery or rehabilitation:** The final stage of illness is recovery or rehabilitation. This stage can be quite variable, depending on the nature of the illness. For some illnesses, recovery is a relatively quick process. For other illnesses, recovery may be a long and difficult process. In some cases, the individual may never fully recover from their illness.

It is important to note that these stages are not necessarily linear, and individuals can move back and forth between stages depending on their experiences and circumstances. Additionally, individual differences, cultural factors, and healthcare system variations can influence the manifestation of these stages.

IMPACT OF ILLNESS ON THE PATIENT AND FAMILY

The impact of illness extends beyond the physical symptoms experienced by a patient and can have far-reaching effects on both the patient and their family. When a person becomes ill, it can significantly disrupt their life and alter their relationships, emotions, and overall well-being. Additionally, family members and caregivers are often deeply affected by the illness as they navigate the challenges of supporting their loved one through their health journey.

Understanding the various dimensions of this impact is crucial in order to provide comprehensive care and support to both the patient and their family. In this discussion, we will explore the emotional, financial, social, and relational implications of illness on the patient and their family, highlighting the complexities and challenges that arise in these circumstances.

Here are some key areas where the impact is often felt:

- **Emotional impact:** Dealing with an illness can evoke a range of emotions for the patient, such as fear, sadness, anger, frustration, or even a sense of loss. They may experience anxiety about their condition, uncertainty about the future, or the psychological strain of managing symptoms. Family members also go through emotional turmoil as they worry about the well-being of their loved one, experience empathy for their suffering, and grapple with their own feelings of helplessness or grief.

- **Impact on body image:** Illnesses and their treatments can often result in physical changes that may impact body image. These changes can include weight loss or gain, hair loss, scarring, changes in skin texture or color, changes in mobility or physical abilities, or the need for medical devices like prosthetics or ostomy bags. These alterations can lead to feelings of self-consciousness, dissatisfaction, or a loss of confidence in one's physical appearance.

- **Lifestyle changes:** Illness often necessitates significant changes in the patient's lifestyle. They may have to adjust their daily routines, modify their diet and exercise habits, or adhere to a complex medication regimen. These changes can be disruptive and challenging, requiring the patient to adapt and find new ways of managing their daily life. Family members may need to provide support in implementing these changes and adjust their own routines to accommodate the patient's needs.

- **Financial burden:** Serious illnesses can place a significant financial strain on both the patient and their family. Medical expenses, including consultations, treatments, medications, and hospital stays, can accumulate rapidly. The costs of specialized equipment or home modifications may also be incurred. In some cases, the patient or their family members may need to take time off work or reduce their working hours to provide care, resulting in a loss of income.

- **Impact on roles and responsibilities:** Illness can disrupt the established roles and responsibilities within a family. The patient may require assistance with daily activities, such as bathing, dressing, or managing household chores. This may necessitate a shift in caregiving responsibilities among family members. The patient may also become dependent on others for transportation to medical appointments or require emotional support, altering the dynamics within the family.

- **Caregiver burden:** Family members who take on the role of caregivers may experience physical, emotional, and mental strain. The demands of providing care, managing medications, coordinating appointments, and dealing with the unpredictability of the illness can lead to exhaustion and burnout. Caregivers may neglect their own self-care and health, impacting their well-being and ability to provide optimal care for the patient.
- **Social impact:** Illness can lead to social isolation for both the patient and their family. The patient's condition may restrict their ability to engage in social activities or attend gatherings due to physical limitations or concerns about their health. This isolation can impact their mental well-being and strain their relationships with friends and extended family members. Family members may also experience social isolation as their focus and availability revolve around the patient's needs.
- **Impact on psychological well-being:** The psychological well-being of both the patient and their family members can be affected by the illness. Patients may experience increased stress, anxiety, or depression as they navigate their health challenges. Family members may also face emotional strain, juggling their own emotions while providing support and care for the patient. It's important to address the mental health needs of both the patient and their family members during the course of the illness.

It is worth noting that the impact of illness can vary depending on the nature and severity of the condition, available support systems, and individual resilience. Healthcare professionals and support networks play a crucial role in providing comprehensive care, addressing the physical, emotional, and social needs of both the patient and their family, and helping them navigate the challenges that arise from illness.

HEALTH-ILLNESS MODELS

Health-illness models are frameworks or theories that provide a way to understand and conceptualize the relationship between health and illness. These models help in examining the factors that contribute to the onset, progression, and management of illness, as well as the promotion of health. Here are a few commonly known health-illness models:

Illness-Wellness Continuum

John W. Travis first envisioned the illness-wellness continuum in 1972. He published it in 1975, and it quickly became an important tool for understanding wellness. The continuum represents wellness as a process, not a static state. It shows that people can move along the continuum in either direction, depending on their choices and behaviors.

The illness-wellness continuum is a conceptual framework that illustrates the spectrum of health, ranging from optimal wellness to severe illness. It suggests that health is not simply the absence of illness but exists on a continuum with varying degrees of well-being. The continuum emphasizes that individuals can move back and forth along this spectrum based on their choices, behaviors, and circumstances.

The illness-wellness continuum is a linear model that ranges from premature death on the left to high-level wellness on the right. The center of the continuum represents a neutral state of health, where there are no signs or symptoms of illness (**Fig. 8.2**). It suggests that individuals exist on a spectrum between these two extremes, with various levels of health and well-being in between.

In this model, the opposite directions of the continuum meet at a neutral point. Progressing to the right of this neutral point signifies an increase in wellness, achieved through awareness, education, and personal growth.

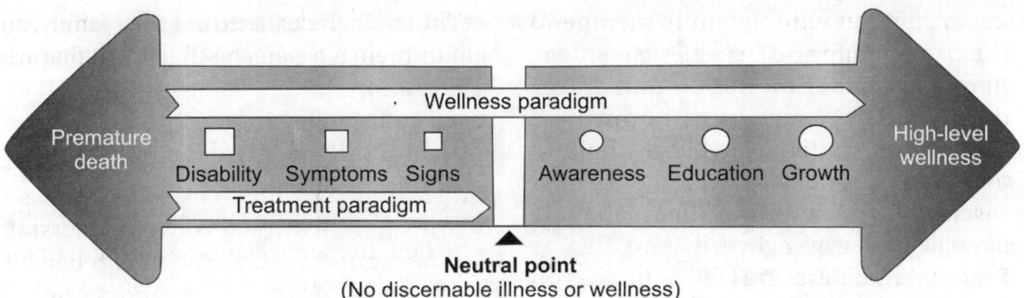

Fig. 8.2: Illness-wellness continuum.

Conversely, moving to the left indicates a decrease in wellness due to various disabilities, signs, and symptoms of illness.

The Illness-Wellness Continuum demonstrates that there exist numerous degrees of wellness, just as there are various degrees of illness. It showcases the relationship between the treatment paradigm and the wellness paradigm.

The treatment paradigm, which encompasses approaches like medications, herbs, surgery, psychotherapy, and acupuncture, can bring individuals to the neutral point, where disease symptoms are alleviated.

On the other hand, the wellness paradigm can be employed at any position on the continuum and assists individuals in progressing towards higher levels of wellness. It encourages individuals to surpass the neutral point and strive to move as far to the right as possible. The wellness paradigm does not aim to replace the treatment paradigm found on the left side of the continuum, but rather to work in synergy with it. While receiving treatment is crucial when one is ill, it is important not to halt progress at the neutral point. Instead, the wellness paradigm should be utilized to advance towards high-level wellness.

The Illness-Wellness Continuum emphasizes the importance of taking a holistic approach to health. It encourages individuals to focus on prevention and proactive self-care measures rather than waiting until they become ill to seek medical attention. It recognizes that even in a state of illness, individuals have the potential to move towards wellness through appropriate interventions and lifestyle changes.

Overall, the continuum serves as a tool for promoting awareness and encouraging individuals to take responsibility for their own health and well-being. It reminds us that health is not simply the absence of disease but a dynamic state that can be influenced by our choices and actions.

Health Belief Model

Health Belief Model (HBM) was developed in the 1950s by social psychologists Irwin Rosenstock and Godfrey Hochbaum. The Health Belief Model is a psychological framework that aims to explain and predict individuals' health-related behaviors by considering their beliefs, perceptions, and attitudes. This model suggests that people's beliefs about health problems, perceived benefits of action and barriers to action, and self-efficacy explain engagement (or lack of engagement) in health-promoting behavior. The HBM has six key constructs:

1. **Perceived susceptibility:** This refers to an individual's belief about their vulnerability to a particular health condition or illness. If someone perceives themselves as being at risk, they are more likely to take preventive actions.
2. **Perceived severity:** This component reflects an individual's assessment of the seriousness and potential consequences of the health condition or illness. The greater the perceived severity, the more

motivated individuals are to engage in health-promoting behaviors.

3. **Perceived benefits:** Individuals weigh the perceived benefits of adopting a specific health behavior. If they believe that a behavior will effectively reduce their susceptibility or severity of illness, they are more likely to engage in it.

4. **Perceived barriers:** This factor focuses on the obstacles or perceived costs associated with adopting a particular health behavior. Barriers can include financial costs, time constraints, fear of side effects, or lack of knowledge. High perceived barriers may discourage individuals from taking action.

5. **Cues to action:** These are external events or triggers that prompt individuals to engage in a particular health behavior. Cues can be internal, such as experiencing symptoms, or external, such as reminders from healthcare professionals or media campaigns.

6. **Self-efficacy:** This component involves an individual's belief in their ability to successfully perform the recommended health behavior. Higher self-efficacy increases the likelihood of taking action.

This model has been applied to various health-related behaviors, such as vaccination, screening tests, medication adherence, and lifestyle changes. By understanding individuals' beliefs and perceptions, healthcare professionals can design interventions that address specific factors influencing health behaviors, thereby promoting positive health outcomes.

Health Promotion Model

The Health Promotion Model (HPM) is a nursing theory developed by Nola J. Pender (1982; revised, 1996), a nursing theorist and professor. The model focuses on understanding and promoting individuals' positive health behaviors and well-being. It provides a framework that incorporates various factors influencing health-related behaviors and emphasizes the importance of personal empowerment and self-efficacy.

The model is designed to explain the factors that influence a person's decision to engage in health-promoting behaviors. The HPM is based on the following assumptions:

- Health is a positive dynamic state, not simply the absence of disease.
- Health promotion is a process of enabling people to increase their control over their health and improve their well-being.
- Health-promoting behaviors are voluntary actions that people take to improve their health.

Components of Health Promotion Model

The HPM identifies four major categories of factors that influence health-promoting behavior:

- Individual characteristics and experiences
- Behavior-specific cognitions and affect
- Perceived behavioral control
- Behavioral outcome

Individual characteristics and experiences include a person's age, gender, race, ethnicity, socioeconomic status, lifestyle, and health beliefs. Behavior-specific cognitions and affect include a person's knowledge about a particular health behavior, their beliefs about the benefits and risks of the behavior, and their emotional response to the behavior. Perceived behavioral control refers to a person's belief that they have the ability to successfully perform a health behavior. Behavioral outcome is the actual performance of the health behavior.

The HPM suggests that these four categories of factors interact with each other to influence a person's decision to engage in health-promoting behavior. For example, a person who is motivated to improve their health (individual characteristic) may be more likely to seek out information about healthy eating (behavior-specific cognition). If the person believes that they can successfully change their eating habits (perceived behavioral control), they are more likely to make healthy food choices (behavioral outcome).

CHAPTER SUMMARY

1. Health is a complex and multifaceted concept that goes beyond the absence of disease and encompasses physical, mental, and social dimensions.
2. Health is influenced by various factors, including genetics, lifestyle choices, socioeconomic status, access to healthcare, and environmental conditions.
3. Health is a multidimensional concept with dimensions such as physical health, mental and emotional well-being, social health, spiritual health, intellectual health, occupational health, and environmental health.
4. Determinants of health are factors that influence an individual's health status and well-being.
5. Wellness and well-being are related concepts that focus on achieving optimal health and overall satisfaction in various aspects of life.
6. The concept of illness is broader than disease, encompassing the overall impact of a health condition on a person's physical, emotional, social, intellectual, developmental, and spiritual functioning.
7. Illness is a complex phenomenon influenced by biological, psychological, social, and cultural factors.
8. Edward A Suchman's model of illness behavior describes five stages individuals go through when experiencing and responding to illness.
9. Illness not only affects the patient's physical health but also has wide-ranging impacts on their emotions, body image, lifestyle, finances, roles and responsibilities, and social relationships.
10. Health-illness models provide frameworks for understanding the relationship between health and illness.

REVIEW QUESTIONS

1. Define health and discuss the dimensions of health.
2. Explain the impact of illness on patient and family.
3. Define illness and describe stages of illness.
4. Discuss on health belief model.

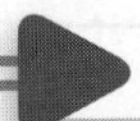 **BIBLIOGRAPHY** 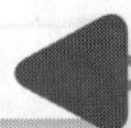

1. Ahern TJ, Kelleher KJ. The impact of illness on family caregivers: A review and analysis of the literature. J Fam Soc Work. 2009;13(3):233-52. doi:10.1080/10522150902727939
2. American Public Health Association. Guide to community preventive services: The guide to community preventive services. Atlanta, GA: Centers for Disease Control and Prevention; 2011.
3. Becker M, Maiman L. Sociobehavioral determinants of compliance with health and medical care recommendations. Med Care. 1975;13(1):10.
4. Breitbart W, Kupfer DJ. The biopsychosocial model of illness: Applications to prevention and treatment. In: Friedman MJ, Schwartz MD, Unutzer ST (Eds). Psychological approaches to health care: Applications in clinical practice and prevention: Oxford University Press; 2005. pp. 11-30.
5. Breitbart W, Rosenfeld B, Passik SD. The impact of illness on the patient's family. J Palliat Med. 1999;2(2):193-207. doi:10.1089/jpm.1999.2.193

6. Brockington IF, Feldman PJ. Health: The Basics. Oxford, England: Oxford University Press; 2006.
7. Cox SM, Matschinger H. The illness-wellness continuum: A new approach to conceptualizing mental health. J Ment Health. 2008;17(2):155-66.
8. Coyne JC, Smith RB. Social support, stress, and coping in adaptation to chronic illness. J Consult Clin Psychol. 1991;59(1):56-64.
9. Hoffman S. The illness-wellness model: A framework for understanding and promoting health. Adv Nurs Sci. 2009;32(2):118-27.
10. Larsen PD. The illness experience. In: Lubkin IM, Larsen PD (Eds). Chronic illness: impact and intervention, 8th edition. Boston, Jones & Bartlett; 2013b.
11. Marmot M. Social determinants of health. New York, NY: Oxford University Press; 2005.
12. Pascucci MA, Chu N, Leasure AR. Health promotion for the oldest of old people. Nurs Older People. 2012;24(3):22-8.
13. Pender NJ. Health promotion in nursing practice, 2nd edition. Norwalk, CT: Appleton-Century-Crofts; 1982.
14. Rosenstock IM. The health belief model: Explaining health behavior through expectancies. In: Glanz K, Lewis FM, Rimer BK (Eds). Health behavior and health education: Theory, research, and practice. Jossey-Bass/Wiley; 1990. pp. 39-62.
15. Sharma SK, Mudgal SK, Thakur K, Gaur R, Aggarwal P. Lifestyle behavior of budding health care professionals: A cross-sectional descriptive study. J Family Med Prim Care. 2020;9:3525-31.
16. World Health Organization. Constitution of the World Health Organization. Geneva, Switzerland: World Health Organization; 1948.

Stress and Adaptation

Learning Objectives

- Define stress and its origins, including its historical development from physics to psychology.
- Understand the various types of stress and recognize their impact on individuals' well-being.
- Identify and analyze the different factors that can influence stress and adaptation.
- Explain the concept of homeostasis and its significance in maintaining a stable internal environment despite external changes.
- Describe the stages of General Adaptation Syndrome (GAS) and their implications for the body's response to stressors.
- Analyze the psychological regulation of homeostasis and defense mechanisms, in maintaining mental equilibrium and overall well-being.
- Evaluate the role of stressors and classify them into different types.
- Apply the knowledge of stress and adaptation to identify strategies and interventions for managing stress effectively and promoting resilience and well-being.

INTRODUCTION

Stress and adaptation are two interconnected concepts that play a significant role in our lives. Stress refers to the physiological and psychological responses we experience when we perceive a demand or threat that exceeds our coping abilities. It can arise from various sources, including work, relationships, financial pressures, health issues, and major life changes. While stress is a natural and necessary part of life, prolonged or chronic stress can have detrimental effects on our physical and mental well-being.

Understanding stress and adaptation is crucial for developing effective coping mechanisms and strategies to manage stressors in our lives. By recognizing the signs of stress, practicing self-care, seeking social support, and implementing healthy lifestyle choices, we can enhance our ability to adapt and maintain overall well-being in the face of life's challenges.

STRESS

The concept of stress originates from the field of physics, specifically mechanics, and was later adopted and adapted in psychology. The term "stress" was first introduced in the 17th century by the English physicist and mathematician Robert Hooke.

In the early 20th century, the concept of stress was applied to the field of psychology by the Canadian physiologist Hans Selye. Selye conducted research on the effects of various stressors on the body and observed common physiological responses, regardless of the specific nature of the stressor.

Stress referred as a physiological and psychological response to external or internal demands or pressures, often referred to as stressors. It is a natural reaction that occurs when we perceive a threat, challenge, or change that requires us to adapt or respond. Stress is a subjective experience. What is stressful for one person may not be stressful for another. The way we perceive stress also affects how we respond to it.

DEFINITIONS

Here are some definitions of stress by different authors:

- **Hans Selye (1956):** "Stress is the nonspecific response of the body to any demand for change."
- **Richard Lazarus (1966):** "Stress is a state of cognitive and emotional arousal that occurs when an individual perceives a threat or demand that exceeds his or her resources for coping."
- **Thomas Holmes and Richard Rahe (1967):** "Stress is the accumulation of life changes that require us to adapt."
- **The American Psychological Association (APA):** "Stress is the feeling of being under too much mental or emotional pressure."

TYPES OF STRESS

There are several types of stress that individuals may experience. Here are some common types:

- **Acute stress:** Acute stress refers to short-term stress that is brief in duration and typically caused by specific events or situations. It is a normal and temporary response to immediate challenges or demands. Examples of acute stressors include giving a presentation, taking an exam, or dealing with a traffic jam.
- **Chronic stress:** Chronic stress is long-term stress that persists over an extended period, often resulting from ongoing or recurring stressors. It can be caused by factors such as work pressures, financial difficulties, relationship problems, or chronic health conditions. Chronic stress can have a cumulative and detrimental impact on physical and mental health if not effectively managed.
- **Eustress:** Eustress refers to positive or beneficial stress that motivates and energizes individuals, leading to positive outcomes. It is often associated with challenging but manageable situations that inspire personal growth, excitement, or anticipation. Examples of eustress include starting a new job, planning a wedding, or engaging in a thrilling activity.
- **Distress:** Distress is the opposite of eustress and refers to negative or harmful stress. It occurs when individuals are unable to cope effectively with stressors, leading to feelings of overwhelm, anxiety, and a sense of being unable to control or manage the situation. Distress can have detrimental effects on physical and mental well-being.
- **Secondary traumatic stress:** Secondary traumatic stress, also known as compassion fatigue or vicarious trauma, occurs when individuals experience stress and emotional strain due to witnessing or hearing about the traumatic experiences of others. This can affect professionals in helping roles, such as healthcare workers, therapists, or first responders.

It is important to note that these types of stress are not mutually exclusive, and individuals may experience a combination of them depending on their circumstances. Recognizing and understanding the different types of stress can help individuals better identify and manage their stress levels and promote overall well-being.

IMPACT OF STRESS ON HEALTH

Stress can have a significant impact on both physical and mental health. When the body's stress response is activated frequently or for prolonged periods, it can lead to a range of health problems. Here are some common effects of stress on health:

- **Cardiovascular issues:** Chronic stress is associated with an increased risk of cardiovascular problems such as high blood pressure, heart disease, heart attacks, and stroke. Prolonged stress can lead to elevated heart rate, constricted blood vessels, and elevated levels of stress hormones, which can strain the cardiovascular system.

- **Weakened immune system:** Stress hormones, particularly cortisol, can suppress the immune system, making individuals more susceptible to infections, illnesses, and autoimmune disorders. Chronic stress can also delay wound healing and increase inflammation in the body.
- **Digestive problems:** Stress can affect the digestive system and contribute to issues such as stomach ulcers, acid reflux, irritable bowel syndrome (IBS), and other gastrointestinal disorders. It can disrupt digestion, alter gut bacteria, and lead to changes in appetite and eating behaviors.
- **Musculoskeletal issues:** Stress can manifest in physical symptoms such as muscle tension, headaches, migraines, and body aches. Prolonged stress can contribute to chronic muscle tension, leading to conditions like tension headaches, neck and back pain, and temporomandibular joint (TMJ) disorders.
- **Sleep disturbances:** Stress can interfere with sleep patterns, leading to difficulties falling asleep, staying asleep, or experiencing restful sleep. Sleep disturbances can further exacerbate stress levels and contribute to fatigue, irritability, and impaired cognitive function.
- **Mental health disorders:** Prolonged or chronic stress can contribute to the development or worsening of mental health conditions such as anxiety disorders, depression, and mood disorders. Stress can disrupt neurotransmitter balance, impact brain structure and function, and contribute to emotional instability and cognitive difficulties.
- **Weight gain and loss:** Stress can affect appetite and eating habits, leading to weight gain or weight loss. Some individuals may turn to comfort eating or emotional eating as a coping mechanism, leading to overeating and weight gain. On the other hand, stress can suppress appetite and lead to weight loss in some individuals.
- **Hormonal imbalances:** Stress can disrupt the delicate balance of hormones in the body, affecting various systems. It can lead to menstrual irregularities in women, reduced libido, fertility problems, and disruptions in the endocrine system.
- **Cognitive impairment:** Chronic stress can impair cognitive function, memory, and concentration. It can make it challenging to focus, make decisions, and perform tasks effectively.
- **Increased risk-taking behaviors:** Some individuals may engage in unhealthy coping mechanisms, such as excessive alcohol consumption, drug use, smoking, or other risky behaviors, as a response to stress. These behaviors can further contribute to health problems and increase the risk of accidents and injuries.

STRESSORS

Stressors are the specific events, situations, or conditions that trigger the stress response in individuals. They are the external or internal factors that cause us to perceive a demand or threat, leading to physiological and psychological responses associated with stress. It is important to consider the individual's unique perspective when assessing stressors because what one person finds stressful, another person may not.

DEFINITIONS

Different authors have defined stressors in different ways. Here are a few examples:
- Richard Lazarus defined a stressor as "any event or situation that is appraised as taxing or exceeding a person's resources."
- Hans Selye defined a stressor as "any stimulus that produces a stress response."
- The American Psychological Association defines a stressor as "anything that causes physical or emotional tension."

TYPES OF STRESSORS

Stressors can be classified into various types based on their nature and impact. Here are some common types of stressors:

- **Physical stressors:** These stressors involve physical demands or challenges that require the body to adapt. They can include strenuous physical exertion, exposure to extreme temperatures, physical injuries, or illnesses.
- **Psychological or cognitive stressors:** Psychological or cognitive stressors arise from mental or emotional challenges that individuals face. They can include academic pressures, work-related demands, financial difficulties, time constraints, information overload, or decision-making dilemmas.
- **Social stressors:** Social stressors stem from interactions and relationships with others. They can include conflicts with family members, friends, or colleagues, social pressures, peer pressure, bullying, discrimination, or feeling socially isolated.
- **Environmental stressors:** Environmental stressors refer to external factors in the physical environment that induce stress. They can include noise pollution, air pollution, overcrowding, natural disasters, harsh weather conditions, or living in an unsafe neighborhood.
- **Life events:** Life events can act as stressors, both positive and negative. Positive life events, such as getting married, starting a new job, or having a child, can still induce stress due to the significant changes and adjustments they require. Negative life events, such as the loss of a loved one, divorce, job loss, or financial crises, can cause substantial stress.
- **Daily hassles:** Daily hassles refer to the minor irritations and frustrations encountered in day-to-day life. These stressors may seem insignificant individually but can accumulate and contribute to chronic stress. Examples include traffic congestion, time pressures, household chores, technology malfunctions, or dealing with difficult people.
- **Internal stressors:** Internal stressors are related to an individual's internal thoughts, beliefs, and perceptions. They can include self-imposed pressure, negative self-talk, perfectionism, self-doubt, or unrealistic expectations. Internal stressors can significantly impact an individual's stress levels and well-being.
- **Anticipatory stressors:** Anticipatory stressors are stressors related to future events or situations that individuals perceive as challenging or threatening. They can include exam anxiety, performance anxiety before a presentation or public speaking, or fear of an upcoming medical procedure.

It is important to note that individuals may respond differently to stressors based on their unique characteristics, previous experiences, and coping mechanisms. What may be a stressor for one person may not elicit the same response in another.

ADAPTATION

Adaptation refers to the ability of an individual, organism, or system to adjust and respond effectively to changes in their environment or circumstances. It involves modifying behaviors, strategies, or physical characteristics to better fit the new conditions. Adaptation can occur at various levels, from biological organisms evolving over generations to individuals adapting their behaviors or mindset to cope with specific situations.

In the context of human adaptation, it often refers to the ability to adjust to new or challenging circumstances, such as changes in personal life, work environment, or societal shifts. Adapting allows individuals to effectively deal with stress, overcome obstacles, and thrive in changing conditions.

Adaptation refers to an individual's coping mechanism in response to stress or a potentially threatening situation. It is an ongoing process wherein individuals strive to maintain a balance between their physiological and psychological well-being, whether in response to changes in their internal or external environment. It plays a crucial role in the normal growth and development of individuals, as it involves their capacity to effectively respond to physical, physiological, psychological, and other stressors present in their environment

FACTORS AFFECTING STRESS AND ADAPTATION

Several factors can influence stress and adaptation in individuals. These factors can vary from person to person and may have different degrees of impact. Here are some key factors that can affect stress and adaptation:

- **Individual factors:** Each person's unique characteristics, including their personality traits, coping skills, resilience, and genetic predispositions, can influence their response to stress and their ability to adapt.
- **Life experiences:** Past experiences, such as traumatic events, childhood upbringing, and significant life transitions, can shape an individual's stress response and their ability to cope with future stressors.
- **Social support:** The presence or absence of a supportive network, including family, friends, and social connections, can impact an individual's stress levels and their ability to adapt. Strong social support can provide emotional and practical assistance during challenging times.
- **Environmental factors:** The environment in which an individual lives and works can contribute to their stress levels. Factors such as noise, pollution, overcrowding, socioeconomic conditions, and access to resources can all impact stress and adaptation.
- **Work-related factors:** Job demands, workload, job insecurity, lack of control, work-life balance, and organizational culture can significantly affect an individual's stress levels and ability to adapt to work-related challenges.
- **Cultural factors:** Cultural beliefs, values, norms, and societal expectations play a role in shaping how individuals perceive and respond to stress. Cultural factors can influence coping strategies, social support systems, and the availability of resources for adaptation.
- **Health and lifestyle:** Physical health, nutrition, exercise, and sleep patterns can impact an individual's resilience to stress and their ability to adapt. Poor health or unhealthy lifestyle habits can increase vulnerability to stress.
- **Economic factors:** Financial stress, economic instability, and socioeconomic disparities can contribute to higher stress levels and challenge an individual's capacity to adapt effectively.

It is important to note that these factors are interconnected and can interact with one another. Understanding the specific factors that affect stress and adaptation for an individual can help tailor strategies and interventions to promote better coping mechanisms and resilience.

HOMEOSTASIS

The concept of homeostasis was first introduced by the French physiologist Claude Bernard in the 19th century and further developed by American physiologist Walter Cannon. Homeostasis involves a dynamic balance between various physiological processes, ensuring that important variables such as body temperature, pH levels, blood pressure, and hormone levels remain within a narrow range that is optimal for cellular function.

Homeostasis refers to the body's ability to maintain a stable internal environment despite external changes. It is a vital regulatory process that allows organisms to function properly and adapt to varying conditions or stressors.

GENERAL ADAPTATION SYNDROME

General adaptation syndrome (GAS) is a concept developed by Hans Selye, a pioneering stress researcher. It describes the body's general response to stressors over time.

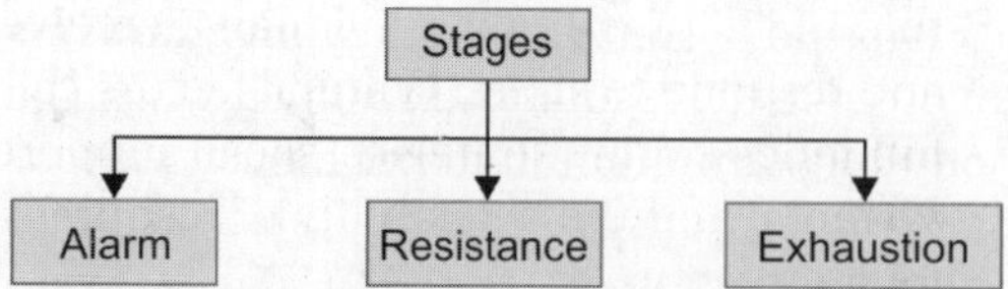

Fig. 9.1: Stages of general adaptation syndrome.

The GAS is a model that explains how the body physiologically reacts to stressors in distinct stages: alarm, resistance, and exhaustion. It can be activated by either a physical or psychological event, and it involves various bodily systems, particularly the neuroendocrine feedback. The response to stress is immediate.

The general adaptation syndrome consists of three stages: alarm, resistance, and exhaustion. Here is a breakdown of each stage (Fig. 9.1):

1. **Alarm stage:** The alarm stage is the initial response to a stressor. When the body perceives a threat or stressor, it activates the fight-or-flight response. The sympathetic nervous system is stimulated, leading to increased heart rate, elevated blood pressure, and the release of stress hormones like cortisol and adrenaline. The body prepares itself to cope with the stressor by mobilizing its resources.

2. **Resistance stage:** If the stressor persists, the body enters the resistance stage. During this stage, the body adapts and attempts to restore homeostasis while continuing to deal with the ongoing stressor. Physiological processes remain heightened, but the body tries to allocate resources to manage the stress. However, if the stressor is chronic or overwhelming, the body's resources may become depleted.

3. **Exhaustion stage:** If the stressor persists for an extended period or if multiple stressors occur simultaneously, the body enters the exhaustion stage. In this stage, the body's resources become depleted, leading to a decline in physiological functioning. The individual may experience fatigue, decreased immune system function, increased vulnerability to illness, and other negative health consequences. If not addressed, chronic stress and exhaustion can lead to long-term health issues.

It is important to note that the general adaptation syndrome is a conceptual model and does not capture the full complexity of individual stress responses. Different individuals may respond differently to stressors, and the duration and intensity of the stages can vary. However, GAS provides a framework for understanding the general physiological responses to stress and the potential consequences of prolonged exposure to stressors. Managing stress effectively and implementing strategies for self-care and resilience can help mitigate the negative impacts of stress and prevent exhaustion.

REGULATION OF HOMEOSTASIS

The regulation of homeostasis involves the coordination of various physiological and psychological processes to maintain a stable internal environment within the body. Here are two key regulatory mechanisms involved in maintaining homeostasis:

1. Physiological

The regulation of physiological homeostasis involves a complex interplay of various control systems within the body. These control systems work together to monitor and adjust the internal environment, ensuring that essential variables remain within a narrow range for optimal functioning. Here are some key mechanisms involved in the regulation of physiological homeostasis:

- **Feedback mechanisms:** Homeostasis is primarily regulated through negative feedback loops. These loops involve three components: a sensor (receptor), a control center (often the brain or endocrine system), and an effector. The sensor detects changes in a specific variable and sends signals to the control center, which compares the current value to the desired set point. If there is a deviation from the set point, the control center activates effectors to bring the variable back to the optimal range.

- **Nervous system regulation:** The nervous system, particularly the autonomic nervous system, plays a vital role in homeostatic regulation. It controls involuntary processes and helps maintain internal balance. For example, in response to a decrease in blood pressure, the autonomic nervous system can stimulate vasoconstriction to raise blood pressure or vasodilation to lower blood pressure.

- **Endocrine system regulation:** The endocrine system secretes hormones that help regulate various bodily functions and contribute to homeostasis. Hormones act as chemical messengers, traveling through the bloodstream to target organs or cells. For instance, the hormone insulin, released by the pancreas, helps regulate glucose levels in the blood.

- **Circulatory system:** The circulatory system, comprised of the heart, blood vessels, and blood, plays a crucial role in transporting oxygen, nutrients, hormones, and waste products throughout the body. It ensures that cells receive essential substances and removes waste materials, contributing to the maintenance of homeostasis.

- **Respiratory system:** The respiratory system helps regulate the balance of oxygen and carbon dioxide in the body, contributing to acid-base balance. Through breathing, the body takes in oxygen and expels carbon dioxide, helping to maintain appropriate levels of these gases in the bloodstream.

- **Renal system:** The kidneys, part of the renal system, are responsible for filtering waste products, maintaining fluid balance, and regulating electrolyte levels. They remove waste and excess substances from the blood while reabsorbing essential materials, ensuring proper composition and volume of bodily fluids.

- **Thermoregulation:** The body maintains its temperature through thermoregulatory mechanisms. When body temperature deviates from the set point, the body can activate processes such as sweating or shivering to restore balance.

These are some of the key mechanisms involved in the regulation of homeostasis. The body constantly monitors and adjusts various variables to ensure internal stability and optimal physiological function. The intricate interplay between different systems and feedback loops allows the body to adapt and respond to changing conditions, maintaining a state of homeostasis.

2. Psychological

Psychological homeostasis plays a vital role in preserving an individual's mental equilibrium and overall well-being. When faced with various stressors—whether physical, social, or psychological—an individual strives to adapt and find balance. Successful adaptation occurs when sufficient internal and external resources are available, enabling the individual to cope effectively and maintain equilibrium.

Psychological regulation of homeostasis refers to the processes and mechanisms involved in maintaining a stable and balanced psychological state within an individual. It involves the regulation of emotions, cognition, behavior, and overall mental well-being. However, if resources are inadequate, maladaptation may occur. Adaptive responses to stressors, such as the interaction between the mind and body, coping strategies, and defense mechanisms, contribute to the maintenance of psychological homeostasis within the body. Here are some key mechanisms involved in the regulation of psychological homeostasis:

Mind and Body Interaction

The mind and body interaction plays a crucial role in the regulation of homeostasis, which is the maintenance of a stable internal environment within the body. Here is how the mind and body interact to regulate homeostasis:

- **Emotional regulation:** Emotions can impact the body's physiological state and disrupt homeostasis. For example, experiencing chronic stress, anxiety, or intense negative emotions can lead to imbalances in heart rate, blood pressure, immune function, and other bodily processes. By regulating emotions through techniques such as mindfulness, relaxation, and emotional expression, the mind can help restore homeostasis.

- **Cognitive regulation:** The mind's cognitive processes, including thoughts, beliefs, and perceptions, can influence the body's physiological responses and impact homeostasis. Negative or distorted thinking patterns, such as catastrophizing or rumination, can contribute to stress and disrupt the body's balance. Cognitive regulation techniques, such as reframing negative thoughts, challenging irrational beliefs, and promoting positive thinking, can aid in restoring homeostasis.
- **Placebo effect:** The mind's beliefs and expectations can influence the body's response to treatments and interventions. The placebo effect, where a person experiences positive health outcomes due to their belief in a treatment's effectiveness, demonstrates the mind's influence on the body's homeostatic mechanisms.

Coping

Coping refers to the cognitive and behavioral actions that an individual undertakes to handle a stressor or challenging situation. It holds significance for both physical and psychological well-being since stress has been linked to various health and psychological consequences. The effectiveness of coping strategies is contingent upon the unique needs of each person, which can be influenced by factors such as age and cultural background. Due to this variability, there is no universal coping strategy that suits everyone or every type of stressor. Additionally, individuals may employ different coping mechanisms at different times, even within the same person.

During times of stress, individuals typically employ a blend of problem-focused and emotion-focused coping strategies. Essentially, when faced with stress, individuals gather information, take steps to modify the situation (problem-focused), and regulate their emotions associated with the stress

(emotion-focused). On certain occasions, individuals may opt to avoid thinking about the situation altogether or alter their thought patterns without directly altering the actual circumstances.

Defense Mechanisms

Defense mechanisms are psychological strategies that individuals unconsciously use to protect themselves from experiencing anxiety, distress, or internal conflicts. These mechanisms operate at an unconscious level and help individuals cope with threatening or uncomfortable thoughts, feelings, or situations. Here are some common defense mechanisms:

- **Repression:** Repression involves pushing distressing or unwanted thoughts, memories, or emotions into the unconscious mind, making them inaccessible to conscious awareness.
- **Denial:** Denial is the refusal to acknowledge or accept a reality or truth that may be too threatening or distressing. It involves avoiding or distorting information that conflicts with one's beliefs or desires.
- **Projection:** Projection involves attributing one's own unacceptable thoughts, feelings, or qualities to others. It allows individuals to externalize their own undesirable traits and project them onto someone else.
- **Rationalization:** Rationalization is the process of creating logical or acceptable explanations or justifications for one's thoughts, actions, or behaviors. It helps individuals protect their self-esteem by providing plausible reasons for their actions or decisions.
- **Displacement:** Displacement occurs when an individual directs their emotions or impulses from one person or object to another that is less threatening or more socially acceptable. It allows for the release of tension or frustration in a safer or more appropriate manner.
- **Sublimation:** Sublimation involves channeling unacceptable or socially inappropriate impulses, such as

aggression or sexuality, into socially acceptable or constructive outlets. For example, redirecting aggressive urges into competitive sports or creative pursuits.

- **Regression:** Regression refers to reverting to earlier, more childlike patterns of behavior or ways of coping. This defense mechanism occurs when individuals face stress or anxiety and retreat to a more familiar and less demanding state.
- **Intellectualization:** Intellectualization involves approaching distressing situations or emotions in a detached and analytical manner. It focuses on logical reasoning and knowledge to distance oneself from the emotional impact of the situation.
- **Reaction formation:** Reaction formation is when an individual expresses thoughts, feelings, or behaviors that are the opposite of their true desires or impulses. It serves as a defense against unacceptable or threatening thoughts or feelings.
- **Undoing:** Undoing is the act of engaging in behaviors or thoughts aimed at negating or reversing previously unacceptable thoughts, actions, or impulses. It is an attempt to alleviate guilt or anxiety associated with those previous actions.

General Adaptation Syndrome

The activation of the GAS occurs indirectly when individuals encounter psychological threats, which vary among individuals and evoke diverse responses. The person's reaction to such threats is influenced by factors such as the intensity and duration of the threat, the presence of concurrent stressors, and whether or not the person anticipated the stressor. Coping with an unforeseen stressor can be particularly challenging. Personal attributes, including the level of personal control, the availability of social support, and feelings of competence, also play a role in shaping the response to a stressor.

▮ STRESS MANAGEMENT

Effective stress management is crucial for maintaining psychological homeostasis.

This involves recognizing and coping with stressors in healthy ways, implementing stress reduction techniques (e.g., relaxation exercises, time management, and problem-solving strategies), and engaging in self-care practices that promote mental well-being.

Stress Management Techniques

Stress management techniques are strategies and practices designed to help individuals effectively cope with and reduce the impact of stress on their physical and mental well-being. Here are several commonly recommended stress management techniques:

- **Relaxation techniques:** Engaging in relaxation techniques can help reduce stress levels and promote a sense of calm. Examples include deep breathing exercises, progressive muscle relaxation, guided imagery, and meditation.
- **Physical activity:** Regular physical exercise is known to release endorphins, which are natural mood boosters. Engaging in activities such as walking, jogging, yoga, or dancing can help reduce stress and improve overall well-being.
- **Time management:** Effective time management can help individuals prioritize tasks, reduce feelings of overwhelm, and improve productivity. This includes setting realistic goals, creating schedules, and learning to delegate tasks when necessary.
- **Social support:** Seeking support from friends, family, or support groups can provide emotional validation, guidance, and a sense of connection. Talking to someone trusted about stressors and challenges can help alleviate emotional burden and provide different perspectives.
- **Positive psychology interventions:** Positive psychology interventions focus on enhancing positive emotions, well-being, and flourishing. These interventions may involve gratitude exercises, acts of kindness, engaging in meaningful activities, and cultivating positive relationships. Such practices promote psychological well-being and contribute

to the regulation of psychological homeostasis.

- **Healthy lifestyle habits:** Adopting a healthy lifestyle can have a positive impact on stress management. This includes getting sufficient sleep, maintaining a balanced diet, limiting caffeine and alcohol intake, and avoiding unhealthy coping mechanisms such as smoking or excessive use of substances.

- **Cognitive reframing:** Cognitive reframing involves consciously changing negative thought patterns and replacing them with more positive or realistic ones. This technique helps individuals reframe stressful situations and develop a more resilient mindset.

- **Self-reflection and self-awareness:** Developing self-awareness and engaging in self-reflection are essential for psychological regulation. It involves gaining insight into one's thoughts, emotions, and behaviors, identifying personal strengths and weaknesses, and cultivating a deeper understanding of oneself. Practices such as meditation, journaling, and therapy can aid in self-reflection and self-awareness.

- **Time for relaxation and self-care:** Taking time for self-care activities that bring joy and relaxation is essential for stress management. Engaging in activities such as reading, hobbies, spending time in nature, or practicing mindfulness can help reduce stress levels and promote overall well-being.

- **Setting boundaries:** Establishing boundaries and learning to say no when necessary can help manage stress by preventing overload and allowing for adequate self-care and rest.

- **Seeking professional help:** In some cases, stress may become overwhelming or chronic, requiring the assistance of a mental health professional. Therapy or counseling can provide individuals with tools and support to effectively manage and reduce stress.

- **Healthy coping strategies:** Developing healthy coping strategies, such as journaling, expressive arts, engaging in hobbies, or seeking professional guidance, can provide outlets for stress and promote emotional well-being.

It is important to remember that different techniques work for different individuals, and it may require some trial and error to find what works best for you. It's also advisable to seek professional help when needed, especially if stress is significantly impacting your daily life or mental health.

ROLE OF NURSE IN STRESS MANAGEMENT

The role of nurses in stress management is crucial, as they play a significant part in supporting individuals in managing stress and promoting overall well-being. Here are some key aspects of a nurse's role in stress management:

- **Assessment:** Nurses are skilled in assessing individuals' stress levels and identifying stressors. Through careful observation and effective communication, they can gather information about the sources and impact of stress on an individual's physical and mental health.

- **Education:** Nurses provide education and information to individuals, families, and communities about stress management techniques. They help raise awareness about the effects of stress on health and well-being and teach strategies to cope with stress effectively.

- **Supportive counselling:** Nurses offer emotional support and engage in therapeutic communication with individuals experiencing stress. They provide a safe and nonjudgmental space for individuals to express their concerns, fears, and anxieties, and offer guidance and coping strategies.

- **Collaboration with interdisciplinary team:** Nurses collaborate with other healthcare professionals, such as psychologists, social workers, and occupational therapists, to develop comprehensive stress management plans for individuals. They contribute their unique nursing perspective and work together to address the multifaceted aspects of stress and its management.

- **Health promotion and prevention:** Nurses play a vital role in promoting health and preventing stress-related conditions. They educate individuals on healthy lifestyle practices, such as exercise, nutrition, and sleep hygiene, which can reduce stress levels and enhance overall well-being.
- **Crisis intervention:** In situations of acute stress or crisis, nurses provide immediate support and intervention. They employ crisis management techniques to stabilize individuals and help them regain a sense of control and stability.
- **Advocacy:** Nurses act as advocates for individuals experiencing stress, ensuring that their needs are met and their rights are respected. They may advocate for appropriate work-life balance, access to resources and support systems, and accommodations that promote stress reduction.
- **Evaluation and follow-up:** Nurses assess the effectiveness of stress management interventions and modify plans as needed. They monitor the progress of individuals in managing stress and provide ongoing support and guidance.
- **Self-care role modelling:** Nurses serve as role models for self-care and stress management. By prioritizing their own well-being and utilizing healthy coping strategies, they inspire and encourage individuals to take care of their own physical and mental health.

Overall, nurses play an integral role in stress management by providing assessment, education, counselling, collaboration, advocacy, and support. Through their expertise and compassionate care, they empower individuals to effectively manage stress, promote resilience, and enhance their overall quality of life.

CHAPTER SUMMARY

1. Stress and adaptation are two interconnected concepts that have a significant impact on our lives.
2. Stress refers to the physiological and psychological responses we experience when we perceive a demand or threat that exceeds our coping abilities.
3. Stress can arise from various sources such as work, relationships, financial pressures, health issues, and major life changes.
4. Stress can be categorized into different types, including acute stress, chronic stress, eustress, distress, and secondary traumatic stress.
5. Stressors, the specific events or situations that trigger the stress response, can be physical, psychological, social, environmental, related to life events, internal, and anticipatory.
6. Adaptation refers to an individual's ability to adjust and respond effectively to changes in their environment or circumstances.
7. Recognizing and understanding stress and adaptation can help individuals better identify and manage their stress levels, develop effective coping strategies, and promote overall well-being.
8. Homeostasis involves maintaining a dynamic balance in the body to keep important variables within an optimal range for cellular function.
9. The regulation of homeostasis involves physiological and psychological mechanisms.
10. The General Adaptation Syndrome consists of three stages: alarm, resistance, and exhaustion.
11. To manage stress effectively, individuals can employ stress management techniques.
12. Nurses play a crucial role in stress management by providing support, education, and interventions to individuals.

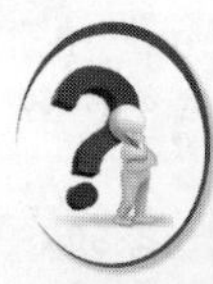

REVIEW QUESTIONS

1. Discuss factors influencing stress and adaptation.
2. Define stress and explain the impact of stress on health.
3. Describe the stress management techniques and role of nurse in stress management.
4. Discuss physiological and psychological regulation of homeostasis.

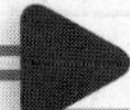 **BIBLIOGRAPHY** 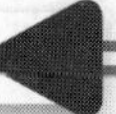

1. Addison WE, Weiten W. Psychology, 10th edition. Boston, MA: Cengage Learning; 2011.
2. American Nurses Association (ANA). Psychiatric–mental health nursing: scope and standards of practice, 2nd edition. Silver Spring, MD, ANA; 2014.
3. American Psychological Association. (2023). Stress. Retrieved from: https://www.apa.org/topics/stress.
4. Banks K, Newman E. Stress management: A comprehensive guide to relieving stress and promoting well-being. New York, NY: Guilford Press; 2011.
5. Berger BG. The portable stress survival guide: Simple strategies for managing stress at work, at home, and in your relationships. New York, NY: Guilford Press; 2012.
6. Caspi O. The stress response: A comprehensive guide to the biology and psychology of stress, coping, and health. New York, NY: Oxford University Press; 2013.
7. Cisler JM, Sigel BA, Kramer TL, Smitherman S, Vanderzee K, Pemberton, J. Cognitive-behavioral therapy for anxiety disorders: A practitioner's guide. New York, NY: Guilford Press; 2014.
8. Cohen S, Kamarck T, Mermelstein R.. A global measure of perceived stress. J Health Soc Behav. 1983;24:385-96.
9. Cohen S, Wills TA. Stress, social support, and the buffering hypothesis. Psychol Bull. 1985;98(2):310-57.
10. Cottrell S. Occupational stress and job satisfaction in mental health nursing: Focused interventions through evidence based assessment. J Psychiatr Ment Health Nurs. 2001;8:157-64.
11. Davies S. Stress and anxiety: A practical guide to coping. London, UK: Jessica Kingsley Publishers; 2015.
12. Diehl J, Opmeer BC, Boer F, Mannarino AP, Lindauer, RJL. Post-traumatic stress disorder: A comprehensive guide to assessment, treatment, and prevention. New York, NY: Guilford Press; 2016.
13. Huether SE, McCance KL. Understanding pathophysiology, 5th edition. St Louis, Mosby; 2012.
14. Ianello P, Balzarotti S. Stress and coping strategies in the emergency room. Emerg Care J.2014;10:72.
15. McEwen BS. Stress and allostatic load: Implications for neuropsychiatric disorders and aging. Arch Gen Psychiatry. 2000;57(1):20-32.
16. Sharma SK, Mudgal SK, Thakur K, Gaur R, Aggarwal P. Lifestyle behavior of budding health care professionals: A cross-sectional descriptive study. J Family Med Prim Care. 2020;9:3525-31
17. Stevens D, Wilcox HC, MacKinnon DF, Mondimore FM, Schweizer B, Jancic D, et al. Post-traumatic stress disorder increases risk for suicide attempt in adults with recurrent major depression. Depress Anxiety. 2013;30(10):940-6.

CHAPTER
10

Healthcare Concept

Learning Objectives

- Define the concept of healthcare and explain its significance in promoting individual and community well-being.
- Identify various factors that influence healthcare delivery, including social, economic, cultural, and environmental factors.
- Describe the different levels of healthcare: primary, secondary, and tertiary, along with their respective roles and functions.
- Identify the facilities associated with each level of care.
- Analyze the benefits and limitations of each level of healthcare in addressing different health needs.
- Describe the structure and organization of the healthcare system in India.
- Identify the major challenges faced by the Indian healthcare system, including accessibility, quality, and disparities.
- Analyze the key healthcare policies and initiatives implemented by the Indian government to improve healthcare services.

INTRODUCTION

The concept of healthcare is a multifaceted and comprehensive approach to maintaining, improving, or restoring the health and well-being of individuals and communities. It encompasses a wide range of practices, services, and interventions that span from preventive measures and health education to diagnosis, treatment, and rehabilitation. The goal of healthcare is to enhance the quality of life, prevent illnesses, alleviate suffering, and promote holistic well-being.

KEY ASPECTS OF THE CONCEPT OF HEALTHCARE

- **Preventive measures:** Healthcare focuses on preventing health issues before they arise. This involves promoting healthy lifestyles, providing vaccinations, conducting screenings, and offering health education to empower individuals with the knowledge and tools to make informed decisions about their health. Preventive healthcare helps reduce the burden of disease and the strain on healthcare systems.
- **Promotion of well-being:** Beyond addressing diseases, healthcare emphasizes holistic well-being. It recognizes that health is not merely the absence of illness but also includes mental, emotional, and social aspects. Healthcare interventions contribute to mental health support, emotional well-being, and overall life satisfaction.

- **Diagnosis and treatment:** Healthcare plays a crucial role in diagnosing illnesses, injuries, and medical conditions. Medical professionals use diagnostic tools, tests, and assessments to identify health issues accurately. Treatment plans are then developed, which may involve medication, surgeries, therapies, or other medical interventions.
- **Holistic approach:** Healthcare acknowledges the interconnectedness of various aspects of health. It considers not only physical health but also mental, emotional, and social well-being. This holistic perspective recognizes that factors like lifestyle, environment, and social determinants influence an individual's health.
- **Patient-centered care:** Healthcare is centered around the needs, preferences, and values of the individual. It encourages a partnership between healthcare providers and patients, allowing patients to actively participate in their care decisions and treatment plans.
- **Equity and accessibility:** A fundamental principle of healthcare is equitable access to healthcare services. It advocates for providing healthcare regardless of socioeconomic status, gender, race, or geographical location. This ensures that everyone has the opportunity to achieve optimal health outcomes.
- **Collaboration:** Healthcare involves collaboration among various healthcare professionals, including doctors, nurses, specialists, therapists, and other allied health professionals. Effective teamwork ensures comprehensive care that addresses the various dimensions of an individual's health.
- **Continuous care:** Healthcare is not limited to a single intervention; it often requires ongoing care and management. Chronic conditions, e.g., demand long-term treatment and monitoring to maintain the patient's health and quality of life.
- **Healthcare systems:** Healthcare operates within healthcare systems, which encompass healthcare facilities, providers, organizations, policies, and regulations. These systems ensure the organization and delivery of healthcare services to populations.

FACTORS INFLUENCING HEALTHCARE DELIVERY SYSTEM IN INDIA

The healthcare delivery system in India is influenced by a wide range of factors that collectively shape the accessibility, quality, and effectiveness of healthcare services. These factors are complex and interrelated, reflecting the diverse social, economic, cultural, and political landscape of the country. Here are some of the key factors that influence the healthcare delivery system in India:

- **Socioeconomic disparities:** Socio-economic factors such as income, education, and occupation play a significant role in determining access to healthcare services. India has a wide income disparity, and many individuals from lower socioeconomic backgrounds face barriers in accessing quality healthcare due to financial constraints.
- **Population density and diversity:** India is densely populated and culturally diverse, leading to variations in healthcare needs and preferences across different regions and communities. Healthcare services need to be adaptable and culturally sensitive to cater to the diverse population.
- **Health infrastructure:** Disparities in healthcare infrastructure between urban and rural areas exist. Urban areas tend to have better access to healthcare facilities, while rural areas often face challenges due to inadequate infrastructure, lack of medical professionals, and limited healthcare facilities.
- **Health workforce:** The availability, distribution, and quality of healthcare professionals, including doctors, nurses, and specialists, influence healthcare

delivery. India faces shortages of healthcare professionals, particularly in rural and remote areas, leading to uneven access to care.

- **Public vs private healthcare:** India has a dual healthcare system with both public and private sectors. While public healthcare aims to provide affordable services, it often faces challenges related to inadequate funding, infrastructure, and staff. Private healthcare offers higher quality care but can be expensive and inaccessible for many.

- **Health insurance and financing:** Lack of health insurance coverage and high out-of-pocket expenses can deter individuals from seeking timely and appropriate healthcare. Health financing models, insurance schemes, and government initiatives play a role in determining the financial burden of healthcare on individuals and families.

- **Government policies and initiatives:** Government policies, programs, and initiatives have a significant impact on healthcare delivery. Schemes like Ayushman Bharat aim to provide health coverage for vulnerable populations, while regulatory policies shape the standards and quality of healthcare services.

- **Technological advancements:** Technological advancements have the potential to enhance healthcare delivery, improve diagnosis, treatment, and patient outcomes. However, uneven access to advanced technology between urban and rural areas remains a challenge.

- **Health information systems:** Effective health information systems are crucial for efficient healthcare delivery. The availability and accuracy of patient records, medical history, and health data contribute to better diagnosis and treatment.

- **Cultural beliefs and practices:** Cultural factors influence healthcare-seeking behavior and treatment preferences. Traditional beliefs, practices, and stigma related to certain diseases can impact individuals' willingness to seek medical care.

- **Public awareness and health education:** Lack of awareness about preventive measures, disease management, and available healthcare services can lead to delayed or inadequate care. Health education campaigns can contribute to better health outcomes.

- **Disease burden and epidemiology:** The prevalence of specific diseases, epidemics, and health crises shape the healthcare delivery system's focus and resource allocation. Communicable diseases, non-communicable diseases, and emerging health threats affect healthcare priorities.

- **Pharmaceutical industry:** The availability, affordability, and quality of medicines impact healthcare delivery. The pharmaceutical industry's practices and regulations influence drug accessibility and affordability.

- **Global health policies and collaborations:** Global health initiatives, partnerships, and collaborations influence healthcare delivery in India. International aid, research, and best practices sharing contribute to addressing healthcare challenges.

- **Political factors:** Political decisions and governance influence healthcare policies, funding allocation, and overall healthcare system development.

In summary, the healthcare delivery system in India is influenced by a complex interplay of factors ranging from socioeconomic disparities and infrastructure challenges to policy decisions, cultural beliefs, and technological advancements. Addressing these factors requires a comprehensive approach involving government interventions, healthcare sector reforms, community engagement, and collaboration between various stakeholders.

LEVELS OF HEALTHCARE SYSTEM

The healthcare system operates at different levels, each with specific roles, functions, and responsibilities. These levels are designed to provide a comprehensive and organized approach to healthcare delivery, catering to individuals' varying medical needs. The three main levels of healthcare are primary, secondary, and tertiary care.

1. Primary Healthcare

- **Role and function:** Primary healthcare serves as the first point of contact for individuals seeking medical care. It focuses on providing comprehensive and basic healthcare services to maintain overall well-being, prevent diseases, and manage common health issues.
- **Services provided:** Primary healthcare encompasses a wide range of services, including health promotion, disease prevention, routine check-ups, immunizations, screenings, basic diagnostics, treatment of common illnesses and injuries, maternal and child health, family planning, and health education.
- **Setting:** Primary healthcare is usually delivered in community-based settings such as clinics, local health centers, doctor's offices, and sometimes through mobile health units.
- **Providers:** General practitioners, family physicians, nurse practitioners, physician assistants, and community health workers are typically involved in delivering primary healthcare services.
- **Importance:** Primary healthcare is vital for promoting good health, preventing diseases, and addressing health concerns at an early stage. It emphasizes the importance of preventive measures and plays a crucial role in improving community health.
- **Role of nurses in primary healthcare (primary level):**
  - *Health promotion and education:* Nurses in primary care educate individuals and communities about healthy lifestyles, disease prevention, and health promotion. They emphasize the importance of regular check-ups, vaccinations, and healthy behaviors.
  - *Preventive care:* Nurses administer vaccinations, conduct health screenings, and promote early detection of health issues. They work to identify risk factors and provide counseling to mitigate health risks.
  - *Patient assessment:* Nurses perform thorough assessments of patients' health status, including physical, mental, and emotional well-being. They gather information, conduct physical examinations, and identify health concerns.
  - *Health counseling:* Nurses provide health counseling and support, addressing patients' questions, concerns, and fears. They offer guidance on adopting healthier lifestyles and managing chronic conditions.
  - *Treatment and basic care:* Nurses deliver basic medical treatments, administer medications, and provide care for patients with common illnesses and injuries. They monitor patients' progress and offer guidance on self-care.
  - *Maternal and child health:* Nurses provide prenatal care, postnatal care, childbirth assistance, neonatal care, and child immunizations. They support expectant mothers and families throughout the pregnancy journey.
  - *Community engagement:* Nurses actively engage with communities to assess health needs, develop health programs, and conduct health education campaigns. They foster partnerships with local organizations to improve community health.

2. Secondary Healthcare

- **Role and function:** Secondary healthcare involves more specialized and advanced medical care beyond the scope of primary care. It focuses on diagnosing, managing, and treating complex health conditions that require specialized medical expertise and technology.
- **Services provided:** Secondary healthcare includes services such as specialty consultations, diagnostic tests (MRI, CT scans), specialized surgeries, intermediate

medical interventions, and short-term hospitalization for more severe illnesses.

- **Setting:** Secondary healthcare is provided in hospitals with specialized departments, advanced medical equipment, and medical specialists.
- **Providers:** Specialists like cardiologists, dermatologists, orthopedic surgeons, gastroenterologists, and other subspecialists play a significant role in delivering secondary healthcare services.
- **Importance:** Secondary healthcare provides specialized treatment options and advanced medical interventions to ensure accurate diagnosis and effective management of various medical conditions. It helps bridge the gap between primary care and tertiary care.
- **Role of nurses in secondary healthcare (secondary level):**
  - *Specialized care*: Nurses in secondary care assist in the delivery of specialized care, such as preparing patients for surgeries and procedures, monitoring patients in recovery, and administering specialized treatments.
  - *Patient monitoring*: Nurses closely monitor patients' conditions, administer medications, and manage symptoms. They collaborate with specialized healthcare teams to ensure proper patient care.
  - *Education and support*: Nurses educate patients about their conditions, treatment options, and postprocedure care. They offer emotional support and address concerns during the recovery process.
  - *Coordination*: Nurses coordinate patient care across departments, ensuring that test results, treatments, and consultations are properly managed and communicated to the patient and healthcare team.
  - *Pain management*: Nurses play a significant role in managing pain and discomfort, ensuring patients' comfort

and well-being during their recovery process.

  - *Wound care*: Nurses manage wound care and ensure that patients' incisions or injuries are properly cleaned, dressed, and monitored for signs of infection.

3. Tertiary Healthcare

- **Role and function:** Tertiary healthcare deals with highly specialized medical care and advanced treatments for complex and critical health conditions. It often involves long-term management and rehabilitation for severe illnesses and injuries.
- **Services provided:** Tertiary healthcare encompasses services such as major surgeries, organ transplants, intensive care unit (ICU) treatments, advanced cancer therapies, management of chronic diseases, and specialized rehabilitation.
- **Setting:** Tertiary healthcare is delivered in specialized hospitals and medical centers equipped with cutting-edge technology, state-of-the-art facilities, and specialized medical teams.
- **Providers:** Highly skilled medical specialists, subspecialists, surgeons, and multidisciplinary medical teams are responsible for providing tertiary healthcare services.
- **Importance:** Tertiary healthcare addresses the most complex and critical health conditions, offering advanced treatments that significantly impact patient outcomes, enhance quality of life, and ensure long-term care for chronic conditions.
- **Role of nurses in tertiary healthcare (tertiary level):**
  - *Critical care:* Nurses in tertiary care settings work in intensive care units (ICUs) and specialized wards. They provide care for patients with critical conditions, closely monitoring vital signs and administering complex treatments.
  - *Complex procedures:* Nurses assist in complex medical procedures and surgeries, ensuring that patients are

prepared, monitored, and cared for during and after the procedure.

- *Patient advocacy:* Nurses advocate for patients' needs, preferences, and rights within the complex tertiary healthcare environment. They ensure that patients receive the best possible care and are informed about their options.
- *Rehabilitation:* Nurses assist in the rehabilitation of patients who have undergone major surgeries or treatments. They help patients regain strength, mobility, and independence.
- *Patient and family education:* Nurses provide comprehensive education to patients and their families about complex conditions, treatments, and long-term care plans. They support patients in understanding their health journey.
- *End-of-life care:* In palliative care and hospice settings, nurses provide compassionate care to patients nearing the end of life. They offer comfort, symptom management, and emotional support to both patients and their families.

CENTRAL LEVEL HEALTH ORGANIZATION IN INDIA

The health institutions within a nation form the fundamental workforce for human well-being. India comprises 28 states and 8 Union territories within its union. According to the constitution, states possess substantial autonomy in concerns pertaining to providing healthcare services to the populace. Consequently, each state has established its distinct framework for delivering healthcare, operating separately from the federal government.

The healthcare structure in India consists of three tiers: the central level, the state level, and the district level (**Fig. 10.1**).

HEALTH ADMINISTRATION AT THE CENTRAL LEVEL

The official organs of the health system at the national level consist of three units:
1. Union Ministry of Health and Family Welfare.
2. The Directorate General of Health Services.
3. The Central Council of Health and Family Welfare.

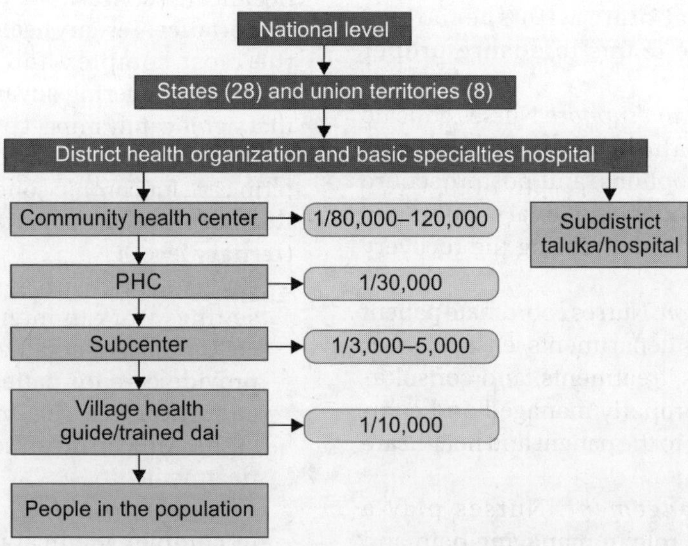

Fig. 10.1: Healthcare structure and organization in India.

Union Ministry of Health and Family Welfare

The leadership of the Union Ministry of Health and Family Welfare comprises a Cabinet Minister, a Minister of State, and a Deputy Health Minister.

These positions are politically appointed and encompass a twofold duty: carrying out political functions and overseeing administrative tasks related to health matters. At present, the federal health ministry encompasses the subsequent divisions (**Fig. 10.2**):

- Department of Health
- Family Welfare Department
- Indian System of Medicine and Homoeopathy Department.

Department of Health

Within the Health Department, a secretary to the Government of India serves as the chief executive, supported by joint secretaries, deputy secretaries, and an extensive administrative team.

Functions

A. **Union List:**
  - Management of global health partnerships and oversight of port-related quarantine activities.
  - Supervision of key central health institutions like the All India Institute of Hygiene and Public Health in Kolkata and the National Institute for Control of Communicable Diseases in Delhi.
  - Encouragement of research via research centers and similar entities.
  - Control and advancement of medical, nursing, and affiliated healthcare professions.
  - Creation and upkeep of standards for pharmaceutical products.
  - Census, along with the compilation and dissemination of additional statistical information.
  - Monitoring of both the arrival and departure of individuals across borders.
  - Control of labor practices within the operations of mines and oil fields.

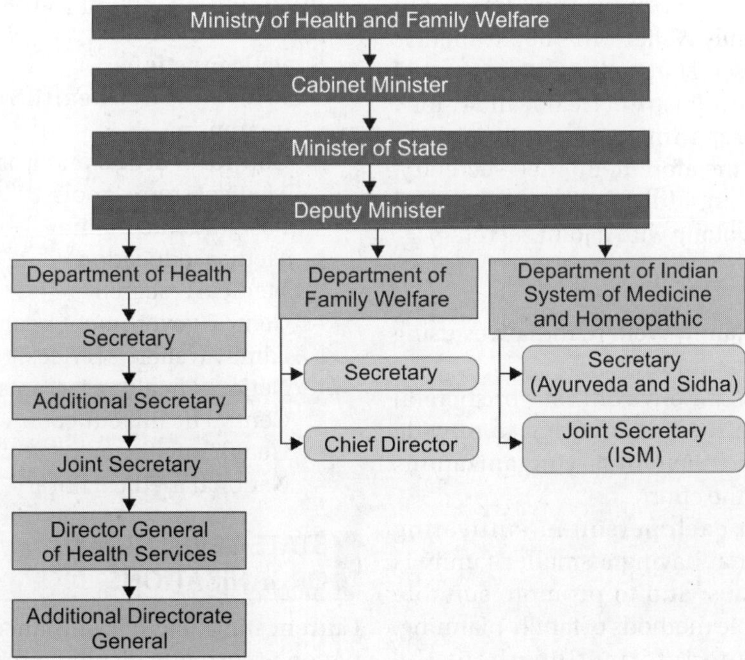

Fig. 10.2: Healthcare organization at central level.

B. **Concurrent list:** The duties enumerated in the concurrent list are shared responsibilities between the central and state governments. Both the federal and state authorities possess concurrent legislative authority. These responsibilities encompass:
- Halting the spread of communicable illnesses between different entities.
- Halting the contamination of food products.
- Oversight of pharmaceuticals and toxic substances.
- Recordkeeping of vital demographic information.
- Ensuring the well-being of laborers.
- Management of nonmajor ports.
- Formulating plans for economic and societal health advancements.
- Implementation of measures for population management and family planning.

Department of Health and Family Welfare

Established in 1966 under the Ministry of Health and Family Welfare, this department is headed by the secretary to the Government of India within the Ministry of Health and Family Welfare. The Department of Family Welfare is overseen by the aforementioned secretary, supported by an additional secretary and commissioner, along with a joint secretary.

Function

- To arrange family welfare initiatives using family welfare centers.
- To establish an environment of societal approval for the initiative and to provide assistance to all voluntary organizations invested in the effort.
- To instruct each person in cultivating the belief that having a smaller family is advantageous, and to promote suitable and agreeable methods of family planning.
- To distribute information about the utilization of family planning extensively and to make available service facilities close to the community.

The Department of Indian System of Medicine and Homeopathy

Established in March 1995, this department has consistently advanced. The focus was on executing various introduced schemes, including education, drug standardization, improving the accessibility of raw materials, research and development, information dissemination, education and communication, and incorporating ISM and Homeopathy into national healthcare.

Most of the functions of this ministry are executed through an independent body known as Directorate General of Health Services (DGHS). The DGHS acts as the primary consultant to the Union Government for matters encompassing both medical and public health domains.

Functions

- **General functions:** The general functions are surveys, planning, coordination, programming and appraisal of all health matters in the country.
- **Specific functions:**
  - International health relations and quarantine
  - Control of drug standards
  - Medical store depots
  - Postgraduate training
  - Medical education
  - Medical research
  - Central government health scheme
  - Family welfare services
  - National health programs
  - Central health education bureau
  - Health intelligence
  - National medical library

STATE-LEVEL HEALTH ORGANIZATIONS

Current state health governance In India, the nation is currently divided into 28 states, and each individual state maintains its distinct

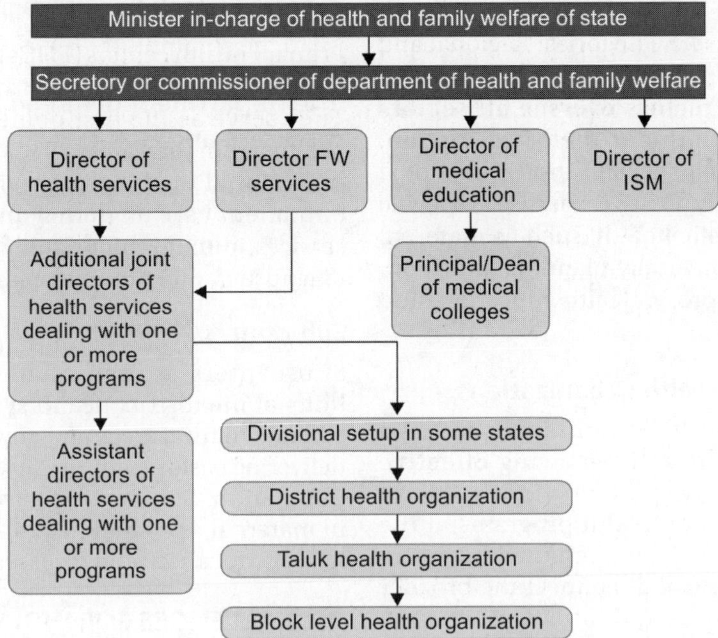

Fig. 10.3: Healthcare organization at state level.

health administration structure. In every state, this administrative sector encompasses the State Ministry of Health and a Health Directorate **(Fig. 10.3)**.

State Ministry of Health

The State Ministry of Health is under the leadership of a minister responsible for Health and Family Welfare, along with a Deputy Minister in charge of the same portfolio. In certain states, the Health Minister might also oversee additional areas of responsibility. The health secretariat serves as the official body for the State Ministry of Health, helmed by a secretary who receives support from Deputy Secretaries and a considerable administrative workforce.

Functions

- Provision of rural healthcare through essential requirements initiative
- Advancement of medical programs
- MCH, family planning, and immunization initiatives
- Initiatives concerning NMIP (malaria) & NFCP (filarial)
- Activities encompassing NLEP, NTCP, NPCB, and measures against communicable illnesses like diarrheal diseases, KFD, JE
- Implementation of school health initiatives, nutritional efforts, and the nationwide goiter control program
- Delivery of laboratory services and establishment of vaccine production units
- Implementation of health education and training endeavors, curative services, and national AIDS control program

State Health Directorate

The head of health services assumes the primary role as the foremost technical consultant to the state government in matters related to medical science and public well-being. This individual also holds the duty of orchestrating and supervising all health-related endeavors. The Director of Health and Family Welfare is supported by an appropriate cadre of deputies and assistants.

The Deputy and Assistant Directors of Health come in two categories: Regional and Functional.

Regional directors oversee all sectors of public health under their jurisdiction, regardless of their specialization. Functional directors typically possess expertise in specific domains of public health, such as maternal and child health, family planning, nutrition, tuberculosis, leprosy, health education, and more.

District-level Health Organizations

District-level health organizations in India play a critical role in ensuring effective healthcare delivery, coordination, and implementation of health programs at the grassroots level. These organizations are the frontline units that connect the broader healthcare policies and initiatives with the local communities. They are responsible for addressing the health needs of the population within their respective districts. Here's a detailed overview of district-level health organizations in India.

District Medical and Health Officer/ Chief Medical and Health Officer

The District Medical and Health Officer (DMHO) or Chief Medical and Health Officer (CMO) is the administrative head of the district-level health organization. They are responsible for overall planning, implementation, and supervision of health programs and services within the district. The DMHO/CMO coordinates activities, manages resources, and ensures the effective functioning of health facilities.

Community Health Centers

Community health centers (CHCs) are designed to provide secondary healthcare services. They are more specialized than PHCs and offer facilities for surgeries, diagnostics, obstetric care, and specialized treatments. CHCs serve as referral centers for PHCs and help bridge the gap between primary and tertiary care.

Primary Health Centers

Primary health centers (PHCs) are the cornerstone of the district-level health system. They serve as the first point of contact for healthcare in rural areas. PHCs provide a range of essential healthcare services, including outpatient care, maternal and child health services, immunization, family planning, basic diagnostics, and preventive interventions.

Sub-centers

Sub-centers are the smallest functional units of the district health system. They are situated in rural areas and are responsible for delivering basic healthcare services to the local population. Sub-centers play a crucial role in maternal and child health, immunization, health education, and disease prevention.

CHALLENGES FOR INDIAN HEALTHCARE SYSTEM

The Indian healthcare system faces several significant challenges that impact accessibility, quality, and disparities in healthcare delivery. Some of the major challenges include:

- **Inadequate infrastructure and resources:** Many healthcare facilities, especially in rural areas, lack proper infrastructure, medical equipment, and trained healthcare professionals. This leads to suboptimal care and limited access to essential medical services.
- **Regional disparities:** There are significant healthcare disparities between urban and rural areas as well as across different states. Urban areas tend to have better healthcare infrastructure, while rural and remote areas often struggle with limited access to quality healthcare services.
- **Uneven distribution of healthcare workforce:** India faces a shortage of doctors, nurses, and other healthcare professionals, which is exacerbated by the unequal distribution of the workforce. Urban areas have a higher concentration of healthcare providers, leaving rural areas underserved.
- **Affordability and financial barriers:** High out-of-pocket healthcare expenses pose a major challenge. Many people

face financial hardships due to medical expenses, and lack of health insurance coverage exacerbates this issue.

- **Quality of care:** The quality of healthcare services varies widely across the country. Inadequate training, outdated practices, and lack of standardized protocols can lead to subpar medical care in certain areas.

- **Lack of preventive care:** The healthcare system has historically focused more on curative rather than preventive care. This leads to a heavier burden of diseases that could have been prevented through early interventions and health education.

- **Urbanization and overcrowding:** Rapid urbanization have led to overburdened healthcare facilities in urban areas, resulting in long waiting times and compromised patient care.

- **Noncommunicable diseases (NCDs):** The prevalence of noncommunicable diseases like diabetes, cardiovascular diseases, and cancer is increasing. These chronic conditions require long-term management and pose a significant challenge to the healthcare system.

- **Maternal and child health:** Despite improvements, maternal and child mortality rates remain high in certain regions. Inadequate access to skilled birth attendants, prenatal care, and postnatal care contribute to this challenge.

- **Health information systems:** Incomplete and outdated health data hampers effective planning and decision-making. A robust health information system is essential for accurate assessment of healthcare needs and resource allocation.

- **Lack of health literacy:** Limited awareness and health literacy among the population hinder their ability to make informed decisions about their health and seek appropriate medical care.

- **Public-private mix:** The dominance of the private sector can lead to variations in healthcare quality and affordability. While the private sector plays a significant role, regulating it to ensure quality care is a challenge.

- **Emerging infectious diseases and pandemics:** The healthcare system's capacity to respond to emerging infectious diseases and pandemics, as highlighted by the COVID-19 pandemic, has revealed vulnerabilities in terms of preparedness, infrastructure, and coordination.

KEY HEALTHCARE POLICIES TO IMPROVE HEALTHCARE SERVICES

The Indian government has implemented several key healthcare policies and initiatives over the years to improve healthcare services, enhance accessibility, and address various health challenges. Here is an analysis of some of the prominent policies and initiatives:

- **National Health Mission (NHM):** Launched in 2013 by merging the National Rural Health Mission (NRHM) and National Urban Health Mission (NUHM), NHM aims to provide accessible, affordable, and quality healthcare to rural and urban populations. It focuses on maternal and child health, reproductive health, immunization, communicable diseases, and more. NHM also emphasizes strengthening healthcare infrastructure at the grassroots level.

- **Ayushman Bharat—Pradhan Mantri Jan Arogya Yojana (PMJAY):** Launched in 2018, PMJAY aims to provide health insurance coverage to economically vulnerable families for secondary and tertiary care hospitalization. It covers more than 50 crore beneficiaries and offers financial protection against catastrophic health expenses.

- **Reproductive, Maternal, Newborn, Child and Adolescent Health (RMNCH+A):** This initiative focuses on improving maternal and child health, reducing infant mortality and maternal mortality rates, and enhancing the overall well-being of mothers and children. It integrates various health services and interventions at different life stages.

- **Mission Indradhanush:** Launched in 2014, this immunization program aims to achieve full immunization coverage for all children and pregnant women by reaching unvaccinated and partially vaccinated areas. It targets seven vaccine-preventable diseases.

- **Pradhan Mantri Surakshit Matritva Abhiyan (PMSMA):** This initiative aims to provide free antenatal care to pregnant women and ensure safe motherhood through early detection of complications and timely medical interventions.

- **Swachh Bharat Mission (SBM):** While primarily a sanitation initiative, SBM also has significant health implications. Improved sanitation and hygiene practices contribute to reducing waterborne diseases and improving overall health outcomes.

- **Janani Shishu Suraksha Karyakram (JSSK):** Under this initiative, pregnant women and sick infants receive free and cashless healthcare services, including transport and medicines, to ensure their well-being during critical times.

These policies and initiatives reflect the government's commitment to addressing various health challenges, improving healthcare access, enhancing the quality of services, and promoting public health. However, while these efforts are commendable, challenges such as implementation gaps, unequal distribution of resources, and the need for sustained funding and monitoring still need to be addressed to achieve comprehensive and equitable healthcare for all citizens.

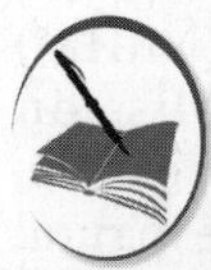

CHAPTER SUMMARY

1. Primary healthcare forms the foundation, focusing on preventive and basic care.
2. Secondary healthcare adds specialized expertise, diagnostics, and treatments.
3. Tertiary healthcare offers the highest level of expertise for critical and complex conditions.
4. A well-structured healthcare system integrates all levels of care to provide a holistic and effective approach to healthcare delivery.
5. Collaboration among primary, secondary, and tertiary care ensures early diagnosis, timely treatment, prevention of complications, and optimal patient outcomes.
6. The central level of the Indian healthcare system is integral to the nation's well-being.
7. The healthcare structure consists of three tiers: central, state, and district levels.
8. The central level includes the Union Ministry of Health and Family Welfare, the Directorate General of Health Services (DGHS), and the Central Council of Health and Family Welfare.
9. Department of health is headed by a Secretary, this department oversees international health relations, central health institutes, research, medical and nursing professions, drug standards, census, and more.
10. Department of Health and Family Welfare focuses on family welfare programs, social acceptance, and family planning education, dissemination, and service facilities.
11. Department of Indian System of Medicine and Homoeopathy emphasizes implementing schemes related to education, drug standardization, raw materials, research, and incorporating traditional medicine into national health care.
12. Each state has its own health administration, with a State Ministry of Health and a Health Directorate.
13. The State Ministry is led by a Minister and Deputy Minister, and the Directorate is responsible for various health initiatives at the state level.
14. District-level health organizations are headed by a District Medical and Health Officer or Chief Medical and Health Officer.
15. The Indian healthcare system faces challenges and the Indian government has introduced policies to improve healthcare services, including the National Health Mission (NHM), Ayushman Bharat—Pradhan Mantri Jan Arogya Yojana (PMJAY), Reproductive, Maternal, Newborn, Child and Adolescent Health (RMNCH+A), Mission Indradhanush, and more.

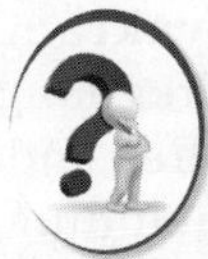

REVIEW QUESTIONS

1. Explain what healthcare entails and its broader meaning beyond medical treatment.
2. Discuss various factors that influence healthcare delivery system in India.
3. Define each level and explain their roles in the healthcare system.
4. Explain the division of the Indian healthcare system into central, state, and district levels.
5. Describe the major challenges faced by the Indian healthcare system.
6. Analyze the government's efforts to promote healthcare system in India.

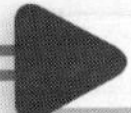 ## BIBLIOGRAPHY 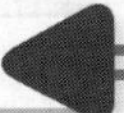

1. Addressing the challenges of the Indian Healthcare System—opinions [Internet]. [cited 2023, Aug 2]. Available from: https://www.tatatrusts.org/insights/opinions/addressing-the-challenges-of-the-indian-healthcare-system.
2. Berwick DM, Nolan TW, Whittington J. The triple aim: Care, health, and cost. Health Aff. 2008;27(3): 759-69.
3. Das J, Kwan A, Daniels B, Satyanarayana S, Subbaraman R, Bergkvist S, et al. Use of standardised patients to assess quality of healthcare in Nairobi, Kenya: A pilot, cross-sectional study with international comparisons. Lancet Glob Health. 2018;6(6):e668-79.
4. Gupta A, Singhal S. Healthcare disparities in India: A review. Indian J Public Health. 2019;63(4): 279-84.
5. Kasthuri A. Challenges to Healthcare in India—The Five A's. Indian J Community Med. 2018;43(3): 141-3.
6. Kruk ME, Gage AD, Arsenault C, Jordan K, Leslie HH, Roder-DeWan, S et al. High-quality health systems in the sustainable development goals era: Time for a revolution. Lancet Glob Health. 2018;6(11): e1196-252.
7. Kumar A. Indian healthcare delivery system: Challenges and opportunities. J Health Manag. 2020;22(1):83-95.
8. Kumar R. Impact of National Health Mission of India on Infant and Maternal Mortality: A logical framework analysis. J Health Manag. 2021;23(1):155-65.
9. National Health Policy. (2017). Ministry of Health and Family Welfare, Government of India. http://164.100.158.44/showfile.php?lid=4275.
10. Organisational chart: Ministry of Health and Family Welfare: GOI [Internet]. [cited 2023, Aug 1]. Available from: https://main.mohfw.gov.in/about-us/organisational-chart.
11. Parida SR. Health Organization and Health Services in India [Internet]. 2021 [cited 2023, Aug 1]. Available from: https://nurseinnursing.com/organization-and-administration-of-health-services-in-india-at-different-levels/.
12. Park K. Park's Textbook of Preventive and Social Medicine. Banarsidas Bhanot Publishers; 2019.
13. Primary health care [Internet]. World Health Organization; [cited 2023, Aug 2]. Available from: https://www.who.int/health-topics/primary-health-care#tab=tab_1.
14. Reddy KS, Patel V, Jha P (Eds). Towards achievement of universal health care in India: A call to action. Public Health Foundation of India; 2018.
15. Sharma SK, Mudgal SK, Thakur K, Gaur R, Aggarwal P. Lifestyle behavior of budding health care professionals: A cross-sectional descriptive study. J Family Med Prim Care. 2020;9:3525-31.
16. Who's who: Ministry of Health and Family Welfare: GOI [Internet]. [cited 2023, Aug 1]. Available from: https://main.mohfw.gov.in/about-us/whos-who.

Development: Human Needs and Problems

👉 Learning Objectives

- Define and differentiate between growth and development.
- Understand the importance of growth and development in the context of human life.
- Identify the key characteristics and milestones associated with growth and development.
- List and explain the fundamental principles that underlie the process of growth and development.
- Identify and describe the factors that influence and impact an individual's growth and development.
- Analyze the interplay between genetic, environmental, social, and cultural factors in shaping human development.
- Describe the various stages of growth and development from infancy to old age.
- Understand the distinct physical, cognitive, and psychosocial characteristics associated with each stage.
- Explain various theoretical models and frameworks used to understand human development.
- Identify the basic needs of individuals at different stages of development, including physiological, safety, social, and self-esteem needs.
- Recognize common developmental challenges and problems that individuals may encounter at various stages.
- Explain role of nurses for health promotion of individual at different developmental stages.

INTRODUCTION

Growth and development are essential processes that occur throughout the lifespan of living organisms, including humans. They involve a series of complex changes and transformations that result in an organism's physical, intellectual, emotional, and social maturation. It is important to understand that growth and development are interconnected and influence each other. Physical growth, e.g., can impact cognitive and social development, as changes in the body can affect the individual's exploration of the environment and interactions with others. Similarly, cognitive and social experiences can shape physical and emotional development.

GROWTH: CONCEPT AND MEANING

Growth, in a general sense, refers to the process of increasing in size, quantity, or volume over time. It involves a measurable and visible change in physical attributes, such as height, weight, or dimensions, or an increase in the number or size of cells, tissues, or structures within an organism.

In biological terms, growth is a fundamental characteristic of living organisms. It is a complex and dynamic process driven by genetic, hormonal, and environmental factors. Growth can occur at different levels, from the cellular level to the level of the whole organism.

At the cellular level, growth involves cell division, where cells multiply and increase in number through mitosis. During this process, a single parent cell divides into two daughter cells, each containing the same genetic material. This proliferation of cells contributes to the overall growth of tissues and organs.

Growth can also refer to an increase in the size and complexity of an organism's body. In humans, for instance, growth is most prominent during childhood and adolescence, where significant changes occur in height, weight, bone structure, and muscle mass. These physical changes are influenced by various factors, including genetics, nutrition, hormones, and overall health.

DEFINITIONS

- James Tanner defined "Growth is an increase in size and weight due to an increase in cell number, size, or both." Tanner's definition emphasizes the quantitative aspects of growth, indicating that it involves an increase in both the number and size of cells.
- Robert J Havighurst defined "Growth refers to the qualitative and quantitative changes in an individual's behavior, thoughts, and feelings." Havighurst's definition expands the concept of growth beyond physical attributes, highlighting the qualitative changes in psychological aspects such as behavior, thoughts, and emotions.
- John W Santrock defined "Growth refers to physical changes that occur from conception to maturity." Santrock's definition focuses specifically on physical changes throughout the lifespan, encompassing the period from conception to adulthood.
- Paul Baltes defined "Growth refers to the process of increasing in size, quantity, or complexity, including physical, cognitive, and socio-emotional dimensions." Baltes'

definition provides a comprehensive perspective, considering growth across multiple dimensions, including physical, cognitive, and socio-emotional aspects.

DEVELOPMENT: CONCEPT AND MEANING

The concept of development is multifaceted and can be understood from various perspectives. In general, development refers to a process of progressive and positive change, advancement, or improvement that occurs over time. It involves a series of transformations in different aspects of an individual, society, or system, leading to growth, maturation, and enhancement of capabilities.

Human development refers to the lifelong process of growth, maturation, and progressive change in individuals. It encompasses the physical, cognitive, emotional, and social aspects of a person's life from conception to death. Human development recognizes that individuals have the potential to learn, develop skills, and acquire knowledge, which allows them to adapt and navigate the challenges and opportunities presented by their environment.

The concept of human development emerged as a multidisciplinary field of study that integrates insights from psychology, biology, sociology, anthropology, and other related disciplines. It aims to understand and optimize the potential and well-being of individuals across their lifespan.

Here are some key components of human development:

- **Physical development:** Physical development involves the changes in the body's structure, size, and functioning. It encompasses biological growth, motor skills development, and changes in physical appearance, such as height, weight, and sexual maturation.
- **Cognitive development:** Cognitive development refers to the growth and progression of mental processes and abilities. It involves the acquisition of knowledge, language development, problem-solving

skills, memory, attention, reasoning, and abstract thinking. Cognitive development is influenced by genetic factors, environmental stimuli, and social interactions.

- **Emotional development:** Emotional development focuses on the understanding, expression, and regulation of emotions. It involves the development of emotional awareness, empathy, self-esteem, emotional resilience, and the ability to manage and cope with various emotions effectively.
- **Social development:** Social development pertains to the acquisition of social skills, values, and behaviors that enable individuals to interact and engage with others in their social environment. It involves the development of social norms, roles, relationships, communication skills, and the ability to cooperate, share, and engage in social interactions.
- **Moral development:** Moral development refers to the formation of ethical values, principles, and decision-making abilities. It involves the understanding of right and wrong, empathy, moral reasoning, and the development of a sense of justice and fairness.

DEFINITIONS

- **G Stanley Hall:** "Development is a progressive series of changes that occur in an orderly, predictable pattern from conception to death, encompassing physical, cognitive, and psychosocial aspects."
- **Jean Piaget:** "Development is the construction of an increasingly complex and organized cognitive structure through the processes of assimilation and accommodation, leading to higher levels of knowledge and understanding."
- **Erik Erikson:** "Development is a lifelong process of psychosocial growth and identity formation, where individuals face and resolve a series of psychosocial crises or conflicts at different stages of life."
- **Lev Vygotsky:** "Development is the result of social interactions and cultural influences, where individuals internalize and acquire higher mental functions through the Zone of Proximal Development (ZPD) and scaffolding."
- **Sigmund Freud:** "Development involves a series of psychosexual stages where the individual's energy is focused on different erogenous zones, and successful resolution of conflicts at each stage leads to healthy personality development."

DIFFERENCES BETWEEN GROWTH AND DEVELOPMENT

The terms growth and development are often used interchangeably, but there are some important differences between the two. Growth refers to the physical changes that occur in an organism, such as an increase in size, weight, and height. Development, on the other hand, refers to the changes that occur in an organism's behavior, cognition, and emotions. **Table 11.1** summarizes the key differences between growth and development.

PRINCIPLES OF GROWTH AND DEVELOPMENT

- **Continuous process:** Growth and development occur in a continuous and ongoing manner throughout the lifespan.
- **Individual differences:** Each individual experiences growth and development at their own pace, influenced by various factors such as genetics, environment, and personal characteristics.
- **Sequential and orderly:** Growth and development generally follow a predictable sequence and occur in a specific order, with later stages building upon earlier ones.
- **Proximodistal and cephalocaudal:** Development typically proceeds from the center of the body outward (proximodistal) and from head to toe (cephalocaudal).
- **Differentiation and integration:** As individuals grow and develop, there is a process of differentiation (specialization of skills and functions) and integration

Table 11.1: Differences between growth and development.

Aspect	Growth	Development
Definition	Increase in size, quantity, or volume	Progressive and positive change over time
Nature	Quantitative	Qualitative
Focus	Physical attributes	Multiple aspects (physical, cognitive, social)
Scope	Size, weight, dimensions	Skills, knowledge, capabilities, behaviors
Measurement	Measurable (height, weight, etc.)	Not easily measurable
Process	Linear and continuous	Complex and multidimensional
Factors	Genetics, nutrition, environment	Genetics, environment, experiences, social factors
Duration	Can be temporary or permanent	Lifelong process
Example	Increase in height, weight, and muscle mass	Cognitive advancement, emotional maturation, social skills development

(coordination of various skills and functions).

- **Nature and nurture:** Both genetic and environmental factors interact to influence growth and development. Nature refers to the influence of genetics, while nurture refers to the impact of the environment and experiences.
- **Sensitive periods:** There are critical or sensitive periods during development when individuals are particularly receptive to certain experiences or learning opportunities.
- **Multidimensional:** Growth and development encompass multiple dimensions, including physical, cognitive, emotional, and social aspects.
- **Influenced by socio-cultural context:** Sociocultural factors, such as family, peers, culture, and society, play a significant role in shaping an individual's growth and development.
- **Interplay of stability and change:** Development involves a dynamic interplay between stability (maintenance of characteristics) and change (acquisition of new abilities or behaviors) throughout life.
- **Cumulative:** Development builds upon prior learning and experiences, with each stage providing a foundation for subsequent growth.

These principles provide a framework for understanding the patterns, processes, and factors that contribute to human growth and development. They highlight the complexity, individuality, and dynamic nature of the developmental journey.

FACTORS INFLUENCING GROWTH AND DEVELOPMENT

Numerous factors influence growth and development, shaping an individual's physical, cognitive, emotional, and social development. These factors can be broadly categorized into the following domains:

Genetic Factors

Inherited traits and genetic makeup play a significant role in determining an individual's growth and development. Genetic factors contribute to physical characteristics, susceptibility to certain diseases or conditions, and potential abilities or talents.

Environmental Factors

- **Prenatal environment:** The conditions and influences experienced in the womb, such as maternal nutrition, exposure to toxins, and prenatal care, can impact fetal development.
- **Physical environment:** The quality of living conditions, access to healthcare, sanitation, nutrition, and exposure to hazards can affect growth and development.

- **Socioeconomic factors:** Economic resources, social status, education, and access to opportunities can influence development outcomes.
- **Cultural and social factors:** Cultural norms, values, beliefs, parenting styles, social support networks, and cultural practices shape an individual's development.
- **Nutrition:** Adequate nutrition is essential for physical growth and cognitive development.
- **Stimulation and enrichment:** Opportunities for learning, cognitive stimulation, and exposure to enriching experiences promote cognitive, social, and emotional development.
- **Stress and adversity:** High levels of chronic stress, adverse childhood experiences, trauma, and negative environmental factors can impact development.

Parental and Caregiver Influence

- **Parenting style:** The style of parenting, including levels of warmth, responsiveness, discipline, and support, can impact various aspects of development.
- **Caregiver-child interaction:** The quality of interaction, attachment, and responsiveness between caregivers and children can influence social and emotional development.
- **Availability of supportive relationships:** Positive and nurturing relationships with caregivers, family members, and peers contribute to healthy development.

Biological Factors

Hormonal influences, brain development, and the maturation of body systems play a role in physical growth and cognitive development.

Educational Opportunities and Learning Environment

Access to quality education, appropriate learning materials, and supportive learning environments can facilitate cognitive and academic development.

Healthcare and Medical Factors

Adequate healthcare, immunizations, disease prevention, and timely medical interventions contribute to healthy growth and development.

Socioeconomic Factors

Socioeconomic status, income, and access to resources can impact the availability of opportunities and resources for optimal growth and development.

It is important to note that these factors do not act independently but often interact and influence each other. Additionally, the relative importance of each factor can vary based on cultural context, individual circumstances, and the specific stage of development.

STAGES OF GROWTH AND DEVELOPMENT

The stages of growth and development refer to the various periods or phases that individuals go through as they mature physically, intellectually, emotionally, and socially. While there are different theories and models proposed by psychologists and researchers, the following stages are commonly recognized:

Prenatal Stage

This stage begins at conception and ends with birth. It is a critical period of development when the embryo and fetus undergo rapid growth and differentiation. Prenatal development is divided into three trimesters, each marked by specific milestones and the formation of major organs and body systems.

Infancy

Infancy is commonly divided into different sub-stages:
- **Neonatal stage:** Birth to 1 month
- **Early infancy:** 1 month to 6 months
- **Late infancy:** 6 months to 1 year

This stage spans from birth to approximately 1 year of age. Infants experience remarkable physical growth and development. They learn to roll over, sit, and crawl. Cognitive development includes acquiring object permanence (understanding that objects exist even when out of sight) and early language skills. Infants also form attachments with their primary caregivers and start to develop trust and a sense of security.

Early Childhood

This stage typically ranges from 1 to 6 years of age. It can be further divided into:
- **Toddlerhood:** 1–3 years
- **Preschool years:** 3–6 years

This stage covers ages 1 to 6 years. Children continue to grow physically and refine their motor skills. They engage in imaginative play, develop more complex language abilities, and acquire basic literacy and numeracy skills. Socially, they begin to interact with peers, learn to share, and develop empathy. Early childhood is a period of rapid brain development and learning.

Middle Childhood

This stage spans from 6 to 11 years of age. Children become more independent and gain further control over their bodies and motor skills. They develop logical thinking and problem-solving abilities, expand their knowledge through formal education, and develop friendships. Middle childhood is a critical period for socialization, moral development, and the formation of self-esteem.

Adolescence

This stage occurs during the teenage years and spans from approximately 12 to 18 years of age. Adolescence can be further divided into:
- **Early adolescence:** 12–14 years
- **Middle adolescence:** 15–17 years
- **Late adolescence:** 18 years and beyond

This stage occurs during the teenage years, typically from 12 to 18 years of age. Adolescents experience significant physical changes due to puberty, including sexual maturation and growth spurts. They undergo cognitive changes, such as developing abstract thinking and introspection. Socially, they navigate peer relationships, establish their identity, and strive for independence while still relying on family support. Emotional and social challenges, along with the exploration of values and beliefs, are common during this stage.

Early Adulthood

This stage encompasses the late teens to the mid-30s. Individuals experience significant life transitions, such as pursuing higher education, starting careers, forming intimate relationships, and potentially becoming parents. Early adulthood is characterized by establishing personal and financial independence, making important life choices, and exploring various roles and responsibilities.

Middle Adulthood

This stage spans from the mid-30s to around 65 years of age. People typically focus on career development, maintaining relationships, and contributing to society. Physical changes associated with aging become more noticeable, but individuals often gain stability and wisdom. They may face the challenges of balancing work and family responsibilities, navigating midlife transitions, and reflecting on their accomplishments and goals.

Late Adulthood

This stage begins around 65 years of age and continues until the end of life. It can be further categorized into:
- **Early old age:** 65–74 years
- **Middle old age:** 75–84 years
- **Late old age:** 85 years and beyond

This stage begins around 65 years of age and continues until the end of life. Older adults may experience physical decline, retirement, and the loss of loved ones. However, many find meaning and satisfaction in their relationships, engage in leisure activities, and maintain their cognitive abilities. Late adulthood can be a time of reflection, wisdom, and continued personal growth.

It is important to remember that these stages are not rigid or fixed. Development is a dynamic and individualized process influenced by various factors, including genetics, environment, culture, and personal experiences. Nonetheless, understanding the general patterns of growth and development can provide valuable insights for individuals, parents, educators, and healthcare professionals.

■ DEVELOPMENTAL MODEL

A developmental model for growth and development refers to a framework or theory that explains the patterns, stages, and processes through which individuals grow and change over time. These models provide a structured way of understanding and studying various aspects of human development, including physical, cognitive, emotional, and social development. There are several well-known developmental models that focus on different aspects of growth and development. For example:

- Piaget's Theory of Cognitive Development
- Erikson's Psychosocial Theory
- Freud's Psychosexual Development Theory

Piaget's Theory of Cognitive Development

One prominent developmental model used to explain growth and development is Jean Piaget's theory of cognitive development. Piaget's model focuses on the intellectual or cognitive aspects of development and describes how children's thinking processes evolve as they grow. According to Piaget, children progress through four major stages of cognitive development:

- **Sensorimotor stage:** This stage occurs from birth to around 2 years of age. Infants at this stage learn about the world through their senses and motor actions. Initially, they primarily engage in reflexive behaviors, but they gradually develop object permanence (the understanding that objects continue to exist even when out of sight) and the ability to mentally represent objects and events.
- **Preoperational stage:** This stage typically spans from ages 2 to 7 years. Children in the preoperational stage develop symbolic representation, which enables them to use words, images, and symbols to represent objects and ideas. They engage in pretend play and develop language skills. However, their thinking is characterized by egocentrism (difficulty seeing things from others' perspectives) and centration (focusing on one aspect of a situation while neglecting others).
- **Concrete operational stage:** This stage generally occurs between the ages of 7 and 11. Children in this stage become more capable of logical thinking and understanding concrete operations. They can classify objects into different categories, understand conservation (the idea that certain properties of objects remain the same even when their appearance changes), and engage in basic problem-solving. However, abstract or hypothetical reasoning is still challenging for them.
- **Formal operational stage:** This stage typically emerges around age 11 and continues through adulthood. Individuals in this stage develop the ability to think abstractly, reason deductively, and engage in hypothetical and scientific thinking. They can consider multiple perspectives, solve complex problems, and engage in advanced reasoning skills.

Piaget's theory emphasizes the active role of children in constructing their understanding of the world through interactions and experiences. He proposed that development occurs through a process of assimilation (incorporating new information into existing mental frameworks) and accommodation (adapting existing frameworks to incorporate new information).

Erikson's Psychosocial Theory

Erik Erikson's psychosocial theory is a widely recognized and influential developmental model that emphasizes the psychological and social aspects of human development. Erikson proposed that individuals go through eight distinct stages of psychosocial development, each characterized by a unique developmental task or crisis that needs to be resolved. Here is an overview of Erikson's psychosocial stages:

- **Trust vs Mistrust (Infancy, 0–1 year):** The first stage occurs during infancy, where the primary task is to develop a sense of trust in the world and in caregivers. Trust is established through consistent care, meeting basic needs, and a responsive and nurturing environment. Mistrust may develop if the child's needs are not consistently met.

- **Autonomy vs Shame and Doubt (Early Childhood, 1–3 years):** In this stage, children strive for autonomy and independence. They assert their will and develop a sense of control over their bodies and actions. If they are excessively restricted or criticized, they may develop shame and doubt about their abilities.

- **Initiative vs Guilt (Preschool Age, 3–6 years):** During this stage, children explore their environment, take initiative in play, and develop a sense of purpose. They start to plan and initiate activities. If their initiatives are constantly criticized or suppressed, they may experience guilt and self-doubt.

- **Industry vs Inferiority (School Age, 6–12 years):** The focus of this stage is on acquiring new skills, developing competence, and mastering tasks. Children strive for accomplishments in academic, social, and extracurricular activities. If they experience consistent failure or criticism, they may develop feelings of inferiority.

- **Identity vs Role Confusion (Adolescence, 12–18 years):** During adolescence, individuals explore their identity, including their values, beliefs, and life goals. They seek to establish a coherent sense of self and a clear identity. If they are unable to form a strong identity, they may experience role confusion and a lack of direction.

- **Intimacy vs Isolation (Young Adulthood, 18–40 years):** In young adulthood, individuals form close and meaningful relationships, both romantically and with friends. They develop the capacity for intimacy and commit to long-term relationships. If they struggle with forming intimate relationships, they may experience feelings of isolation and loneliness.

- **Generativity vs Stagnation (Middle Adulthood, 40–65 years):** This stage is characterized by a focus on productivity and contributing to society, whether through work, family, or community involvement. Individuals strive to leave a positive impact and develop a sense of generativity. If they feel unproductive or stagnant, they may experience a sense of purposelessness.

- **Integrity vs Despair (Late Adulthood, 65+ years):** The final stage occurs in late adulthood, where individuals reflect on their lives and evaluate their accomplishments. They strive for a sense of integrity and acceptance of their life's journey. If they are filled with regrets and feel a lack of fulfillment, they may experience despair and dissatisfaction.

Erikson's theory emphasizes that successfully navigating each stage contributes to the overall development of a healthy personality and well-being. It underscores the importance of social interactions, relationships, and the resolution of psychosocial challenges in promoting healthy development and a strong sense of self.

Freud's Psychosexual Development Theory

Sigmund Freud's psychosexual development theory is a psychological model that focuses on the influence of early childhood experiences on the development of personality and behavior. Freud proposed that individuals progress through a series of psychosexual stages, each characterized by a primary erogenous zone and a developmental conflict that needs to be resolved. Here is an overview of Freud's psychosexual stages:

- **Oral Stage (Birth to 1 year):** The oral stage is focused on the mouth as the primary source of pleasure and exploration. Infants derive pleasure through activities such as sucking and biting. The main developmental conflict in this stage is the weaning process, where the child needs to transition from breastfeeding or bottle-feeding to other forms of nourishment. If the conflict is not resolved adequately, it may lead to oral fixation or dependency issues in adulthood.

- **Anal Stage (1–3 years):** The anal stage centers around the anus as the erogenous zone. During this stage, children experience pleasure and control through the process of elimination. The main conflict revolves around toilet training and the child's ability to control bowel movements. If toilet training is overly strict or too lenient, it can lead to an anal-retentive personality (rigidity, obsessiveness) or an anal-expulsive personality (disorganized, impulsive) in adulthood.

- **Phallic Stage (3–6 years):** The phallic stage is characterized by the focus on the genital area. Children develop sexual curiosity and become aware of their own gender identity and differences between sexes. The Oedipus complex (boys' desire for their mother and rivalry with their father) and the Electra complex (girls' desire for their father and rivalry with their mother) are central conflicts in this stage. Resolution of these conflicts leads to identification with the same-sex parent and the development of the superego.

- **Latency Stage (6 years to puberty):** The latency stage is considered a period of relative calm and diminished sexual interest. Children primarily focus on developing social and cognitive skills, engaging in hobbies, and forming same-sex friendships. Sexual energy is largely sublimated into other activities during this stage.

- **Genital Stage (Puberty to adulthood):** The genital stage represents the culmination of psychosexual development. It is marked by the reawakening of sexual interests and the emergence of mature adult sexuality. Individuals strive to establish intimate relationships and engage in mutually satisfying sexual experiences.

Freud believed that unresolved conflicts or fixations from earlier stages could have lasting effects on an individual's personality and behavior in adulthood. He proposed that psychoanalysis, a therapeutic method, could help individuals explore and resolve these unconscious conflicts through techniques such as free association, dream analysis, and interpretation of unconscious thoughts and desires.

ASSESSMENT OF GROWTH AND DEVELOPMENT

The assessment of growth and development involves the systematic evaluation of an individual's physical, cognitive, emotional, and social progress across different stages of life. It helps in understanding and monitoring the overall well-being and developmental trajectory of an individual. Here are some common approaches and tools used for assessing growth and development:

Developmental Milestones

Developmental milestones are key skills, behaviors, or abilities that individuals typically acquire at certain ages. They serve as general guidelines for tracking growth and development. Milestones can include physical milestones (e.g., crawling, walking), cognitive milestones (e.g., language development, problem-solving), social milestones (e.g., sharing, taking turns), and emotional milestones (e.g., self-regulation, empathy). Comparing an individual's progress against established milestones can provide insights into their development.

Observational Assessments

Observational assessments involve direct observation of an individual's behavior and interactions in various settings. Professionals, such as educators, psychologists, or healthcare providers, may observe and document a person's skills, behavior patterns, social interactions, and emotional responses. This qualitative data can help identify strengths, areas of concern, and patterns of development.

Standardized Developmental Screening Tools

Standardized developmental screening tools are questionnaires or checklists designed to assess a child's development across multiple domains. Examples include the Ages and Stages Questionnaires (ASQ) and the Denver Developmental Screening Test (DDST). These tools ask parents or caregivers to provide information about their child's skills and behaviors, which is then compared to established norms to identify any potential developmental delays or concerns.

Psychometric Assessments

Psychometric assessments are standardized tests that measure specific aspects of an individual's development, such as cognitive abilities, language skills, or emotional functioning. Examples include intelligence tests (e.g., Wechsler Intelligence Scale for Children, Stanford-Binet Intelligence Scale), language assessments (e.g., Peabody Picture Vocabulary Test), or personality inventories (e.g., Minnesota Multiphasic Personality Inventory for adolescents and adults). These assessments provide quantitative data that can help identify strengths, weaknesses, and potential areas for intervention.

Growth Charts

Growth charts are graphical representations of an individual's physical growth over time. They track measurements such as height, weight, and head circumference and compare them to population-based norms. Growth charts are commonly used in pediatric settings to monitor a child's growth and identify any potential growth abnormalities or delays.

It is important to note that assessment of growth and development should be conducted by trained professionals who consider multiple sources of information, including direct observation, reports from parents or caregivers, and relevant assessment tools. A comprehensive assessment approach ensures a more accurate understanding of an individual's growth and development and helps inform appropriate interventions and support when needed.

BASIC NEEDS OF INDIVIDUALS AT DIFFERENT DEVELOPMENTAL STAGES

The basic needs of individuals vary across different developmental stages as they progress through life. These needs reflect the fundamental requirements for their physical, cognitive, emotional, and social well-being. Here are some of the basic needs typically associated with different developmental stages:

Infancy Stage

During infancy (0–1 year), individuals have specific basic needs that are crucial for their overall well-being and healthy development. These needs can be categorized into physical, emotional, and cognitive domains. Here are the basic needs of individuals during infancy:

Physical Needs

- **Nutrition:** Infants require proper nourishment through breastfeeding or formula feeding to support their growth and development. The World Health Organization recommends initiating breastfeeding within the first half hour after delivery and exclusively breastfeeding for the initial six months after childbirth. They need frequent and regular feeding sessions to meet their nutritional requirements.
- **Sleep:** Infants need sufficient sleep for their growth and brain development. They have varying sleep patterns and require multiple naps throughout the day.
- **Hygiene and safety:** Infants need a clean and safe environment to ensure their physical well-being. This includes regular

bathing, diaper changes, maintaining appropriate room temperature, and keeping hazardous objects out of their reach.

- **Preventing diseases:** In infancy, preventive measures are taken to protect against certain infectious diseases through vaccination. The recommended immunization schedule is followed to ensure the infant receives appropriate vaccines.
- **Elimination:** Typically, breastfed infants have loose, greenish-yellow stools that may contain mucus during the fourth to sixth day after birth, while infants who are formula-fed have firmer stools.
- **Toilet training readiness:** By the age of three months, infants tend to have bowel movements after each feeding. At around seven months of age, bowel movements become more regular. By ten months, infants can be introduced to a potty chair for toilet training.
- **Play:** Play is a natural and spontaneous activity for infants. They engage in different types of play, including social affective play (responding with smiles and cooing to interacting adults), sense pleasure play (exploring and learning from sensory experiences in their environment), and skill play (imitating actions and developing new abilities).

Emotional Needs

- **Bonding and attachment:** Infants need nurturing and responsive caregivers to form secure attachments. They require loving and positive interactions with their caregivers to develop a sense of trust and emotional security.
- **Comfort and soothing:** Infants need to feel comforted and soothed when they experience distress or discomfort. This can be achieved through gentle touch, rocking, cuddling, and soothing sounds or lullabies.
- **Emotional engagement:** Infants benefit from interactions that promote emotional engagement and responsiveness. Smiling, talking, and engaging in age-appropriate play help in fostering emotional connections with caregivers.

Cognitive Needs

- **Sensory stimulation:** Infants require exposure to a variety of sensory experiences to promote cognitive development. This includes visual stimulation, exposure to different sounds, textures, and objects that encourage exploration.
- **Language development:** Infants benefit from exposure to language and communication. They need to hear spoken language, be spoken to, and engage in early communication through cooing, babbling, and gestures.
- **Object exploration:** Infants develop cognitive skills through exploring and manipulating objects in their environment. They need safe and age-appropriate toys and objects to support their cognitive growth.

Toddler Stage

During the toddler stage (1–3 years), individuals continue to have specific basic needs that are important for their overall well-being and development. Toddlers are rapidly growing and experiencing significant milestones in their physical, cognitive, and social-emotional domains. Here are the basic needs of individuals during toddlerhood:

Physical Needs

- **Nutrition:** Toddlers require a balanced and nutritious diet to support their growth and development. This includes a variety of foods from different food groups, appropriate portion sizes, and regular meals and snacks.
- **Sleep:** Sufficient sleep is crucial for toddlers' physical and cognitive development. They generally need around 11–14 hours of sleep, including both night-time sleep and naps, to support their growing bodies and active minds.
- **Safety:** Toddlers need a safe environment that minimizes potential hazards. This

includes childproofing the home, securing furniture, using safety gates, and keeping dangerous objects out of their reach.

Emotional Needs

- **Secure relationships:** Toddlers thrive on secure and nurturing relationships with their caregivers. They need consistent love, attention, and emotional support to develop a sense of trust and security.
- **Emotional expression:** Toddlers are learning to understand and express their emotions. They need opportunities to express their feelings, such as joy, frustration, and sadness, in a supportive and validating environment.
- **Positive reinforcement:** Toddlers benefit from positive reinforcement and encouragement. Praising their efforts, acknowledging their achievements, and offering affectionate gestures help build their self-esteem and confidence.

Cognitive Needs

- **Exploration and play:** Toddlers have a natural curiosity and desire to explore their environment. They need opportunities for active play, both indoors and outdoors, to stimulate their cognitive and motor skills.
- **Language development:** Language acquisition is a significant aspect of toddlerhood. They need exposure to a rich language environment, engaging in conversations, reading books, singing songs, and practicing new words and phrases.
- **Problem-solving:** Toddlers are developing problem-solving skills. They benefit from age-appropriate puzzles, toys, and activities that encourage problem-solving, critical thinking, and decision-making.

Social Needs

- **Social interaction:** Toddlers are becoming increasingly social and enjoy interactions with peers and family members. They need opportunities for social play, group activities, and positive social experiences to develop their social skills and build relationships.
- **Independence:** Toddlers are eager to assert their independence and develop autonomy. They need opportunities to make choices, engage in age-appropriate tasks, and develop self-help skills, such as feeding themselves or dressing with assistance.

Childhood Stage

During childhood, individuals have a range of basic needs that contribute to their overall well-being and development. These needs encompass various domains, including physical, emotional, cognitive, and social aspects. Here are some of the basic needs of childhood:

Physical Needs

- **Nutrition:** Children require a balanced and nutritious diet to support their growth, energy levels, and overall health. This includes adequate intake of essential nutrients, vitamins, and minerals.
- **Exercise and physical activity:** Regular physical activity is crucial for children's physical development, motor skills, and overall health. They need opportunities for active play, sports, and age-appropriate exercise.
- **Rest and sleep:** Sufficient rest and sleep are essential for children's physical growth, cognitive functioning, and emotional well-being. Establishing regular sleep routines and ensuring a comfortable sleep environment is important.

Emotional Needs

- **Love and emotional support:** Children need a nurturing and supportive environment where they feel loved, valued, and emotionally secure. They require affection, praise, encouragement, and empathy from caregivers.
- **Emotional expression:** Children need opportunities to understand and express their emotions in a healthy and constructive

manner. They benefit from learning emotional regulation, coping skills, and problem-solving strategies.

- **Positive relationships:** Building positive relationships with family members, peers, and other significant individuals fosters a sense of belonging, social support, and emotional connection.

Cognitive Needs

- **Education and learning:** Children have a natural curiosity and need access to quality education and learning opportunities. They require stimulating environments, age-appropriate educational materials, and supportive teachers or caregivers.
- **Intellectual stimulation:** Children benefit from engaging in activities that promote critical thinking, problem-solving, creativity, and exploration. They need opportunities to develop their cognitive skills and expand their knowledge base.
- **Language development:** Language acquisition is a critical aspect of childhood. Children need exposure to language-rich environments, communication with others, and literacy experiences to develop their language skills.

Social Needs

- **Peer interaction:** Children need opportunities for positive social interactions and play with peers. Interacting with others helps develop social skills, empathy, cooperation, and a sense of belonging.
- **Community involvement:** Being part of a community and engaging in activities beyond the family unit can foster a sense of social responsibility, cultural awareness, and civic participation.
- **Positive role models:** Children benefit from having positive role models who demonstrate desirable values, behaviors, and attitudes. These role models can inspire and guide children in their social development.

Adolescent Stage

During the adolescent stage, individuals have specific basic needs that are important for their overall well-being, development, and successful transition into adulthood. These needs encompass various domains, including physical, emotional, cognitive, and social aspects. Here are some of the basic needs for adolescents:

Physical Needs

- **Health and nutrition:** Adolescents require a balanced diet, regular exercise, and proper healthcare to support their physical growth, development, and overall health. They need access to nutritious meals, information about healthy lifestyle choices, and preventive healthcare services.
- **Sleep:** Adequate sleep is crucial for adolescents' physical and mental well-being. They require a sufficient amount of quality sleep to support their growth, cognitive functioning, and overall daytime performance.

Emotional Needs

- **Emotional support:** Adolescents need a supportive and caring environment where they feel understood, validated, and accepted. They require emotional support from family, friends, and trusted adults to navigate the challenges of adolescence.
- **Self-identity and autonomy:** Adolescents are developing their sense of self-identity and autonomy. They need opportunities for self-expression, exploration, and the freedom to make age-appropriate choices.
- **Coping skills:** Adolescents need to develop healthy coping strategies to manage stress, emotions, and conflicts effectively. They benefit from learning emotional regulation, problem-solving skills, and resilience-building techniques.

Cognitive Needs

- **Education and skill development:** Adolescents require access to quality education and opportunities for intellectual growth. They need a stimulating learning environment, educational resources, and guidance to develop their academic skills and pursue their interests.

- **Critical thinking and decision-making:** Adolescents need to develop critical thinking skills, the ability to evaluate information, and make responsible decisions. They benefit from learning problem-solving techniques and ethical reasoning.

Social Needs

- **Peer relationships:** Adolescents have a strong need for social interactions and forming relationships with peers. They require opportunities for socializing, participating in group activities, and developing interpersonal skills.
- **Family relationships:** Adolescents still need support and connection from their family. They benefit from positive family relationships, open communication, and a sense of belonging within their family unit.
- **Identity and belonging:** Adolescents are exploring their sense of identity and seeking a sense of belonging. They require opportunities for self-discovery, cultural exploration, and involvement in social groups or communities that align with their values and interests.

Adulthood Stage

During adulthood, individuals have a range of basic needs that contribute to their overall well-being, personal fulfillment, and successful functioning in various life domains. The specific needs may vary based on individual circumstances and cultural factors, but here are some common basic needs during adulthood:

Physical Needs

- **Health and wellness:** Adults require proper nutrition, regular exercise, and adequate rest to maintain physical well-being. They also need access to healthcare services and preventive measures to address any health concerns.
- **Safety and security:** Adults need a safe and secure living environment, protection from harm, and financial stability to meet their basic needs and maintain a sense of security.

Emotional Needs

- **Connection and relationships:** Adults have a need for meaningful relationships, companionship, and social connections. They require emotional support, love, and a sense of belonging from family, friends, and a broader community.
- **Emotional well-being:** Adults need to develop emotional resilience, coping strategies, and self-care practices to manage stress, emotions, and life challenges effectively.

Cognitive Needs

- **Lifelong Learning:** Adults benefit from continued intellectual stimulation and learning opportunities. They need access to educational resources, skill development programs, and personal growth activities.
- **Problem-solving and decision-making:** Adults require cognitive abilities to make informed decisions, solve problems, and navigate various life situations effectively.

Social Needs

- **Meaningful work and productivity:** Adults have a need for fulfilling employment or meaningful work that provides financial stability, a sense of purpose, and personal satisfaction.
- **Social engagement:** Adults benefit from participating in social activities, volunteering, and community involvement. They require opportunities for social interaction, cultural engagement, and recreational pursuits.
- **Intimacy and family:** Many adults have a need for intimate relationships and may desire starting a family or nurturing existing familial bonds.

Personal Fulfillment

- **Autonomy and self-expression:** Adults require a sense of autonomy, personal agency, and the freedom to express their values, beliefs, and identity.
- **Pursuit of meaning and life goals:** Adults have a need for a sense of purpose, meaning, and fulfillment in their lives. They may strive for personal growth, achievement, and making a positive impact in their communities or society.

COMMON PROBLEMS IN DIFFERENT DEVELOPMENTAL STAGES

Throughout various developmental stages, individuals may encounter common problems or challenges that can affect their well-being and overall development. These challenges can arise due to a variety of factors, including biological, psychological, social, and environmental influences. Here is an introduction to some of the common problems faced during different developmental stages:

At Birth

During the time of birth, babies can encounter various common problems, some of which require medical attention and intervention. Here are a few common problems that babies may experience:

- **Respiratory distress:** Some babies may have difficulty breathing or exhibit signs of respiratory distress shortly after birth. This can be caused by conditions such as transient tachypnea of the newborn, meconium aspiration syndrome, or respiratory distress syndrome.
- **Jaundice:** Jaundice is a common condition in newborns characterized by yellowing of the skin and eyes due to elevated bilirubin levels. It typically resolves on its own, but in severe cases, treatment such as phototherapy may be required.
- **Birth injuries:** During the birthing process, babies may experience birth injuries, such as bruising, swelling, or fractures. These injuries are often minor and heal over time,

but in some cases, medical attention may be necessary.

- **Infections:** Newborns are susceptible to various infections, including group B streptococcus (GBS), urinary tract infections, or respiratory infections. Prompt diagnosis and treatment are essential to prevent complications.
- **Low birth weight or prematurity:** Some babies are born with low birth weight or prematurely, which can increase the risk of health issues and require specialized care in a neonatal intensive care unit (NICU).
- **Congenital abnormalities:** Some babies may be born with congenital abnormalities, such as heart defects, cleft palate, or genetic disorders. Early diagnosis and appropriate medical management are important for the well-being of these babies.
- **Feeding difficulties:** Some newborns may experience challenges with breastfeeding or bottle feeding, including difficulties with latching, inadequate milk transfer, or swallowing issues. Support from lactation consultants or healthcare professionals can help address these concerns.
- **Neonatal withdrawal:** Babies born to mothers who used substances during pregnancy may experience neonatal withdrawal symptoms, known as neonatal abstinence syndrome. These babies may require specialized care to manage withdrawal symptoms and promote their well-being.

Infancy Stage

During the infancy stage, which spans from birth to around 2 years of age, infants may encounter various common problems. These challenges can affect their health, development, and overall well-being. Here are some common problems that infants may experience:

- **Feeding difficulties:** Infants may have difficulties with breastfeeding or bottle feeding, including issues with latching, inadequate milk transfer, or swallowing problems. These challenges can lead to poor weight gain and nutritional concerns.

- **Colic:** Colic is characterized by excessive and inconsolable crying in otherwise healthy infants. It usually begins around 2–3 weeks of age and may last for several months. The exact cause of colic is unknown, but it typically improves on its own over time.
- **Sleep problems:** Infants often experience irregular sleep patterns, frequent waking, and difficulties in establishing regular sleep routines. Sleep regression, night waking, and short sleep cycles are common during infancy.
- **Diaper rash:** Due to sensitive skin, infants are prone to develop diaper rash, which is characterized by redness, irritation, and discomfort in the diaper area. It can be caused by prolonged contact with wetness or irritation from certain products.
- **Teething discomfort:** Teething, the eruption of the baby's first teeth, can be accompanied by discomfort, irritability, drooling, and a desire to chew on objects. Some infants may experience more discomfort during this stage.
- **Common illnesses:** Infants are more susceptible to common illnesses such as colds, ear infections, respiratory infections, and gastrointestinal infections. These can cause symptoms such as coughing, sneezing, fever, congestion, and diarrhea.
- **Reflux:** Gastroesophageal reflux (GER) is common in infants and can cause regurgitation of stomach contents, leading to discomfort and irritability. Most cases of reflux resolve on their own as the baby's digestive system matures.
- **Developmental delays:** Some infants may experience developmental delays in areas such as motor skills (rolling, sitting, crawling), communication (babbling, gesturing), or social interactions. Early intervention and support are important in addressing these delays.

Toddler Stage

The toddler stage, typically ranging from ages 1 to 3, is a period of rapid growth and development. During this time, toddlers may encounter various common problems that are a part of their normal development. Here are some common issues that toddlers may experience:

- **Temper tantrums:** Toddlers often display tantrums as they navigate their increasing independence and struggle with communication skills. Tantrums can be triggered by frustration, tiredness, hunger, or a desire for autonomy.
- **Picky eating:** Many toddlers exhibit picky eating habits, showing preferences for certain foods while rejecting others. This behavior is often a result of exploring new tastes and textures and asserting independence.
- **Sleep challenges:** Toddlers may experience sleep difficulties, such as bedtime resistance, night waking, or difficulty staying asleep. Changes in routine, separation anxiety, or developmental milestones can contribute to these sleep challenges.
- **Toilet training issues:** The process of toilet training can be challenging for both toddlers and parents. Accidents, resistance, and difficulty recognizing bodily cues for elimination are common during this stage.
- **Language development delays:** Some toddlers may experience delays in language development, resulting in limited vocabulary or difficulty expressing themselves verbally. However, it's important to note that language development varies among individuals, and each child has their own pace.
- **Exploration and safety concerns:** Toddlers are curious and eager to explore their environment. However, their curiosity can lead to potential safety hazards as they may lack understanding of danger and have limited impulse control.
- **Socialization challenges:** Toddlers are learning to interact with others and develop

social skills. Sharing, taking turns, and playing cooperatively can be challenging during this stage, leading to conflicts with peers.

- **Separation anxiety:** Many toddlers experience separation anxiety when separated from their caregivers. They may exhibit distress or clinginess when being left with unfamiliar people or in new environments.
- **Bumps and falls:** Toddlers are often active and mobile, which puts them at risk for falls and minor injuries as they learn to walk, run, and climb.
- **Boundary testing:** Toddlers are known to test boundaries and assert their independence. They may engage in defiant behaviors, such as saying "no" frequently or challenging rules and limits.

Childhood Stage

The childhood stage, typically ranging from ages 3 to 12, is a period of significant growth and development. During this time, children may encounter various common problems that can impact their physical, emotional, and social well-being. Here are some common issues that children may experience during childhood:

- **Common illnesses:** Children are susceptible to common childhood illnesses such as colds, flu, ear infections, and gastrointestinal infections. These illnesses can cause symptoms such as coughing, sneezing, fever, sore throat, and stomach aches.
- **Allergies:** Many children develop allergies to certain foods, environmental factors (such as pollen or dust mites), or animal dander. Allergies can cause symptoms ranging from mild to severe, including itchy eyes, nasal congestion, skin rashes, and difficulty breathing.
- **Dental problems:** Childhood is a crucial time for dental health. Common dental issues in children include cavities, tooth decay, misaligned teeth, and gum problems. Regular dental check-ups and proper oral hygiene practices are essential.
- **Learning difficulties:** Some children may experience learning difficulties or developmental delays in areas such as reading, writing, math, or attention span. Learning disorders like dyslexia and attention-deficit/hyperactivity disorder (ADHD) are relatively common and may require specialized support.
- **Behavioral issues:** Children may exhibit behavioral challenges such as aggression, defiance, hyperactivity, or difficulty with impulse control. These behaviors can stem from various factors, including environmental influences, emotional struggles, or underlying developmental disorders.
- **Peer pressure:** As children interact more with peers, they may face peer pressure to conform to certain behaviors, attitudes, or social norms. Peer pressure can influence their choices related to friendships, academics, and risky behaviors.
- **Bullying:** Bullying can be a significant issue during childhood, with children experiencing verbal, physical, or psychological aggression from their peers. It can lead to emotional distress, low self-esteem, and academic difficulties.
- **Emotional and mental health:** Children may experience emotional and mental health challenges such as anxiety, depression, mood swings, or adjustment difficulties. These issues can be influenced by factors such as family dynamics, school stress, trauma, or genetic predispositions.
- **Body image and self-esteem:** Some children may develop concerns about body image and self-esteem, especially during the pre-adolescent stage. Media influences, societal expectations, and peer comparisons can contribute to these concerns.
- **Safety issues:** Childhood is a time of exploration, and children may be prone to accidents and injuries. Safety concerns include road safety, water safety, and

awareness of potential hazards in their environment.

Adolescent Stage

The adolescent stage, typically spanning from ages 10 to 19, is a period of significant physical, cognitive, and social development. During this time, adolescents may encounter various common problems that can impact their well-being and transition into adulthood. Here are some common issues that adolescents may experience:

- **Identity and self-esteem:** Adolescents often grapple with questions of identity, trying to understand who they are, their values, and their place in the world. This search for identity can lead to fluctuations in self-esteem and confidence.
- **Peer pressure:** Peer pressure becomes more prominent during adolescence. Adolescents may feel pressure to conform to societal expectations, engage in risky behaviors, or succumb to negative influences from their peers.
- **Body image and eating disorders:** Many adolescents become concerned about their body image and may develop negative body perceptions or engage in disordered eating patterns. This can contribute to the development of eating disorders such as anorexia nervosa or bulimia nervosa.
- **Mental health issues:** Adolescence is a period when mental health disorders may emerge or become more pronounced. Common mental health concerns include depression, anxiety, self-harm behaviors, substance abuse, and mood disorders.
- **Academic stress:** Adolescents face increased academic demands and may experience stress related to schoolwork, exams, and future career choices. The pressure to excel academically can lead to anxiety, burnout, or feelings of inadequacy.
- **Relationships and dating:** Adolescents navigate romantic and interpersonal relationships, which can bring both joy and challenges. They may encounter issues related to communication, conflict resolution, boundaries, and sexual health.
- **Risky behaviors:** Some adolescents may engage in risky behaviors such as experimenting with drugs or alcohol, engaging in unsafe sexual practices, or reckless driving. These behaviors can have serious consequences for their health and well-being.
- **Cyberbullying and online safety:** With increased use of technology and social media, adolescents are vulnerable to cyberbullying, online harassment, and exposure to inappropriate content. They may face challenges in maintaining online privacy and navigating the digital world safely.
- **Peer and family conflict:** Adolescents may experience conflicts with their peers and family members as they assert their independence and develop their own identities. Conflicts can arise from differences in values, expectations, or communication styles.
- **Future planning and transitions:** Adolescents face the task of planning for their future, including decisions about education, career paths, and transitioning into adulthood. This period can bring uncertainty and stress about the future.

Adulthood and Old Stage

During adulthood and old age, individuals may encounter various common problems that can affect their physical health, mental well-being, and overall quality of life. Here are some common issues that people may experience during these stages:

Adulthood

- **Work-life balance:** Balancing the demands of work, family, and personal life can be challenging. Striving for a healthy work-life balance is important to avoid burnout and maintain overall well-being.
- **Relationship challenges:** Maintaining healthy relationships, whether romantic

or friendships, requires effort and effective communication. Issues such as conflicts, breakups, or divorce can occur during this stage.

- **Financial pressures:** Managing finances, including debt, mortgage payments, and saving for retirement, can be stressful during adulthood. Financial pressures can impact overall well-being and quality of life.
- **Parenting responsibilities:** Raising children and managing the responsibilities of parenthood can be demanding, requiring time, energy, and emotional investment.
- **Stress and mental health:** Adulthood is often associated with increased stress levels due to various responsibilities and pressures. Common mental health concerns such as anxiety, depression, and stress-related disorders may arise during this stage.

Old Age Stage

- **Age-related health issues:** With advancing age, individuals are more prone to age-related health conditions, including chronic diseases such as arthritis, diabetes, cardiovascular diseases, and cognitive decline such as dementia or Alzheimer's disease.
- **Physical limitations:** Old age can bring physical limitations and decreased mobility, making daily activities more challenging. Conditions like reduced balance, muscle weakness, and mobility issues may affect independence.
- **Loneliness and social isolation:** Changes in social circles, retirement, and loss of loved ones can contribute to feelings of loneliness and social isolation in old age. Maintaining social connections and engaging in community activities are crucial for mental and emotional well-being.
- **Financial security:** Retirement and financial planning become significant concerns in old age. Adequate financial resources and planning are essential to meet the healthcare and living expenses associated with old age.
- **Changes in mental health:** Older adults may experience mental health issues such as depression, anxiety, or cognitive decline. Early detection and appropriate support are essential to maintain mental well-being.
- **Loss and grief:** Coping with the loss of loved ones, including friends, spouses, or siblings, becomes more common in old age. Dealing with grief and adapting to life changes can be challenging during this stage.
- **Ageism and discrimination:** Older adults may face ageism and discrimination, which can impact their self-esteem, access to healthcare, and opportunities for employment or social engagement.
- **Caregiving and long-term care:** Older adults may require caregiving support or transition to long-term care facilities due to declining health. Navigating the healthcare system and ensuring appropriate care can be complex.

ROLE OF NURSES FOR HEALTH PROMOTION OF INDIVIDUAL AT DIFFERENT DEVELOPMENTAL STAGES

Nurses play a crucial role in health promotion for individuals at different developmental stages. They are involved in providing comprehensive care, education, and support to individuals and their families, enabling them to make informed decisions and adopt healthy behaviors. Here's a breakdown of the role of nurses in health promotion across various developmental stages:

At Birth

- Conduct initial health assessments and screenings for newborns.
- Educate parents on newborn care, including breastfeeding, nutrition, and safe sleep practices.
- Provide guidance on infant immunizations and schedule.

- Support bonding and attachment between parents and newborns.
- Monitor and promote healthy growth and development milestones.
- Offer resources and support for postpartum recovery and mental health.
- Collaborate with other healthcare professionals to ensure comprehensive care for the newborn and family.

Toddler Stage

- Conduct regular health check-ups and assessments for toddlers.
- Educate parents on nutrition and healthy eating habits for toddlers.
- Provide guidance on age-appropriate physical activity and play.
- Promote safety measures to prevent accidents and injuries.
- Offer advice on proper dental care and hygiene practices.
- Support parents in managing behavioral issues and promoting positive discipline strategies.
- Provide resources and information on toilet training and sleep routines.
- Identify and address developmental delays or concerns through screenings and referrals.
- Collaborate with early childhood educators and community organizations to promote early childhood interventions and programs.

Childhood Stage

- Conduct regular health assessments and screenings for children.
- Educate children and parents on healthy eating habits, balanced nutrition, and portion control.
- Promote physical activity and provide guidance on age-appropriate exercise.
- Offer information on the importance of regular immunizations and preventive health measures.
- Provide education on oral health care and hygiene practices.

- Collaborate with schools and communities to develop and implement health promotion programs.
- Address mental health concerns and provide support and resources for children and families.
- Screen for developmental delays, learning disabilities, and vision or hearing impairments.
- Advocate for a safe and healthy school environment, including bullying prevention and injury prevention.

Adolescent Stage

- Provide comprehensive health assessments and screenings for adolescents.
- Offer education on sexual and reproductive health, including contraception, sexually transmitted infections, and healthy relationships.
- Promote mental health awareness and provide support for common adolescent issues such as stress, anxiety, and depression.
- Educate on the risks and consequences of substance abuse and provide resources for prevention and intervention.
- Address body image concerns and promote healthy body image and self-esteem.
- Offer guidance on healthy lifestyle choices, including nutrition, physical activity, and sleep.
- Advocate for comprehensive sexuality education in schools.
- Collaborate with schools and community organizations to develop and implement health promotion programs targeting adolescents.
- Facilitate access to appropriate healthcare services and resources for adolescents.

Adult Stage

- Conduct regular health assessments and screenings for adults.
- Educate on healthy lifestyle choices, including nutrition, exercise, and stress management.

- Provide guidance on disease prevention and early detection, such as cancer screenings and immunizations.
- Support individuals in managing chronic conditions, including medication adherence and self-care practices.
- Offer counseling and resources for mental health concerns, including anxiety and depression.
- Promote healthy relationships and provide education on sexual health.
- Advocate for workplace wellness programs and occupational health and safety.
- Collaborate with community organizations to address health disparities and promote access to healthcare services.
- Provide support and resources for healthy aging and age-related health concerns.
- Facilitate health promotion through patient education, counseling, and referrals to appropriate healthcare professionals.

Old Age Stage

- Conduct comprehensive health assessments and screenings for older adults.
- Provide education on healthy aging practices, including nutrition, exercise, and fall prevention.
- Offer guidance on medication management and promote adherence to prescribed treatments.
- Assess and address cognitive decline and provide support for individuals with dementia or Alzheimer's disease.
- Advocate for the mental health and emotional well-being of older adults.
- Screen for and address age-related health concerns, such as osteoporosis, cardiovascular disease, and diabetes.
- Promote social engagement and connection to prevent isolation and loneliness.
- Collaborate with other healthcare professionals to develop care plans for managing chronic conditions and optimizing quality of life.
- Provide resources and support for end-of-life care planning and palliative care.
- Advocate for the rights and dignity of older adults and ensure their access to appropriate healthcare services.

CHAPTER SUMMARY

1. Growth and development are interconnected processes that occur throughout the lifespan of living organisms, including humans.
2. Growth involves an increase in size, quantity, or volume, while development refers to progressive and positive changes in behavior, cognition, and emotions.
3. Human development is a lifelong process that encompasses growth, maturation, and the acquisition of skills and knowledge.
4. Principles of growth and development are the continuous nature of the process, individual differences, sequential and orderly progression, and the interplay between nature and nurture, among others.
5. Factors influencing growth and development are categorized into genetic, environmental, parental and caregiver influences, biological, educational, healthcare and medical, and socioeconomic factors.
6. The stages of growth and development are starting from prenatal development through infancy, early childhood, middle childhood, adolescence, early adulthood, middle adulthood, and late adulthood.
7. The developmental models are three well-known theories: Piaget's theory of cognitive development, Erikson's psychosocial theory, and Freud's psychosexual development theory.

8. The assessment of growth and development, which involves evaluating an individual's physical, cognitive, emotional, and social progress.
9. The basic needs of individuals vary across different developmental stages as they progress through life.
10. Throughout various developmental stages, individuals may encounter common problems or challenges that can affect their well-being and overall development and these can arise due to a variety of factors, including biological, psychological, social, and environmental influences.
11. Nurses play a key role and are involved in providing comprehensive care, education, and support to individuals and their families, enabling them to make informed decisions and adopt healthy behaviors.

REVIEW QUESTIONS

1. Explain the distinction between growth and development.
2. Explore the factors that influence growth and development.
3. Explain the fundamental needs of an individual at various life stages.
4. Discuss the role of a nurse for health promotion of individual at different developmental stages.
5. Describe the common problems during various life stages.

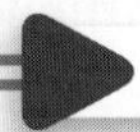 **BIBLIOGRAPHY** 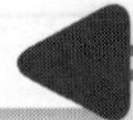

1. Bose K. Concept of human physical growth and development Bose, http://nsdl.niscair.res.in/bitstream/123456789/243/1/PDF+5.5CHAPTER+ON+HUMAN+GROWTH+FOR+CSIR.pdf
2. Bowlby J. A secure base: Parent-child attachment and healthy human development. Basic Books; 1988.
3. Crain WC. Theories of development. Prentice-Hall; 1985, pp. 118–136. Retrieved from http://faculty.plts.edu/gpence/html/kohlberg.htm
4. Department of education and early childhood development. Factors affecting growth, State of Victoria; 2012. <http://www.education.vic.vov.au/Documents/Childhood/Professionals/Support/Factorsaffgrowth.Pdf>
5. Erikson EH. Childhood and society, 2nd edition. WW Norton. New York; 1963.
6. Feldman RS. Development across the life span, 6th edition. Upper Saddle River, NJ: Prentice Hall; 2011. ISBN 0205805914.
7. Freud S. Three essays on the theory of sexuality. Standard Edition. 1905;7:125-245.
8. Gesell A, Ilg FL, Ames LB, Bullis GE. The Child from Five to Ten. Harper; 1940.
9. Ghai OP, Vinod KP, Bagga A. Essential pediatrics, 7th edition. CBS Publishers and Distributers Pvt. Ltd.; 2009. ISBN 9788123917771.
10. Havighurst RJ. Developmental tasks and education. Longman; 1972.
11. Hurlock EB. Developmental psychology—A life-span approaches 5th edition. New Delhi: McGraw-Hill; 1980.
12. Marlow DR, Redding BA. Marlow's Textbook of Pediatric Nursing. South Asian Edition, Elsevier; 2013.
13. Phatak AT, Khurana B. Baroda development screening test for infants. Indian a pediatrics. 1991;28(1):31-37. PMID 1711514.
14. Piaget J. The theory of stages in cognitive structure. New York: McGraw Hill; 1969.
15. Stuart GW, Laraia MT. Principles and practice of pediatric nursing, 7th edition. Mosby: St. Louis; 2000.

Nursing Theories

Learning Objectives

♦ Define the concept of theory in the context of nursing.
♦ Understand the significance of theories in guiding nursing practice, research, and education.
♦ Identify and discuss the key characteristics that distinguish nursing theories from other types of theories.
♦ Analyze the elements that constitute a nursing theory.
♦ Describe the hierarchical structure of nursing theories.
♦ Enumerate the reasons why nursing theories are essential in the nursing profession.
♦ Differentiate between the various levels of nursing theories based on their scope and applicability in clinical practice.
♦ Define the metaparadigms of nursing, which include person, environment, health, and nursing.
♦ Understand how these metaparadigms serve as foundational concepts in nursing theories.

INTRODUCTION

The word "theory" has multiple meanings depending on the context in which it is used. In scientific and academic contexts, the term "theory" carries a more rigorous and well-defined meaning, referring to a comprehensive and well-substantiated explanation of a phenomenon supported by a body of evidence, rigorous testing, and peer review. In this context, a theory is not merely a conjecture or guess but a well-established and widely accepted framework that has withstood scrutiny and has predictive and explanatory power.

A theory serves as a fundamental pillar in various academic disciplines, providing a framework for understanding, explaining, and predicting phenomena. It represents a structured set of principles, concepts, or ideas that are systematically organized to explain specific aspects of the world around us. The development and application of theory are crucial in fields such as nursing, science, social sciences, philosophy, and many others.

NURSING THEORY

The term "nursing theory" is derived from the field of nursing itself. Nursing theory encompasses a collection of concepts, principles, and assumptions that are specific to the discipline of nursing. It is a specialized body of knowledge developed by nurse scholars and theorists to guide nursing practice, education, research, and professional development.

The development of nursing theories has evolved over time, with influential nurse scholars such as Florence Nightingale, Hildegard Peplau, Dorothea Orem, Virginia

Henderson, and many others contributing to the body of nursing knowledge. These theorists have examined and conceptualized various aspects of nursing practice, emphasizing the unique role of nurses in promoting health, preventing illness, and providing compassionate care.

DEFINITIONS

Here are definitions of nursing theory by various authors:

- **Florence Nightingale:** "Nursing theories are an interpretation of observations, a methodical grouping of information to project an explanatory theory that will be predictive, explanatory, and enable further theoretical development."
- **Hildegard E Peplau:** "Nursing theory is a conceptualization of some aspect of nursing that describes, explains, predicts, or prescribes nursing care. It presents the phenomena of interest to nursing in a systematic way, identifies relationships among the phenomena, and describes and explains those relationships."
- **Dorothea Orem:** "Nursing theory is a set of related concepts, definitions, and propositions that explain and predict nursing care phenomena. It provides a systematic framework for nurses to plan, organize, and deliver nursing care based on clients' needs."
- **Martha E Rogers:** "Nursing theory is a view of the person, the environment, health, and nursing, that represents a particular worldview and provides a systematic perspective for understanding nursing phenomena."
- **Madeleine M Leininger:** "Nursing theory is a creative and rigorous structuring of ideas that project a tentative, purposeful, and systematic view of phenomena. It is developed and tested through systematic research, and it guides nursing practice, education, and research."
- **Virginia Henderson:** "Nursing theory is a body of knowledge that assists in defining the essentials of nursing practice and provides a framework for understanding the art and science of nursing. It focuses on promoting, restoring, and maintaining health and meeting the basic needs of individuals."

These definitions showcase the perspectives of prominent nursing theorists who have contributed to the development and advancement of nursing theory. While each definition may emphasize different aspects, they all recognize nursing theory as a systematic, conceptual framework that guides nursing practice, education, and research, aiming to explain, predict, and improve nursing care and patient outcomes.

COMPONENTS OF NURSING THEORY

The components of nursing theory work together to provide a comprehensive and systematic framework for understanding nursing practice, guiding research, and enhancing patient care. Concepts and definitions establish a shared language and understanding, while assumptions shape the theoretical perspective. Relationships illuminate the connections between concepts. Together, these components form the foundation of nursing theory and contribute to the advancement of nursing knowledge and practice. Nursing theory are made up of four main components **(Fig. 12.1)**:

1. **Concepts:** Concepts are the foundational elements of a nursing theory. They represent the key ideas, constructs, or variables that are central to understanding

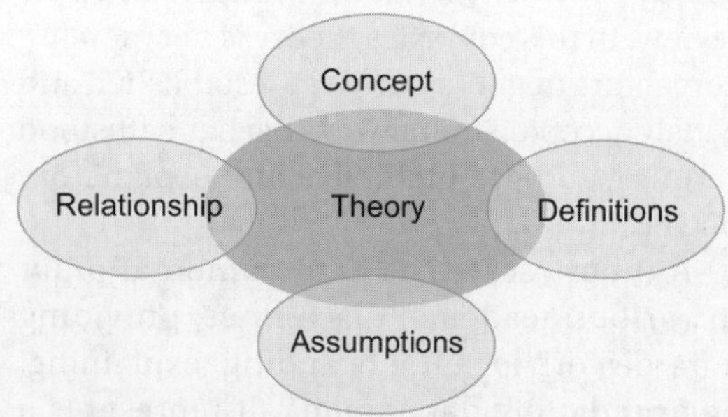

Fig. 12.1: Components of nursing theory.

and explaining nursing phenomena. Concepts in nursing theory can include health, illness, environment, nursing interventions, patient responses, and more. These concepts are defined and described within the theory, providing a shared language and framework for discussing and analyzing nursing practice. For example, in the nursing theory of Dorothea Orem, the concepts of self-care, self-care deficit, and nursing are central to the theory.

2. **Definitions:** Nursing theories provide clear and precise definitions of the concepts included in the theory. These definitions establish a common understanding of the terms used within the theory and ensure clarity in communication. Defining concepts in nursing theory helps to avoid confusion and promotes consistent interpretation and application of the theory's principles. For example, Orem defines self-care as "the activities a person performs on his own behalf in maintaining life, health, and well-being."

3. **Relationships:** Nursing theories establish relationships between the concepts included in the theory. These relationships define how the concepts interact, influence each other, or contribute to the understanding of nursing phenomena. Relationships in nursing theory can be causal (one concept causes another), correlational (concepts are related in a noncausal manner), predictive (concepts can predict outcomes or behaviors), or descriptive (concepts describe aspects of nursing practice or patient experiences). These relationships provide a structure for understanding the complex dynamics and connections within nursing practice. For example, Orem's theory states that there is a reciprocal relationship between self-care and nursing. This means that nurses help people to meet their self-care needs, and in doing so, they also help to promote health.

4. **Assumptions:** Assumptions are foundational beliefs or statements that underlie a nursing theory. They serve as starting points or accepted truths within the theory's framework. Assumptions can relate to the nature of nursing, the nurse-patient relationship, the goals of healthcare, or other aspects specific to the theory. Assumptions guide the development and interpretation of the theory and shape its overall perspective. For example, Orem's theory assumes that people have the capacity for self-care, and that nurses can help people to meet their self-care needs.

CHARACTERISTICS OF NURSING THEORY

Nursing theories possess several key characteristics that distinguish them within the field of nursing. These characteristics highlight the unique nature and purpose of nursing theory. Here are some key characteristics of nursing theory:

- **Holistic perspective:** Nursing theories embrace a holistic perspective, recognizing the interconnectedness of physical, psychological, social, and spiritual aspects of individuals and their environments. They acknowledge the whole person and consider various factors that influence health and well-being.

- **Patient-centered:** Nursing theories prioritize the patient as the central focus. They emphasize understanding and addressing patients' unique needs, experiences, and responses to health and illness. Patient-centeredness is a core principle within nursing theory, guiding the planning and delivery of individualized care.

- **Evidence-based:** Nursing theories are grounded in evidence and promote evidence-based practice. They integrate research findings, empirical evidence, and best practices to inform nursing interventions, decision-making, and care delivery. Evidence-based theories contribute to improving patient outcomes and promoting quality care.

- **Practical application:** Nursing theories emphasize practical application in real-world settings. They provide guidance and frameworks for nursing practice, offering nurses a systematic approach to assess, plan, implement, and evaluate care interventions. Nursing theories bridge the gap between theory and practice, translating knowledge into action.
- **Conceptual clarity:** Nursing theories strive for conceptual clarity, providing clear and precise definitions of concepts and relationships within the theory. They establish a shared understanding and common language among nurses, promoting effective communication and collaboration in nursing practice, education, and research.
- **Adaptability and flexibility:** Nursing theories are adaptable and flexible, recognizing the dynamic nature of healthcare and the evolving needs of patients and communities. They can be applied across various settings, populations, and contexts, allowing for modifications and customization based on specific circumstances.
- **Continual development:** Nursing theories are not static; they continue to evolve and develop. New theories emerge as nursing knowledge expands, and existing theories are refined and revised based on ongoing research and practice. Nursing theory development is an ongoing process that reflects the growth and advancement of the nursing profession.
- **Integration of multiple disciplines:** Nursing theories often integrate concepts and principles from various disciplines such as psychology, sociology, biology, and ethics. They draw from interdisciplinary knowledge to enhance understanding of human health, behavior, and the complex nature of nursing care.
- **Research and evidence generation:** Nursing theories contribute to research in the field of nursing. They guide the development of research questions, study designs, and methodologies, promoting the generation of new knowledge and evidence to advance nursing practice and theory itself.
- **Professional identity and autonomy:** Nursing theories contribute to the professional identity and autonomy of nurses. They articulate the unique role and contributions of nursing within the healthcare system, empowering nurses to advocate for patients, contribute to policy development, and shape the future of the profession.

TYPES OF NURSING THEORIES

There are various types or classifications of nursing theories, each serving a specific purpose within the field of nursing. Here are three common types of nursing theories (Table 12.1):

1. Grand Nursing Theories

Grand nursing theories are comprehensive and abstract in nature, aiming to provide a broad framework for understanding the overall nature and scope of nursing. They often address fundamental concepts such as the nurse-patient relationship, nursing roles, and

Type of theory	Level of abstraction	Scope	Purpose
Grand theory	High	Broad	Provides a framework for understanding the nursing profession and its role in society
Middle-range theory	Medium	Narrow	Can be tested empirically and used to guide research and practice
Practice-level theory	Low	Specific	Designed to guide nurses in the provision of care to specific patient populations or in specific settings

Table 12.1: Differences between the three types of nursing theories.

the promotion of health. Grand theories offer a high level of abstraction and may not provide specific guidance for practice but instead focus on broader concepts and principles. Examples of grand nursing theories include:

- Imogene King's Theory of Goal Attainment
- Sister Callista Roy's Adaptation Model
- Martha Rogers' Science of Unitary Human Beings.

2. Middle-Range Nursing Theories

Middle-range nursing theories are more focused and specific than grand theories. They aim to explain and predict phenomena within a particular area of nursing practice or clinical situation. These theories provide a narrower scope and are more directly applicable to specific nursing interventions, patient populations, or healthcare contexts.

Examples of middle-range nursing theories include:

- Madeleine Leininger's Theory of Culture Care Diversity and Universality
- Patricia Benner's Novice to Expert Theory
- Katharine Kolcaba's Comfort Theory.

3. Practice Nursing Theories

Practice nursing theories are highly specific and practical in nature. They offer guidance and frameworks for nursing interventions, decision-making, and care delivery in day-to-day practice. Practice theories are focused on the application of nursing knowledge to improve patient outcomes and promote effective nursing practice.

Examples of practice nursing theories include:

- Nola Pender's Health Promotion Model
- Hildegard Peplau's Interpersonal Relations Theory
- Jean Watson's Theory of Human Caring.

It is important to note that these classifications are not rigid or mutually exclusive. Many nursing theories can overlap or span multiple types, and theorists may have different interpretations or categorizations. Additionally, nursing theories can evolve over time, with new theories emerging and existing theories being refined or expanded upon.

■ IMPORTANCE OF NURSING THEORIES

Nursing theories are important as they provide a systematic and evidence-based approach to nursing practice, education, research, and the advancement of the nursing profession. They guide nurses in delivering high-quality, patient-centered care and contribute to the improvement of healthcare outcomes. Here is some key importance of nursing theories:

- Provides a foundation for understanding the nature and scope of nursing.
- Guides nursing practice by offering frameworks for assessment, planning, implementation, and evaluation of care.
- Enhances critical thinking and clinical reasoning skills in nurses.
- Promotes evidence-based practice by integrating research findings and best practices.
- Informs nursing education by shaping curriculum development and teaching strategies.
- Advances the profession by contributing to the development of nursing knowledge.
- Supports the development of a professional identity and autonomy for nurses.
- Facilitates effective communication and collaboration among healthcare professionals.
- Guides nursing research by providing a theoretical framework for generating new knowledge.
- Improves patient outcomes by promoting holistic, patient-centered care.

■ METAPARADIGMS OF NURSING THEORIES

The metaparadigms of nursing theories represent the overarching concepts that form the foundation of nursing knowledge and practice. They provide a framework for understanding and analyzing nursing phenomena. The four metaparadigms

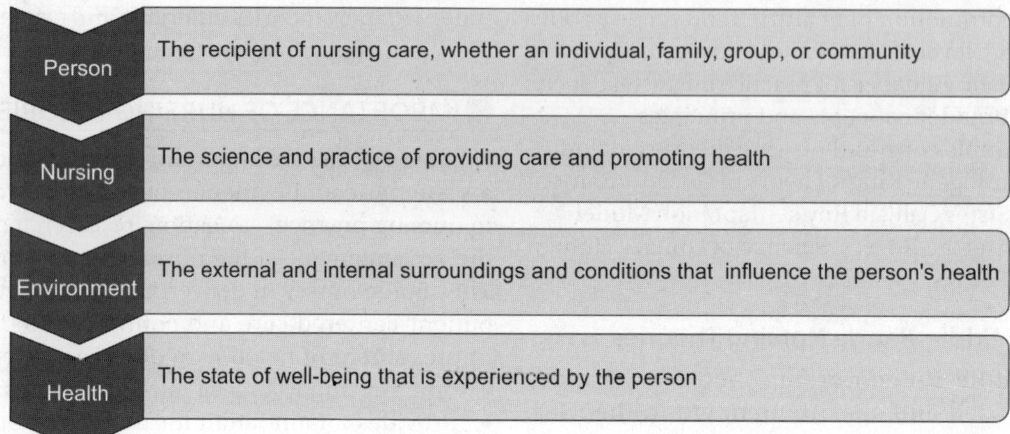

Fig. 12.2: The components of nursing metaparadigm.

commonly identified in nursing theories are (**Fig. 12.2**):

1. **Person:** The person metaparadigm refers to the individual, group, or community receiving nursing care. It encompasses the physical, psychological, social, and spiritual dimensions of the person. Nursing theories acknowledge the uniqueness of each person and recognize the importance of individualized care and holistic well-being.

2. **Environment:** The environment meta-paradigm encompasses the external and internal factors that influence the person's health and well-being. It includes the physical, social, cultural, and organizational context in which nursing care is provided. Nursing theories emphasize the impact of the environment on health outcomes and highlight the importance of creating supportive and conducive healthcare settings.

3. **Health:** The health metaparadigm pertains to the state of well-being of the person. It encompasses physical, mental, and social aspects of health. Nursing theories recognize health as a dynamic and multidimensional concept that extends beyond the absence of disease. They emphasize health promotion, disease prevention, and the attainment of optimal health outcomes.

4. **Nursing:** The nursing metaparadigm focuses on the unique role and responsi-bilities of the nurse. It encompasses the knowledge, skills, and actions that nurses employ to provide care and promote health. Nursing theories highlight the nurse-patient relationship, the art and science of nursing practice, and the importance of evidence-based interventions. They also recognize the ethical and professional standards that guide nursing practice.

These metaparadigms provide a comprehensive framework for understanding the essential components of nursing theories. They guide the development of theories and serve as a basis for assessing and evaluating nursing practice, education, and research. The metaparadigms of nursing theories emphasize the interrelatedness of the person, environment, health, and nursing, highlighting the holistic and patient-centered nature of nursing care. By incorporating these metaparadigms, nursing theories promote a comprehensive and integrated approach to addressing the health and well-being of individuals, families, and communities.

CHAPTER SUMMARY

1. Nursing theory is a specialized body of knowledge within the field of nursing, encompassing concepts, principles, and assumptions specific to nursing practice.
2. Nursing theory serves as a comprehensive and systematic framework for understanding, explaining, and predicting nursing phenomena.
3. Nursing theories are developed by nurse scholars and theorists to guide nursing practice, education, research, and professional development.
4. The components of nursing theory include concepts, definitions, relationships, and assumptions.
5. Nursing theories can be classified into three types: grand nursing theories, middle-range nursing theories, and practice nursing theories.
6. Nursing theories possess several key characteristics, including a holistic perspective, patient-centeredness, evidence-based grounding, and practical applicability.
7. The metaparadigms of nursing theories represent the fundamental concepts of person, environment, health, and nursing.

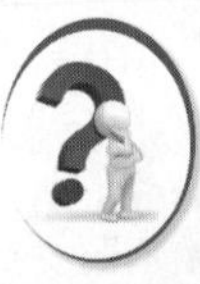

REVIEW QUESTIONS

1. Define "theory" in the context of nursing fields. Explain the significance of nursing theory in the field of nursing.
2. Discuss the four main components of nursing theory.
3. Describe the key characteristics of nursing theories that distinguish them within the field of nursing.
4. Evaluate the importance of nursing theories in guiding nursing practice and patient care.
5. Explain the metaparadigms of nursing theories. Provide examples of how each metaparadigm influences nursing care and patient-centered practice.

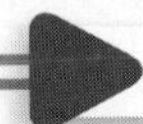 ## BIBLIOGRAPHY 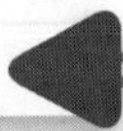

1. Alligood MR (Ed). Nursing theory: Utilization and application, 5th edition. St. Louis, Missouri: Elsevier Mosby; 2014.
2. Association of Colleges of Nursing. (2019). The essentials of master's education in nursing. Retrieved from: https://www.aacnnursing.org/Education-Resources/AACN-Essentials.
3. Chinn P, Kramer M. Integrated Theory and Knowledge Development in Nursing, 8th edition. St. Louis: Mosby; 2010.
4. Chinn PL, Kramer MK. Integrated theory and knowledge development in nursing, 9th edition. Elsevier; 2015.
5. Johnson DE. Johnson's behavioral system model and its applications: A theoretical perspective. Nurs Sci Q. 2014;27(4):312-20.
6. McEwen M, Wills EM. Theoretical basis for nursing, 5th edition. Lippincott Williams & Wilkins; 2019.

7. Meleis AI. Theoretical nursing: Development and progress, 6th edition. Wolters Kluwer; 2018.

8. Neuman B. The Neuman systems model. In: Parker ME (Ed). Nursing theories and nursing practice. FA Davis; 2010. pp. 195-208.

9. Parse RR. The human becoming theory: A guide to research in nursing. Thousand Oaks, CA: Sage Publications; 2000.

10. Peplau HE. Interpersonal relations in nursing: A conceptual framework. Nurs Sci Q. 1997;10(2):66-72.

11. Rogers ME. Nursing: Science of unitary human beings. In: Parker ME (Ed). Nursing theories in practice. National League for Nursing; 1990. pp. 93-108.

12. Roy C. The Roy adaptation model. In: Parker ME (Ed). Nursing theories and nursing practice. FA Davis; 2009. pp. 111-27.

13. Watson J. Nursing: The philosophy and science of caring. Nurs Clin North Am. 1979;14(3):375-87.

Nursing Process: Assessment and Nursing Diagnosis

Learning Objectives

- Explain the importance of the nursing process in guiding systematic and holistic patient care.
- Identify the core characteristics of the nursing process.
- Describe the primary purposes of the nursing process.
- Recognize the role of the nursing process in enhancing patient outcomes and improving the quality of nursing practice.
- Identify and describe the different steps of the nursing process.
- Define nursing assessment and its significance in gathering comprehensive patient data.
- Identify the purposes of nursing assessment.
- Differentiate between the various types of nursing assessment.
- Describe the systematic steps involved in conducting a nursing assessment.
- Define nursing diagnosis and its role in identifying patients' actual or potential health problems.
- Differentiate between medical and nursing diagnoses and describe the process of formulating nursing diagnoses.
- Identify common errors and challenges that can occur during the diagnostic process in nursing.
- Discuss strategies and guidelines to minimize errors and enhance the accuracy of nursing diagnoses.

INTRODUCTION

The history of the nursing process can be traced back to the late 1950s and early 1960s when nursing leaders and educators recognized the need for a more systematic and organized approach to patient care. Prior to the development of the nursing process, nursing care was often based on trial and error and lacked a standardized framework for delivering care. By the 1980s, the nursing process had become an integral part of nursing education and was widely incorporated into nursing curricula. It became a standard approach to patient care in various healthcare settings.

Since its inception, the nursing process has continued to evolve, incorporating new research, technology, and best practices. Today, it remains a fundamental aspect of nursing practice, guiding nurses in providing patient-centered care and promoting positive patient outcomes.

The nursing process is a systematic and organized method that nurses use to provide optimal patient care. It serves as the foundation for nursing practice and guides nurses in delivering patient-centered care, promoting health, preventing illness, and assisting patients and their families to cope with health challenges.

DEFINITIONS

- Dorothea Orem, a prominent nursing theorist, described the nursing process as a self-care framework. She believed that nurses should assist patients in performing self-care activities to maintain their health, prevent illness, and manage health challenges.
- Betty Neuman, a nursing theorist known for her work in systems theory, defined the nursing process as a series of organized steps to assess the impact of stressors on patients and devise appropriate nursing interventions to support their stability and well-being.
- Ida Jean Orlando, a prominent nurse theorist, defined the nursing process as a deliberate and systematic process of understanding patient behavior, identifying patient needs, and using the nurse-patient relationship to meet those needs. She emphasized the importance of nursing actions and interventions based on the unique needs of each patient.

CHARACTERISTICS OF NURSING PROCESS

The nursing process possesses several key characteristics that make it an effective and essential approach to patient care. These characteristics ensure that nursing care is systematic, patient-centered, evidence-based, and continuously evolving. The main characteristics of the nursing process include:

- **Systematic:** The nursing process follows a structured and organized approach, with a series of logical steps that nurses follow to provide care. Each step builds upon the previous one, creating a cohesive and comprehensive method for delivering patient care.
- **Patient-centered:** Patient-centered care is a fundamental aspect of the nursing process. It recognizes the individuality and unique needs of each patient, considering their preferences, values, and beliefs when developing care plans and making healthcare decisions.
- **Holistic:** The nursing process takes a holistic approach to patient care, considering not only the physical health but also the emotional, social, cultural, and spiritual aspects of the patient. This comprehensive view ensures that all aspects of the patient's well-being are addressed.
- **Evidence-based:** The nursing process emphasizes the use of evidence-based practice, meaning that nursing interventions and decisions are grounded in the best available research and clinical evidence. This ensures that patients receive care that is based on proven effectiveness and safety.
- **Dynamic:** The nursing process is a dynamic and ongoing process. It recognizes that patient conditions and needs can change rapidly, requiring nurses to continually reassess, reevaluate, and adapt their care plans to meet the evolving needs of the patient.
- **Collaborative:** Collaboration is essential in the nursing process. Nurses work together with patients, their families, and other members of the healthcare team to gather information, set goals, and implement interventions. This interprofessional collaboration ensures a well-rounded and coordinated approach to patient care.
- **Problem-solving:** The nursing process involves critical thinking and problem-solving skills. Nurses assess patient problems, identify nursing diagnoses, and develop interventions to address these issues effectively.
- **Outcome-oriented:** The nursing process is goal-oriented, with clearly defined outcomes for patient care. Nurses set measurable and achievable goals in the planning phase and evaluate the success of the care provided based on these outcomes.
- **Culturally sensitive:** The nursing process respects and incorporates cultural diversity. Nurses consider cultural beliefs, values, and

practices when providing care to ensure it is culturally sensitive and appropriate for the patient.

PURPOSES OF NURSING PROCESS

The nursing process serves several important purposes in providing effective patient care. Here are the key purposes of the nursing process:

- Facilitates systematic and organized care delivery.
- Promotes individualized patient-centered care.
- Identifies patient's unique health needs and concerns.
- Assists in setting clear and achievable patient goals.
- Guides evidence-based nursing interventions.
- Promotes holistic assessment of patients (physical, emotional, social, and spiritual aspects).
- Enhances critical thinking and clinical decision-making skills of nurses.
- Facilitates effective communication among healthcare team members.
- Allows for ongoing evaluation and modification of care plans.
- Supports continuity of care during transitions across healthcare settings.
- Fosters patient and family involvement in care planning and decision-making.
- Improves patient outcomes and quality of care provided.

STEPS OF NURSING PROCESS

The nursing process is a systematic five-step approach **(Fig. 13.1)** that requires critical thinking and is utilized by professional nurses to apply the most current evidence in patient care, promoting overall well-being and managing responses to health and illness. The five key steps, presented below:

1. Assessment

- Gather comprehensive and relevant patient data through interviews, observations,

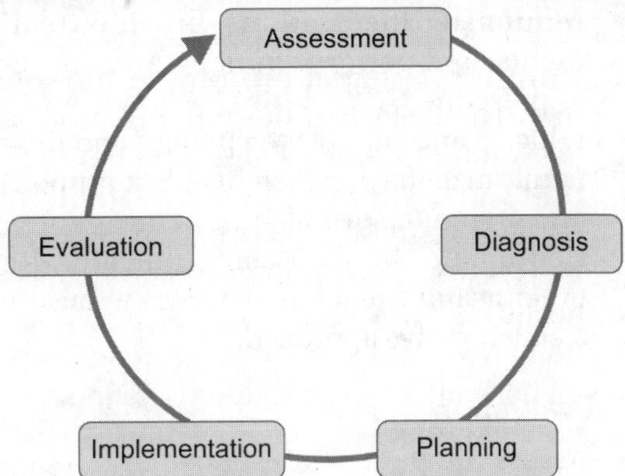

Fig. 13.1: Steps of nursing process.

physical examinations, and review of medical records.
- Identify the patient's health needs, concerns, and potential risks.
- Consider the patient's physical, emotional, social, cultural, and spiritual aspects during the assessment.

2. Diagnosis

- Analyze and interpret the collected data to formulate nursing diagnoses.
- Differentiate nursing diagnoses from medical diagnoses. Nursing diagnoses focus on the patient's response to health conditions.
- Use standardized nursing diagnosis classifications (e.g., NANDA International) to identify appropriate nursing diagnoses.

3. Planning

- Collaborate with the patient, their family, and other healthcare team members to set patient-centered goals and outcomes.
- Develop a comprehensive care plan that outlines nursing interventions to address the identified nursing diagnoses and achieve the established goals.
- Ensure that the care plan is evidence-based and reflects best practices.

4. Implementation

- Put the care plan into action by delivering the planned nursing interventions.

- Administer medications, provide treatments, and perform nursing procedures as prescribed.
- Educate and support the patient and their family in managing their health conditions and promoting overall well-being.
- Coordinate care and communicate with other healthcare team members to ensure a collaborative approach.

5. Evaluation

- Assess the patient's response to nursing interventions and the achievement of established goals and outcomes.
- Compare the actual outcomes with the expected outcomes outlined in the care plan.
- Identify the effectiveness of the care provided and the need for any modifications to the care plan.
- Continuously reassess and repeat the nursing process as necessary to meet the changing needs of the patient.

NURSING ASSESSMENT

It serves as the fundamental guide for providing patient care, emphasizing a patient-centered approach that considers the whole person. This holistic approach enhances patient assessment and education, emphasizes the importance of involving the patient's family, encourages patient compliance with interventions, and leads to improved patient outcomes.

According to the Quality and Safety Education for Nurses (QSEN) institute (2014), patient-centered care involves acknowledging the patient or their representative as the primary decision-maker and an active participant in receiving compassionate and well-coordinated care, which is tailored to respect their preferences, values, and requirements. Therefore, assessment becomes a crucial initial phase in gathering comprehensive information about the patient's health status and concerns, achieved through a collaborative and therapeutic relationship between the nurse and the patient.

DEFINITIONS

- Carpenito-Moyet define "Nursing assessment is the systematic and continuous collection of information about the patient's health status and patient and family concerns, as well as the analysis and synthesis of that information."
- Marilynn E Doenges, Mary Frances Moorhouse, and Alice C. Murr define "Nursing assessment is a critical step in the nursing process, encompassing the systematic collection, verification, organization, interpretation, and documentation of data relevant to the patient's health and situation."
- Betty J Ackley and Gail B Ladwig define "Nursing assessment is the process of collecting comprehensive data about a patient's health status through physical examination, patient interviews, and analysis of medical records, to identify the patient's needs, problems, and strengths."

PURPOSES OF NURSING ASSESSMENT

The nursing assessment serves several important purposes in providing comprehensive and individualized patient care. Here are the key purposes of nursing assessment:
- Identify the patient's current health status and overall well-being.
- Obtain comprehensive data about the patient's physical, emotional, social, and spiritual aspects.
- Identify any existing health problems, potential risks, and areas of concern.
- Establish a baseline for monitoring changes in the patient's health over time.
- Facilitate the formulation of nursing diagnoses and the development of care plans.
- Support evidence-based decision-making and the selection of appropriate nursing interventions.

- Promote effective communication and collaboration among healthcare team members.
- Enhance patient and family involvement in care planning and decision-making.
- Identify the patient's preferences, values, and needs for a patient-centered approach to care.
- Monitor the effectiveness of nursing interventions and patient responses to treatments.
- Promote patient safety by identifying potential hazards and contraindications.
- Facilitate the evaluation of patient outcomes and the overall quality of care provided.

TYPES OF ASSESSMENT

Nursing assessments are a crucial part of patient care, and there are several types of nursing assessments that nurses conduct to gather information about patients' health status and needs. Here are some common types of nursing assessments:

- **Comprehensive assessment:** This is the most extensive type of assessment, usually conducted when a patient is admitted to a healthcare facility or when their condition changes significantly. It involves a thorough evaluation of the patient's physical, psychological, social, and spiritual health, as well as their medical history and current symptoms.
- **Initial assessment:** This assessment is performed at the beginning of a patient's stay in a healthcare setting. It focuses on gathering essential information to establish a baseline for the patient's health and to identify any immediate health concerns.
- **Ongoing/continuing assessment:** This type of assessment is performed regularly during a patient's stay to monitor their progress, detect changes in their condition, and evaluate the effectiveness of the care provided.
- **Focused/problem-specific assessment:** In situations where a patient presents with a specific health issue or complaint, this type of assessment is conducted to concentrate on the relevant problem and gather information related to it.
- **Emergency/triage assessment:** This assessment is performed in emergency situations to rapidly assess a patient's condition and determine the priority of care based on the severity of their injuries or illnesses.
- **Time-lapsed assessment:** This assessment involves comparing the patient's current health status to the baseline data collected during a previous assessment to identify any changes or trends in their condition over time.

STEPS OF ASSESSMENT

Assessment involves purposeful and methodical gathering of data concerning a patient's current and historical health status, as well as their functional capabilities and coping strategies in the past and present. Nursing assessment comprises two steps:

- Acquiring information from primary sources, such as the patient, and secondary sources, including Acquiring information family, friends, healthcare providers, and medical records.
- Analyzing and validating the data to ensure a comprehensive and accurate patient database.

Acquiring Appropriate Information

The data comprises information gathered from both the client and various sources concerning their health and medical condition. This data serves as the foundation for nursing or medical diagnosis. Careful consideration is given to selecting the relevant data to be collected from the patient. This involves determining the appropriate identifying the sources from which this data will be obtained and type of data to gather.

Sources of Information

Various sources of information are utilized to conduct a thorough nursing assessment. Some common sources include:

- **Patient:** Direct communication with the patient is a primary source of information. Nurses conduct interviews to gather subjective data, understand the patient's health history, current symptoms, and personal preferences. A physical assessment involves observing and examining the patient's body for signs of physical health or abnormalities. It provides objective data on the patient's physical condition.
- **Family members or significant others:** Input from family members or close friends can offer valuable information about the patient's health history, lifestyle, and support system.
- **Medical records:** Reviewing the patient's medical records provides valuable data, including past medical history, laboratory test results, imaging reports, and previous treatment plans.
- **Healthcare team members:** Collaborating with other members of the healthcare team, such as physicians, therapists, and social workers, allows nurses to gain insights into the patient's overall care plan and progress.
- **Community resources:** Nurses may explore community resources that may impact the patient's health, such as support groups, home health services, or social assistance programs.
- **Patient's own records:** Patients may keep their health records or medication lists, which can be helpful for obtaining accurate information.
- **Patient diaries or journals:** In certain cases, patients may maintain diaries or journals that provide insight into their health experiences and emotional well-being.
- **Scientific literature:** Nurses refer to evidence-based research and medical literature to stay updated on best practices, treatment guidelines, and nursing interventions.

Using a combination of these sources, nurses can conduct a comprehensive and accurate nursing assessment, enabling them to develop individualized care plans and provide patient-centered care.

Types of Data

Subjective data and objective data are two types of information collected during the nursing assessment process to gain a comprehensive understanding of a patient's health status. Let's define each type and provide some examples:

Subjective Data

Subjective data refers to information that is based on the patient's perceptions, feelings, and experiences. It is typically communicated by the patient and is not directly measurable or observable by others. Subjective data is obtained through patient interviews and discussions. Nurses need to be attentive and empathetic when gathering subjective data to understand the patient's perspective accurately. Here are some examples of subjective data:

- **Patient's pain level:** "I have a throbbing pain in my right knee."
- **Feelings of nausea:** "I feel nauseous and queasy after eating breakfast."
- **Emotional state:** "I am feeling anxious and worried about my upcoming surgery."
- **Sleep patterns:** "I have been having trouble sleeping, and I feel restless at night."
- **Quality of life:** "I feel weak and unable to perform my daily activities."

Objective Data

Objective data refers to measurable and observable information about a patient's health status that can be obtained through physical examinations, laboratory tests, and direct observations. Unlike subjective data, objective data can be verified by others and does not rely on the patient's perception. Nurses use various assessment techniques to gather objective data, including physical assessments and diagnostic tests. Here are some examples of objective data:

- **Vital signs:** Blood pressure of 120/80 mm Hg, heart rate of 78 beats per minute and respiratory rate of 18 cycles per minute. Oral temperature reading of 98.6°F.

- **Laboratory results:** Hemoglobin level of 12 g/dL and blood glucose level of 110 mg/dL.
- **Physical examination findings:** Swollen and tender left ankle with limited range of motion.
- **Wound assessment:** A 2 × 3 cm superficial abrasion on the right forearm with mild bleeding.
- **Observation:** Patient grimacing while walking and holding their abdomen.

In nursing practice, both subjective and objective data are vital for making accurate assessments, diagnosing health conditions, planning interventions, and evaluating patient outcomes. The combination of these two types of data allows nurses to provide individualized and evidence-based care for each patient.

Methods of Information Collection

Nursing assessment involves collecting comprehensive data about a patient's health status, needs, and concerns. Various methods and techniques are used in nursing assessment to obtain a holistic understanding of the patient's condition. Some common methods of nursing assessment include:

Patient Interviews

Direct communication with the patient is a fundamental method of gathering subjective data. Nurses conduct interviews to obtain information about the patient's health history, current symptoms, lifestyle, and personal preferences.

Nursing Health History

During the first or early interaction with a patient, you collect a nursing health history, which is a crucial element of a comprehensive assessment. The health history forms, whether manual or electronic, are typically organized in a structured manner. However, as you conduct a patient-centered interview, you discern which aspects of the history necessitate thorough exploration and which

can be addressed with less detail. The extent of the history depends on factors such as time availability and the patient's priorities. A comprehensive history encompasses all dimensions of health enabling you to create a comprehensive care plan. The components of a nursing health history may vary depending on the setting, patient population, and specific healthcare needs. However, some common components typically included in a nursing health history are as follows:

- **Biographical information:** This includes the patient's name, age, gender, contact information, occupation, and marital status.
- **Chief complaint/reason for seeking healthcare:** The primary reason why the patient is seeking medical attention or healthcare services.
- **Present health concerns/current symptoms:** A detailed description of the patient's current symptoms, including their onset, duration, severity, and any aggravating or alleviating factors.
- **Past medical history:** This covers the patient's past illnesses, surgeries, hospitalizations, and significant medical events.
- **Family history:** Information about the health conditions and medical history of the patient's immediate family members.
- **Social history:** This includes the patient's living situation, support system, employment status, educational background, and lifestyle habits (e.g., smoking, alcohol consumption).
- **Medications:** A list of all prescription and over-the-counter medications the patient is currently taking, including dosages and frequency.
- **Allergies:** Any known allergies to medications, foods, or environmental factors.
- **Immunization history:** Information about the patient's vaccination history and immunization status.
- **Psychosocial history:** This includes an evaluation of the patient's mental health,

emotional well-being, coping strategies, and support system.

- **Cultural and spiritual history:** An exploration of the patient's cultural beliefs, values, and spiritual practices that may influence their healthcare decisions and preferences.
- **Developmental history (for pediatric patients):** Information about the child's growth, development, milestones, and any developmental concerns.

Physical Examination

Physical assessments involve observing and examining the patient's body to gather objective data. This includes assessing vital signs, general appearance, skin condition, cardiovascular system, respiratory system, and other body systems. Various techniques are used during a physical examination, depending on the body system being assessed. Here are some common techniques of physical examination:

- **Inspection:** Inspection involves a visual examination of the patient's body to observe any visible abnormalities, signs, or symptoms. During this technique, the healthcare professional carefully observes the patient's skin, posture, gait, movements, and overall appearance. The process may involve using a penlight or otoscope to examine body cavities like the mouth, ears, and nose. Inspection is the first step of physical examination and provides valuable initial information related to health status of the patient.
  Example: Inspecting the patient's skin for rashes, lesions, bruises, or discolorations.
- **Palpation:** Palpation is the use of touch to assess various parts of the body for texture, temperature, tenderness, masses, or pulsations. It involves gentle pressure applied with the fingers or hands. Palpation can be light, deep, or bimanual (using both hands). This technique helps healthcare professionals identify abnormalities in tissues and organs that may not be apparent during visual inspection.

Example: Palpating the patient's abdomen to feel for organ enlargement or tenderness.

- **Percussion:** Percussion is the technique of tapping the body's surface with the fingertips to create sound waves. The resulting sounds help evaluate the density and location of underlying organs or structures. The two main types of sounds produced during percussion are resonance (heard over normal lung tissue) and dullness (heard over solid organs or fluid-filled areas).

Example: Percussing the chest to assess lung resonance and identify areas of abnormal dullness.

- **Auscultation:** Auscultation involves listening to internal body sounds using a stethoscope. By placing the stethoscope on the patient's skin, the healthcare professional can hear sounds produced by the heart, lungs, bowel, and blood vessels. This technique helps detect abnormal heart sounds, lung sounds, bowel sounds, and vascular bruits.

Example: Auscultating the heart to identify abnormal heart murmurs or irregular rhythms.

Validating and Analyzing the Data

Assessment entails the ongoing interpretation of information, which is a vital aspect of critical thinking within the assessment process. Skillful and continuous interpretation and validation of assessment data guarantee the acquisition of a comprehensive database. Ultimately, this progression leads to the second step of the nursing process, where clinical decisions are made concerning the patient's care. These decisions manifest as nursing diagnoses or collaborative problems that demand coordinated treatment involving multiple healthcare disciplines.

- **Data validation:** The process of validating data is essential to ensure its accuracy and authenticity. This involves verifying the collected data to eliminate errors and biases. To achieve this, both subjective and objective cues are identified and analyzed.

Proper and validated instruments are used for physical examinations, and statements made by patients or their significant others are clarified. Additionally, cross-referencing with medical records, sharing and consulting with team members, and comparing findings with existing literature and research reports are undertaken to ensure consistency with normal findings.

- **Analyzing/interpretation of data:** When engaging in critical interpretation of assessment information, you aim to identify any abnormal findings, recognize the need for further observations to clarify data, and initiate the process of identifying the patient's health problems. This process is known as clinical reasoning. As you progress, you start noticing patterns within the data, which guide you to collect additional information and clarify existing data. These patterns create meaningful and coherent clusters of information, known as data clusters. These clusters help in clearly identifying the patient's health problems.

Documentation of Data

Recording assessment findings and problem interpretations is essential, as failing to do so means this information is lost and unavailable to other caregivers. Lack of specificity in the documentation may result in vague impressions for the reader. This information serves as a baseline for identifying patient health issues, planning and implementing care, and evaluating the patient's response to interventions. Conclusions drawn from this data will eventually become nursing diagnoses; hence, they must be factual and accurate. Here are some key points to consider regarding the documentation of data in nursing assessment:

- Document the outcomes of the nursing health history and physical examination in a clear and concise manner, using appropriate language.
- Utilizing standardized forms, particularly electronic ones, facilitates entering assessment data as the patient responds to inquiries.
- It is crucial to maintain a timely and succinct record that can be accessed by other healthcare professionals, as it ensures continuity of care.
- To ensure factual documentation, develop the habit of reporting all observations succinctly.
- Focus on presenting facts and be descriptive whenever possible.
- Precisely report anything sensed.
- When recording objective information, use precise terminology, such as indicating the patient's weight (e.g., 77.2 kg or 170 lbs) and describing physical exam findings (e.g., "abdomen is soft and nontender to palpation").
- When documenting subjective information, use quotation marks.
- Avoid making generalizations or forming judgments in written communication while entering data.
- Only pertinent data directly related to the patient's health status, diagnosis, and care should be documented. Avoid irrelevant or extraneous information.
- Ensure that the documentation is legible and easy to read to avoid misinterpretation.

NURSING DIAGNOSIS

Introduction

In the nursing assessment process (as explained above), you gather information from various sources about the patient. As you collect and analyze this data, you start to recognize certain cues that create patterns of information. These patterns can indicate the patient's current health status and their inclination towards wellness and health promotion. Alternatively, these patterns may reveal existing health issues the patient is facing. Accurately identifying these patterns leads to diagnostic conclusions.

A diagnosis is a clinical judgment based on the information gathered during the assessment. These diagnostic conclusions encompass problems that are primarily addressed by nurses (referred to as nursing diagnoses) and also those requiring collaborative efforts from multiple healthcare disciplines (known as collaborative problems).

The nursing diagnosis, as the second step of the nursing process, categorizes health issues falling under the purview of nursing care, specifically those problems that nurses can address and handle.

DEFINITION

- **North American Nursing Diagnosis Association (NANDA):** NANDA defines nursing diagnosis as "a clinical judgment about individual, family, or community responses to actual or potential health problems/life processes. Nursing diagnoses provide the basis for selection of nursing interventions to achieve outcomes for which the nurse has accountability" (NANDA-I, 2015).
- **Lynda Juall Carpenito:** According to Carpenito, nursing diagnosis is "a clinical judgment concerning a human response to health conditions/life processes, or vulnerability for that response, by an individual, family, group, or community" (Carpenito, 2016).
- **Marjory Gordon:** Gordon defines nursing diagnosis as "a judgment based on a process of analysis of data in which the nurse identifies actual or potential health problems (actual or potential alterations in health) and determines nursing interventions to deal with the identified health problems" (Gordon, 1994).
- **Betty J Ackley and Gail B Ladwig:** Ackley and Ladwig describe nursing diagnosis as "a clinical judgment concerning a human response to health conditions/ life processes, or vulnerability for that response, by an individual, family, group, or community. A nursing diagnosis provides the basis for selection of nursing interventions to achieve outcomes for which the nurse has accountability" (Ackley & Ladwig, 2020).

MEDICAL AND NURSING DIAGNOSIS

A medical diagnosis is established by evaluating physical signs, symptoms, a patient's medical history, and diagnostic test results to identify a specific disease or condition. Once determined, a medical diagnosis remains unchanged as long as the condition persists. Physicians have the authority to manage and treat the diseases and conditions specified in medical diagnoses, and they are qualified to perform surgical procedures.

A nursing diagnosis is a professional judgment made by a nurse, which involves assessing a human response to health conditions or life processes, or identifying vulnerability to such responses in individuals, families, or communities. Nurses are authorized and competent to address these nursing diagnoses in their practice. Nursing diagnoses can be cantered on identifying existing health issues, promoting health, or identifying potential risks.

Nursing diagnoses are dynamic and change as per the evolving requirements of the patient, ensuring that care remains responsive to the patient's ever-changing health status.

There are basic differences between medical and nursing diagnosis **(Table 13.1)**.

TYPES OF NURSING DIAGNOSIS

In nursing practice, nursing diagnoses are categorized into various types based on their focus and purpose. Here are five types of nursing diagnoses:

1. **Actual nursing diagnosis:** An actual nursing diagnosis refers to a current and existing health problem or condition that is present and identified through assessment data. Nurses use this diagnosis to guide their interventions and provide targeted care to address the identified problem.

   Example: Acute pain related to surgical incision as evidenced by patient's verbal

Table 13.1: Differences between nursing and medical diagnosis.

Aspect	Nursing diagnosis	Medical diagnosis
Scope	Nursing practice	Medical practice
Focus	Patient's response to health problems, life processes, or vulnerabilities	Specific disease or medical condition affecting the patient
Purpose	Guide nursing care and interventions	Form the basis for medical treatment and management
Provider	Usually determined by nurses	Determined by physicians or healthcare providers
Nature of information	Subjective and objective data	Objective data based on signs, symptoms, and diagnostic tests
Examples	Impaired mobility, ineffective coping, risk for falls	Pneumonia, type 2 diabetes, hypertension

reports of pain (e.g., pain score of 8 on a scale of 0–10).

2. **Risk nursing diagnosis:** A risk nursing diagnosis indicates a potential health problem or vulnerability to a certain condition that the patient is at risk of developing. Nurses use this diagnosis to implement preventive measures and reduce the likelihood of the potential problem occurring.

   Example: Risk for impaired skin integrity related to immobility and incontinence as evidenced by bedridden status and history of pressure ulcers.

3. **Health promotion nursing diagnosis:** A health promotion nursing diagnosis focuses on the patient's motivation and readiness to improve their overall health and well-being. Nurses use this diagnosis to provide education and support to promote and enhance the patient's health.

   Example: Readiness for Enhanced Nutrition related to expressed willingness to adopt a balanced diet and engage in regular physical activity.

4. **Wellness nursing diagnosis:** A wellness nursing diagnosis identifies a patient's optimal health status and strengths. Nurses use this diagnosis to support and maintain the patient's current state of well-being.

   Example: Readiness for enhanced sleep pattern related to the patient's consistent sleep schedule and healthy sleep hygiene practices.

5. **Syndrome nursing diagnosis:** A syndrome nursing diagnosis refers to a cluster of related nursing diagnoses that frequently occur together. It helps nurses recognize patterns of health problems and tailor interventions accordingly.

   Example: Fatigue syndrome related to disturbed sleep pattern, increased physical activity, and emotional stress.

■ DIAGNOSTIC PROCESS

The process of diagnosis necessitates the application of critical thinking skills. By utilizing your knowledge, experience, critical thinking mindset, and intellectual standards, you can effectively gather and analyze assessment data to determine nursing diagnoses. Consistently applying critical thinking in this manner will enhance your proficiency in making nursing diagnoses, leading to better competence in patient care.

The process of diagnostic reasoning entails utilizing the assessment data collected from a patient to logically justify a clinical judgment, specifically a nursing diagnosis in this context. This diagnostic process originates from the assessment process and involves a series of decision-making steps (depicted in **Fig. 13.2**).

Data Clustering

The process of analyzing and interpreting assessment data starts with organizing all the patient's information into coherent and

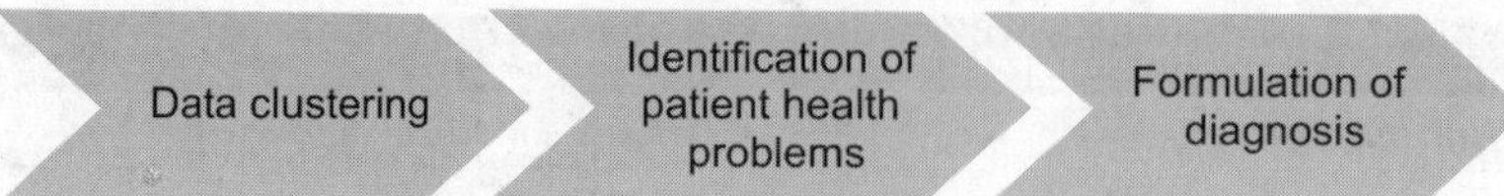

Fig. 13.2: Nursing diagnostic process.

usable data clusters. A data cluster is an assembly of cues, which are the indications or manifestations gathered during the assessment. These cues may consist of objective (quantifiable or observable) or subjective (reported by the patient) elements, and they can also encompass risk factors. By analyzing these cues in conjunction with one another, healthcare professionals can begin to draw diagnostic conclusions about the patient's health condition.

In nursing, data analysis and interpretation entail recognizing patterns among the grouped data, comparing them with established benchmarks, and reaching a well-grounded determination regarding the patient's reaction to a health issue. The North American Nursing Diagnosis Association International (NANDA-I) classification of nursing diagnoses serves as the benchmark for the anticipated patterns of data corresponding to each particular nursing diagnosis. These criteria are exemplified by defining characteristics or risk factors, as mentioned earlier. Defining characteristics refer to the observable cues collected during the assessment that cluster together as manifestations of a problem-focused or health promotion nursing diagnosis. These defining characteristics help nurses in formulating accurate nursing diagnoses and developing appropriate care plans tailored to each patient's unique needs.

Data Interpretation

During the analysis of defining characteristics or risk factors clusters, the patient's responses to health conditions are taken into account. This interpretation helps in choosing from multiple potential diagnoses that could be applicable to the patient. There are often several possible diagnoses or explanations

to consider. By comparing the defining characteristics or risk factors in the patient's data with the various diagnoses in NANDA-I, a more accurate selection can be made. To ensure precision, it is important to thoroughly review all characteristics or risk factors, discard irrelevant ones, and confirm the relevant ones that align with the patient's condition.

When examining patterns of defining characteristics, it is essential to juxtapose the patient's data with established standards for normal and healthy patterns. Utilize accepted norms, such as values from laboratory tests and diagnostic assessments, professional recommendations, and known physiological or anatomical limits, as a reference for comparison and evaluation. Throughout this process, assess whether the grouped signs and symptoms are typical for the patient, taking into account their present health status and medical history, and whether they fall within the range of expected healthy responses. Identify any defining characteristics that deviate from healthy norms to pinpoint particular health problems or areas of concern.

Formulating a Nursing Diagnostic Statement

Once you have organized and interpreted the clustered assessment data, your goal is to choose the appropriate nursing diagnostic statement. To craft an accurate nursing diagnostic statement, you must identify the correct diagnostic label along with its associated defining characteristics or risk factors, and if applicable, a related factor.

A nursing diagnosis consists of three main components: the problem (diagnostic label), the etiology (related factors or causes), and the defining characteristics (signs and symptoms). These components help nurses communicate the patient's healthcare needs and guide the development of appropriate nursing interventions. Here is a description of each component:

- **Problem (diagnostic label):** The problem, also known as the diagnostic label, describes the health issue or alteration in the patient's health status that the nurse has identified. It is written in clear and concise terms and represents the essence of the nursing diagnosis. The problem is usually stated in terms of the patient's response to their health condition rather than the medical condition itself. For example, instead of stating "pneumonia," a nursing diagnosis might be "ineffective airway clearance related to excessive mucus production and airway inflammation."

- **Etiology (related factors or causes):** The etiology identifies the underlying factors or causes that contribute to the patient's problem or health alteration. It explains why the patient is experiencing the specific nursing diagnosis. The etiology helps to determine the appropriate nursing interventions to address the problem effectively. It is essential to choose factors that are within the nurse's scope of practice and that can be influenced by nursing care. In the example above, the etiology includes "excessive mucus production and airway inflammation."

- **Defining characteristics (signs and symptoms):** The defining characteristics are the clinical cues or evidence that support the presence of the nursing diagnosis. These are the observable and measurable signs and symptoms that the nurse has assessed during the patient's assessment. The defining characteristics provide evidence for the existence of the problem and help differentiate it from other possible nursing diagnoses. Continuing with the previous example, defining characteristics may include "cough with yellow sputum," "wheezing," and "crackles heard on lung auscultation."

The acronym PES, which stands for problem, etiology, and symptoms, is a useful tool for constructing a three-part nursing diagnosis. For example:

1. Nursing diagnosis (**Problem**): Ineffective airway clearance
2. Related factors (**Etiology**): Excessive mucus production and airway inflammation
3. Defining characteristics (**Signs and symptoms**): Cough with yellow sputum, Wheezing, Crackles heard on lung auscultation

Nurses use nursing diagnoses to develop individualized care plans and interventions tailored to the patient's specific healthcare needs, aiming to improve patient outcomes and overall well-being.

ERRORS OF NURSING DIAGNOSIS PROCESS

The nursing diagnosis process is a critical step in the nursing care planning, but like any complex task, it can be susceptible to errors. Some common errors that can occur during the nursing diagnosis process include errors during data collection, clustering, interpretation, and formulating diagnostic statement. Some common errors that can occur during the nursing diagnosis process include:

- **Errors during data collection:** One of the fundamental steps in nursing diagnosis is data collection. Errors can arise if the nurse fails to gather comprehensive and accurate information about the patient's health status, leading to incorrect or incomplete diagnoses.

- **Errors during data clustering:** Mistakes happen when data clustering is done prematurely, inaccurately, or neglected altogether. Premature clustering refers to the act of assigning a nursing diagnosis before all relevant data is grouped together.

- **Errors during interpretation of data:** Even when data is collected properly, there is a risk of misinterpreting the information. This can result from assumptions, biases, or a lack of understanding of specific clinical indicators.

- **Errors during formulating nursing diagnosis:** Nurses may make errors in identifying the appropriate nursing diagnosis for a patient. This could be due to a lack of knowledge or experience, leading to a misalignment between the diagnosis and the patient's actual health condition.

GUIDELINES TO REDUCE ERRORS IN THE DIAGNOSTIC PROCESS

To reduce errors in the nursing diagnostic statement and enhance the accuracy of the nursing diagnosis process, nurses can follow these guidelines:

- Gather comprehensive and accurate patient data from multiple sources.
- Base diagnoses on evidence, research, and best practices.
- Focus on recognizing the patient's reaction, not the medical condition they have been diagnosed with.
- Formulate a NANDA-I diagnostic statement rather than simply stating the symptom observed.
- Look for a treatable underlying cause or risk factor instead of focusing on a clinical sign or a chronic issue that doesn't have a nursing intervention.
- Identify a problem resulting from the treatment or diagnostic study, rather than concentrating on the treatment or study itself.
- Focus on identifying the patient's issues rather than any challenges you might face with nursing care.
- Identify the patient's problem instead of solely focusing on nursing interventions.
- Identify the patient's problem rather than the desired goal of care.
- Make impartial and professional judgments instead of being influenced by prejudice.
- Refrain from making legally problematic statements. Avoid implicating blame, negligence, or malpractice, as they could lead to potential lawsuits.
- Clearly specify the problem and its underlying cause to avoid circular statements that lack direction for nursing care.
- Include only one patient problem in the diagnostic statement for clarity and precision.
- Refrain from making a diagnosis before all relevant data is considered.
- Remain objective and avoid personal assumptions when interpreting data.
- Involve the patient to understand their concerns and preferences.

DOCUMENTATION

Documentation of nursing diagnosis is a crucial aspect of the nursing process, as it helps communicate the identified patient problems, their underlying causes, and the planned nursing interventions to other healthcare professionals. Proper documentation ensures continuity of care, facilitates effective communication among the healthcare team, and provides a record of the patient's progress over time. When documenting nursing diagnoses, the following points should be considered:

- **Clear and concise language:** Use clear and concise language to describe the nursing diagnoses and related factors or risk factors.
- **Standardized terminology:** Use standardized nursing diagnostic language, such as NANDA-I taxonomies, to maintain consistency and clarity in documentation.
- **Link to assessment data:** Include relevant assessment data to support the nursing diagnoses and demonstrate evidence-based reasoning.
- **Avoid medical diagnoses:** Document nursing diagnoses based on the patient's response to their health condition rather than using medical diagnoses.
- **Patient-centered approach:** Focus on the patient's needs and problems, and involve the patient in the documentation process when possible.
- **Avoid jargon and abbreviations:** Use plain language and avoid jargon or abbreviations

that might be unclear to other healthcare professionals.

- **Date and time:** Always include the date and time of documentation to track the progression of the patient's condition and interventions.
- **Relevance to care plan:** Ensure that the documented nursing diagnoses align with the overall care plan and nursing interventions.
- **Collaborative documentation:** If appropriate, collaborate with other healthcare team members to document relevant information and ensure a comprehensive record.

- **Updates and revisions:** Regularly update the nursing diagnoses as the patient's condition changes and revise the care plan accordingly.
- **Privacy and confidentiality:** Adhere to patient privacy and confidentiality guidelines while documenting nursing diagnoses.
- **Legibility:** Write legibly to prevent misinterpretation of the documented information.
- **Consistency:** Maintain consistent and standardized documentation practices throughout the healthcare facility or organization.

CHAPTER SUMMARY

1. Today, nursing process is a fundamental aspect of nursing practice, guiding nurses in providing patient-centered care and promoting positive patient outcomes.
2. The nursing process is characterized by several key features, making it an effective and essential approach to patient care.
3. The nursing process considers the patient's physical, emotional, social, cultural, and spiritual aspects, taking a holistic approach to care.
4. The nursing process serves several essential purposes including facilitating systematic and organized care delivery, promoting individualized patient-centered care, identifying patient needs, setting achievable goals, guiding evidence-based nursing interventions, and fostering effective communication among healthcare team members.
5. The nursing process consists of five main steps: assessment, diagnosis, planning, implementation, and evaluation.
6. Nursing assessment involves gathering comprehensive and relevant patient data through interviews, observations, physical examinations, and medical record reviews.
7. The assessment process aims to identify the patient's health needs, concerns, and potential risks, taking a patient-centered and holistic approach.
8. Subjective data is based on the patient's perceptions and feelings and is gathered through patient interviews.
9. Objective data is measurable and observable and is obtained through physical examinations, laboratory tests, and direct observations.
10. To ensure accurate and valid data, the nursing assessment involves data validation and analysis.
11. Documentation of the nursing assessment findings is a crucial aspect of the process, ensuring continuity of care and providing a baseline for developing care plans and evaluating patient responses to interventions.
12. Nursing diagnosis, which is the second step in the nursing process.
13. Nursing diagnosis involves analyzing data collected during the nursing assessment to recognize patterns of information that indicate the patient's health status and health promotion needs or reveal existing health issues.
14. There are five types of nursing diagnoses: Actual nursing diagnosis, Risk nursing diagnosis, Health promotion nursing diagnosis, Wellness nursing diagnosis, and syndrome nursing diagnosis.

15. The diagnostic process involves critical thinking skills and decision-making steps.
16. To reduce errors in the diagnostic process, nurses can follow guidelines such as gathering comprehensive and accurate data, focusing on patient responses, utilizing standardized language, involving the patient in decision-making, and avoiding bias.
17. Proper documentation of nursing diagnoses is crucial for communication, continuity of care, and tracking patient progress over time.

REVIEW QUESTIONS

1. Define nursing process and discuss the characteristics of the nursing process.
2. Explain the steps of the nursing process and purposes of the nursing process.
3. Define nursing assessment and describe the steps of nursing assessment.
4. Define nursing diagnosis and differentiate between nursing and medical diagnosis.
5. Discuss the sources of diagnostic errors and how to avoid these errors when formulating nursing diagnosis.

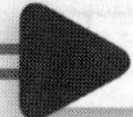 **BIBLIOGRAPHY** 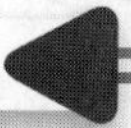

1. Ackley BJ, Ladwig GB. Nursing Diagnosis Handbook: An Evidence-Based Guide to Planning Care, 12th edition. St. Louis, MO: Elsevier; 2021.
2. Ball JW, Dains JE, Flynn JA, Solomon BS, Stewart, RW. Seidel's Guide to Physical Examination, 9th edition. St. Louis, MO: Elsevier; 2018.
3. Bates B, Bickley LS. Bates' Guide to Physical Examination and History Taking, 12th edition. Philadelphia, PA: Wolters Kluwer; 2017.
4. Carpenito-Moyet LJ. Nursing diagnoses: Application to clinical practice, 14th edition. Philadelphia, Lippincott, Williams & Wilkins; 2013.
5. Carpenito-Moyet LJ. Nursing diagnosis: Application to clinical practice, 14th edition. Philadelphia, Lippincott, Williams & Wilkins; 2013.
6. Carpenito-Moyet LJ. Nursing Diagnosis: Application to Clinical Practice, 15th edition. Philadelphia, PA: Wolters Kluwer; 2017.
7. Doenges ME, Moorhouse MF, Murr AC. Nurse's Pocket Guide: Diagnoses, Prioritized Interventions, and Rationales, 15th edition. Philadelphia: FA Davis Company; 2019.
8. Elwyn G, Dehlendorf C, Epstein RM, Marrin K, White J, Frosch DL. Shared decision making and motivational interviewing: achieving patient-centered care across the spectrum of health care problems. Ann Fam Med. 2014;12(3):270-5.
9. Gordon M. Nursing diagnosis: Process and application, 3rd edition. St Louis, Mosby; 1994.
10. Lunney M. Use of critical thinking in the diagnostic process. Int J Nurs Terminol Classif. 2010;21(2):82.
11. Müller-Staub M, Needham I, Odenbreit M, Lavin MA, van Achterberg T. Implementing nursing diagnostics effectively: cluster randomized trial. J Adv Nurs. 2008;63(3):291-301.
12. NANDA International (NANDA-I): Nursing diagnoses: Definitions and classification, 2012–2014. Oxford, Wiley-Blackwell; 2012.
13. Neuman B. The Neuman Systems Model, 3rd edition. Upper Saddle River, NJ: Prentice Hall; 1995.
14. Orem DE. Nursing: Concepts of Practice, 7th edition. St. Louis, MO: Mosby; 2001.
15. Orlando IJ. The Dynamic Nurse-Patient Relationship. New York: GP Putnam's Sons; 1961.
16. Seaback WW. Nursing process: Concepts and application. Clifton Park, NY: Delmar, Cengage Learning; 2013.
17. Wilkinson JM. Nursing process and critical thinking. Upper Saddle River, NJ: Pearson; 2012.

Nursing Process: Planning, Implementation and Evaluation

◾ PLANNING

Introduction

In the nursing process, the third step is planning, which involves several key actions. First, the nurse identifies the patient's nursing diagnoses. Next, the nurse prioritizes these diagnoses and decide patient-centered goals along with expected outcomes. Based on the identified diagnoses, appropriate nursing interventions are chosen for each one. Collaboration with the patient, family (if applicable), and the healthcare team is essential to determine the urgency of the identified problems and to prioritize the patient's needs.

Critical thinking, deliberate decision-making, and problem-solving skills are crucial during the planning phase. The most important principle in planning is to create a personalized care plan that addresses the unique needs of the client. To achieve this, close communication with the patient, their family, and the healthcare team is essential, and ongoing consultation with team members may be necessary.

Definitions

Planning, as a step of the nursing process, involves various definitions and perspectives from different authors. Below are some definitions provided by authors and nursing experts:

- Ackley and Ladwig (2014) define "Planning is the third step in the nursing process where the nurse prioritizes nursing diagnoses and collaborative problems, sets patient-centered goals and expected outcomes, and selects appropriate nursing interventions for each diagnosis."

- According to Suhonen and colleagues (2011), "planning in the nursing process requires critical thinking applied through deliberate decision making and problem solving. The nurse individualizes a plan of care for the patient's unique needs by closely communicating with patients, their families, and the healthcare team. The nursing diagnoses identified direct the selection of individualized nursing interventions and the goals and outcomes the nurse aims to achieve."
- Doenges, et al. (2016) define, "Planning in the nursing process involves the formulation of a comprehensive plan of care that addresses the patient's nursing diagnoses and healthcare needs."
- Carpenito-Moyet (2017) proposed, "Planning is a critical step in the nursing process where the nurse establishes a roadmap for care delivery. This involves setting achievable goals and outcomes based on the nursing diagnoses and formulating evidence-based nursing interventions."
- **Dorothy E Johnson (1968):** "Planning is the process of setting goals and developing a plan of care."

PURPOSES

Planning in the nursing process serves several important purposes that contribute to effective patient care and positive outcomes. Some of the key purposes of planning in the nursing process include:

- **Goal setting:** Planning allows nurses to set clear and achievable patient-centered goals. These goals are based on the identified nursing diagnoses and collaborative problems and are designed to address the specific needs and concerns of the patient.
- **Individualized care:** Through planning, nurses develop a personalized care plan tailored to unique needs of the client, preferences, and circumstances. This individualized approach ensures that the patient receives the most appropriate and effective care possible.

- **Optimizing resource allocation:** Planning helps nurses allocate their time, resources, and efforts efficiently. By identifying and prioritizing nursing interventions, nurses can focus on the most critical aspects of care and utilize available resources effectively.
- **Continuity of care:** A well-thought-out plan of care ensures continuity in patient care. It provides a roadmap for all healthcare team members to follow, facilitating seamless communication and coordination in delivering care across different shifts and disciplines.
- **Promoting safety:** Planning involves considering potential risks and implementing measures to ensure patient safety. By proactively addressing safety concerns, nurses can prevent adverse events and enhance patient well-being.
- **Facilitating collaboration:** Planning requires collaboration with patients, their families, and the healthcare team. This teamwork fosters a patient-centered approach, enhances communication, and promotes a shared understanding of the goals and interventions.
- **Enhancing critical thinking:** Developing a comprehensive plan of care necessitates critical thinking skills. Nurses must analyze data, make informed decisions, and adapt the plan as needed, promoting professional growth and expertise.
- **Measuring progress:** The plan of care serves as a benchmark for monitoring the patient's condition and allows nurses to make adjustments as needed and track the patient's response to treatment.
- **Empowering patients:** Involving patients in the planning process empowers them to take an active role in their care. When patients understand their goals and interventions, they are more likely to comply with treatment plans and engage in self-care.
- **Ethical decision making:** Planning requires ethical considerations, ensuring that the care provided respects patients'

autonomy, dignity, and cultural beliefs. Ethical decision-making is fundamental to maintaining the trust and well-being of patients.

Overall, planning in the nursing process plays a pivotal role in providing high-quality care, fostering collaboration, and promoting positive patient outcomes. It combines evidence-based practice, critical thinking, and patient-centered approaches to optimize healthcare delivery and improve the overall patient experience.

PLANNING PROCESS

The planning part of the nursing process encompasses several steps that guide nurses in developing a comprehensive and individualized plan of care for their patients. The steps of planning in the nursing process typically include.

Setting Priorities

In nursing practice, a patient typically has several nursing diagnoses and issues. When attending to multiple patients, it becomes essential for the nurse to adeptly determine the order of importance for their needs in order to deliver safe, efficient, and effective care. This process of prioritization entails organizing nursing diagnoses and patient problems based on their urgency and importance, establishing a preferred sequence for implementing nursing interventions. Prioritization helps the nurse focus on the most critical issues that need immediate attention.

Nursing diagnoses can be classified into different priority levels based on the urgency and importance of the patient's needs. The three common priority classifications for nursing diagnoses are:

1. **High priority:** These are nursing diagnoses that require immediate attention and intervention because they pose a significant threat to the patient's health. Failure to address high-priority issues promptly could lead to severe consequences. Examples of high-priority nursing diagnoses include:

patient experiencing severe respiratory distress, patient with unstable blood pressure (e.g., dangerously high or low).

2. **Intermediate priority:** Nursing diagnoses with intermediate priority are important but not immediately life-threatening. They still require timely intervention to prevent deterioration or further complications. Examples of intermediate-priority nursing diagnoses include: patient with impaired mobility, patient with a compromised immune system or an open wound needs preventive measures to reduce the risk of infection.

3. **Low priority:** These nursing diagnoses are less urgent and do not pose an immediate threat to the patient's health. They may be addressed after high and intermediate priority needs are met. Examples of low-priority nursing diagnoses include: patient with disturbed sleep pattern, patient lacking in health knowledge.

It is important to note that priority classification can change as the patient's condition evolves, and nursing interventions are implemented. Regular reassessment and communication with the healthcare team help ensure appropriate adjustments to the priority levels of nursing diagnoses. The priority classifications assist nurses in organizing their care delivery and directing their efforts to achieve the best possible outcomes for the patient.

Establishing Measurable Goals and Expected Outcomes

After you have identified the nursing diagnoses of your patients, it is essential to consider what you aim to accomplish and how you will recognize the desired outcomes.

In the planning stage, you establish specific goals and expected outcomes for every nursing diagnosis. These goals serve as a clear guide for determining the appropriate interventions to provide optimal care for the patient. Additionally, they facilitate the evaluation of intervention effectiveness.

A goal is a broad statement that outlines the intended transformation in the patient's condition, perception, or behavior. On the other hand, an expected outcome refers to a measurable change in the patient's behavior, physical condition, or perception, which needs to be accomplished to successfully reach the goal. It serves as a specific and observable indicator of progress towards reaching the broader goal. Examples of expected outcomes:

"Within 24 hours, the patient will move from the bed to a chair with minimal assistance."

"By the end of the day, the patient will take 10 steps with the assistance of a physical therapist."

Nurses set clear and measurable goals and expected outcomes in collaboration with the patient and their family. These goals and expected outcomes are specific, achievable, relevant, and time-bound.

Writing goals and expected outcomes: Writing well-formulated goals and expected outcomes is of utmost importance as they play a critical role in directing your nursing care. By setting patient-centered goals that are relevant to nursing diagnoses, the expected outcomes define the precise desired responses in different facets of the patient's health, including physiological, psychological, social, developmental, or spiritual dimensions. This comprehensive approach ensures a holistic and individualized approach to patient care. Usually, it is standard practice to develop multiple expected outcomes for each nursing diagnosis and goal to comprehensively address the patient's health issues.

Use SMART criteria to ensure that your goals and expected outcomes are well-defined and achievable (**Fig. 14.1**).

- **Specific:** Clearly state what you want to achieve.
- **Measurable:** Include quantifiable criteria to evaluate progress.

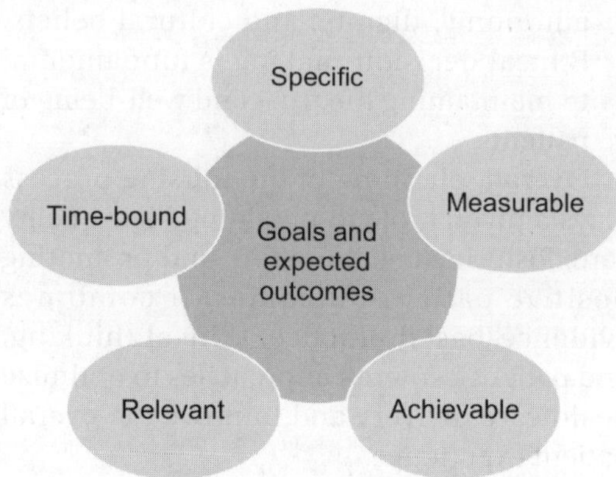

Fig. 14.1: SMART criteria for well-defined goals and expected outcomes.

- **Achievable:** Set realistic and attainable outcomes.
- **Relevant:** Ensure the outcomes are relevant to the patient's needs and the nursing diagnosis.
- **Time-bound:** Set a specific timeframe for achieving the outcomes.

Types of Goals

The timeframe for setting goals depends on factors such as the nature of the problem, its cause, the patient's overall health condition, and the treatment environment.

- **Short-term goal:** This type of goal indicates a particular behavior or response that you expect the patient to achieve within a brief period, usually less than seven days. In acute care settings, goals may be set for just a few hours to address immediate needs.
- **Long-term goal:** On the other hand, a long-term goal denotes an objective behavior or response that you anticipate the patient to accomplish over an extended period, often spanning several days, weeks, or even months. These goals address more comprehensive and lasting changes in the patient's health and well-being.

Selecting Evidence-based Interventions

In the planning phase, you analyze and decide on nursing interventions necessary to achieve the goals and expected outcomes of your patient. After identifying nursing diagnoses, goals and outcomes are established.

During this stage, you carefully choose interventions aimed at helping the patient progress from their current health status to the level specified in the established goal, as indicated by the expected outcomes. To select appropriate nursing interventions, you utilize the most pertinent and reliable evidence related to the patient's health issues and exercise sound clinical decision.

Types of Nursing Interventions

Nursing interventions are the actions and activities that nurses perform to provide care and support to patients in various healthcare settings. These interventions are based on evidence-based practice, nursing knowledge, and clinical judgment to promote positive patient outcomes. There are different types of nursing interventions, and they can be classified into three categories:

1. **Independent nursing interventions:** Independent nursing interventions are actions that nurses can initiate and perform autonomously without requiring a physician's order or supervision. These interventions are based on nursing knowledge, expertise, and evidence-based practice. Nurses are trained and authorized to implement independent interventions to meet the unique needs of their patients e.g., providing patient education and health promotion, monitoring and assessing vital signs, assisting with activities of daily living (ADLs).

2. **Dependent nursing interventions:** Dependent nursing interventions are actions that nurses perform based on the physician's orders or under the direction and supervision of other healthcare professionals. These interventions require a healthcare provider's authorization and typically relate to medical treatments, diagnostic procedures, or changes in the patient's care plan. Examples of dependent nursing interventions include: administering intravenous (IV) medications or fluids, dressing changes, assisting with medical procedures like biopsies, lumbar punctures, or intubation as directed by a healthcare provider.

3. **Interdependent or collaborative nursing interventions:** Interdependent nursing interventions are collaborative actions that nurses perform in conjunction with other healthcare professionals. These interventions involve working together as a team to address the patient's needs comprehensively. Collaboration is essential in interdependent interventions, and effective communication among team members is crucial for seamless patient care. Examples of interdependent nursing interventions include: interdisciplinary rounds, coordinating care transitions, collaborating with specialists.

By employing these three types of nursing interventions—independent, dependent, and interdependent—nurses can provide comprehensive and patient-centered care that addresses the diverse needs of their patients.

Selection of Intervention

The selection of nursing interventions is a critical aspect of the nursing process, as it directly impacts patient outcomes and the quality of care provided. When choosing nursing interventions, nurses consider several important criteria to ensure that the interventions are appropriate, effective, and individualized for each patient's unique needs. Some of the key criteria for selecting nursing interventions include:

- **Relevance to nursing diagnoses:** Nursing interventions should directly address the identified nursing diagnoses and collaborative problems. Each intervention should be specifically tailored to meet the patient's health issues and goals.

- **Evidence-based practice:** Nurses rely on evidence-based practice, which involves integrating the best available evidence from research studies, clinical guidelines, and expert consensus into their decision-making. Evidence-based interventions have been shown to be effective and safe in similar patient populations.

- **Appropriateness to the patient's condition:** Interventions suited to the current health status, medical history, and overall condition of the patient. They must consider factors such as age, cultural background, comorbidities, and any other relevant patient-specific factors.
- **Feasibility and resources:** Nurses assess whether the chosen interventions are feasible to implement in the specific healthcare setting and with the available resources. This includes considering the availability of equipment, personnel, and time required for each intervention.
- **Patient preferences and informed consent:** Nurses help patients in the process of decision-making, seeking their input and considering their preferences and values. Obtaining informed consent before implementing interventions is essential, particularly for procedures or treatments with potential risks.
- **Ethical considerations:** Nurses make ethical decisions regarding interventions, ensuring that the interventions respect the patient's autonomy, dignity, and rights. They also consider any cultural or religious beliefs that may impact the choice of interventions.
- **Compatibility with interdisciplinary care:** In settings with a multidisciplinary healthcare team, nurses select interventions that are compatible with the overall care plan and that align with the contributions of other team members.
- **Realistic and achievable:** Interventions should be realistic and achievable within the context of the current condition of your patient and resources available. Unrealistic interventions can lead to frustration and hinder progress.

Nurses choose appropriate nursing interventions for each nursing diagnosis to achieve the established goals and outcomes.

These interventions are based on the best available evidence, clinical guidelines, and the nurse's expertise.

Plan Nursing Care

Once the appropriate nursing interventions have been chosen, they must be organized and documented in a specific format known as a nursing care plan. This plan is created for each nursing diagnosis, outlining the actions and steps required to address the patient's needs effectively.

A nursing care plan comprises nursing diagnoses, goals or expected outcomes, specific nursing interventions, and an evaluation section. This structure enables nurses to quickly identify a patient's clinical needs and current condition. When there are changes in the patient's status, the plan is updated accordingly. While preprinted standardized care plans and electronic health record (EHR) care plans follow a consistent format, each plan can be tailored to address the patient's unique needs. The nursing care plan functions as a centralized document, detailing the patient's diagnoses and problems, the corresponding plan of care for each issue, and the outcomes for monitoring and assessing the patient's progress.

System for Nursing Care Plan

In nursing practice, various systems and approaches are used for planning nursing care. These systems provide structured frameworks to ensure comprehensive and patient-centered care delivery. Some common systems for planning nursing care include:

- **Standardized care plans:** Standardized care plans are preprinted or computer-generated care plans that follow established protocols for specific medical conditions or common nursing diagnoses. These plans offer a standardized approach to care and can save time while ensuring evidence-based practices.
- **Electronic health records (EHR):** Electronic health records are digital systems

that integrate patient health information, including nursing care plans, into a single platform. EHRs streamline communication among healthcare team members, promote real-time updates, and facilitate access to patient data.

- **Nursing Kardex:** A nursing Kardex is a concise and organized summary of essential patient information that is commonly used in healthcare settings, especially in nursing units. It is a quick reference tool that provides an at-a-glance view of a patient's current condition, care plan, and important care-related information. The Kardex is usually kept at the nursing station or carried by nurses during their rounds to facilitate efficient patient care.

- **Critical pathways/clinical pathways:** Critical pathways, also known as clinical pathways, are interdisciplinary care plans that outline the sequence and timing of interventions across different healthcare disciplines. They aim to promote multidisciplinary collaboration, standardize care practices, and reduce variations in care.

- **Collaborative care models:** Collaborative care models involve healthcare professionals from various disciplines working together to develop a comprehensive care plan. This approach ensures holistic care that addresses the patient's physical, emotional, and social needs.

Documentation and Communication

Documentation and communication are crucial aspects of the planning phase in the nursing process. Proper documentation ensures that all relevant information related to the patient's care is recorded accurately and comprehensively, while effective communication facilitates the exchange of vital patient data among healthcare team members.

Part of the planning process involves transferring crucial information from one nurse to another during care transitions, such as the end of a shift, patient transfers to different units, or discharges to other healthcare settings. Handoff reporting provides a valuable opportunity to inquire, clarify, and confirm crucial information regarding the patient's progress and ongoing care needs. It is a standard practice used by nurses to communicate the patient's care plan to the incoming healthcare personnel. During a handoff report, it is essential to provide accurate, current, and relevant information to the next nurse taking over the patient's care. The handoff phase is crucial for ensuring continuity of care and preventing errors or delays in delivering nursing interventions for the patient.

Consulting with Other Healthcare Professionals

Consulting with other healthcare professionals during the planning phase of the nursing process is a vital aspect of providing comprehensive and effective patient care. Collaboration among different healthcare team members ensures that a holistic approach is taken to address the patient's complex needs.

Consulting with other healthcare professionals during this phase of the nursing process fosters teamwork, facilitates a comprehensive care approach, and enhances patient outcomes. It emphasizes the importance of a collaborative and integrated approach to patient care, with each professional contributing their expertise to create a well-rounded and patient-centered care plan.

IMPLEMENTATION

Introduction

Once the nursing process reaches the fourth step, known as Implementation, it formally commences following the development of a comprehensive care plan. This care plan should be founded on well-defined and relevant nursing diagnoses, allowing for the initiation of appropriate interventions geared towards aiding the patient in attaining their health-related goals and expected outcomes. A nursing intervention refers to any treatment administered by a nurse, based on their clinical judgment and knowledge, with the primary objective of improving patient outcomes.

Implementation, as the fourth step of the nursing process, refers to the formal initiation of a care plan following the development of clear and relevant nursing diagnoses. In this stage, the nurse implements interventions intended to support the patient in achieving the predetermined goals and expected outcomes essential for improving or maintaining their health status. These nursing interventions are guided by clinical judgment and knowledge, and they may involve both direct and indirect care measures targeted at individuals, families, and/or the community.

Direct care interventions involve administering treatments and providing care through direct interactions with patients. For instance, administering medications, inserting a urinary catheter, giving discharge instructions, or offering counseling during times of grief are examples of direct care interventions. These interventions are carried out directly on the patient to address their specific needs.

On the other hand, indirect care interventions are measures conducted away from the patient, but they are done for the benefit of the patient or a group of patients. This includes tasks such as managing a patient's environment to ensure safety and infection control, documentation of patient information, and collaborating with other healthcare professionals as part of an interdisciplinary team. Although these interventions do not involve direct patient interaction, they play a crucial role in supporting and optimizing patient care.

DEFINITIONS

- Potter et al. (2021) proposes, "Implementation is the phase in the nursing process where the nurse puts the care plan into action. It involves performing nursing interventions that are tailored to the individual patient's needs and based on evidence-based practices."
- **Dorothy E Johnson (1968):** "Implementation is the process of carrying out the nursing care plan."
- **Margaret A Newman (1979):** "Implementation is the process of carrying out the nursing interventions that have been planned."
- **Patricia Benner (1984):** "Implementation is the process of putting the nursing care plan into action and evaluating its effectiveness."

FACTORS INFLUENCING THE IMPLEMENTATION

The step of implementation in the nursing process can be influenced by various factors. Some of the key factors that can impact the implementation phase are:

- **Patient's condition and response:** The patient's health status and their response to previous interventions can significantly influence the implementation of the care plan. You must continuously assess the condition of your patient and adapt the interventions accordingly.
- **Healthcare setting:** The type of healthcare setting, such as a hospital, community, or long-term care facility, can impact the resources available, the team structure, and the workflow, all of which can influence the implementation of nursing interventions.
- **Available resources:** The availability of resources, including staffing, equipment, medications, and technology, can affect the nurse's ability to implement the care plan effectively.
- **Interdisciplinary collaboration:** Effective collaboration with other healthcare professionals, such as physicians, therapists, and social workers, is crucial during implementation. A coordinated approach ensures that all aspects of the patient's care are addressed.
- **Time constraints:** Nurses often face time constraints due to heavy workloads and busy schedules. Time limitations can impact the thoroughness and timely implementation of interventions.

- **Nurse's knowledge and skills:** The nurse's level of knowledge, experience, and proficiency in performing specific interventions can influence the quality of implementation.
- **Patient's preferences and values:** Patient-centered care involves considering the patient's preferences, cultural belief, and values when implementing interventions.
- **Family and support system:** The involvement and support of the patient's family and caregivers can affect the success of implementation, especially in home care or community settings.
- **Healthcare policies and guidelines:** Institutional policies, clinical guidelines, and evidence-based practices can guide and sometimes restrict the implementation of certain interventions.
- **Ethical and legal considerations:** Ethical dilemmas and legal considerations may arise during implementation, particularly when making decisions about the care and treatment.

▮ IMPLEMENTATION PROCESS

The implementation process involves a series of steps to put the care plan into action and deliver nursing interventions effectively. While the specific steps may vary depending on the context and healthcare setting, the general steps of the implementation process in nursing include.

Reassessment and Reviewing Existing Plan

Before implementation can begin, the nurse conducts a comprehensive reassessment of the patient's health status, needs, and preferences. Reassessment serves to confirm the nursing diagnoses, evaluate the care plan's relevance, and ascertain the ongoing suitability of nursing interventions for the patient's condition. Should there be any changes in the patient's status, rendering the current nursing diagnosis and interventions inadequate, adjustments to the care plan become necessary. By conducting thorough reviews and making necessary modifications, nurses can ensure the timely implementation of appropriate nursing interventions, ultimately catering to the patient's evolving requirements.

Organizing and Preparation

The nurse organizes the necessary resources, such as medications, equipment, and supplies, required to carry out the planned interventions. Adequate preparation ensures a smooth implementation process. Here are some aspects which need preparation during implementation:

- **Time management:** Time management is a critical aspect of the implementation process in nursing. Effective time management in implementation enables nurses to provide timely and high-quality care, leading to better patient outcomes and overall satisfaction with the healthcare experience.
- **Personnel:** By effectively managing personnel during the implementation process, healthcare organizations can optimize patient care delivery, enhance patient outcomes, and create a positive and supportive work environment for their staff.
- **Environment:** Environment preparation in implementation involves setting up the physical and organizational conditions to facilitate the smooth and effective execution of nursing interventions and the overall care plan. Properly preparing the environment can enhance patient safety, streamline workflows, and improve the overall quality of care. Controlling noise, temperature, and lighting in healthcare settings is crucial for creating an environment that maximizes patient comfort and promotes healing.
- **Patient:** Patient preparation in implementation involves engaging and preparing the patient for the nursing interventions and care plan that will be implemented. It is essential to inform and involve the patient in their care to ensure their cooperation and active participation,

leading to better outcomes and patient satisfaction. Patient preparation in implementation fosters a patient-centered approach to care, promoting active involvement and cooperation. By providing education, addressing concerns, and ensuring patient comfort, nurses can help patients feel more empowered and engaged in their healthcare journey, ultimately contributing to improved health outcomes.

Anticipating and Preventing Complications

As a nurse, it is crucial to remain vigilant about the potential risks associated with a patient's illness and the treatments they receive. Should the patient's condition evolve, be prepared to adjust the chosen interventions accordingly. Evaluate the advantages of the treatment in relation to the potential risks and implement preventive measures to mitigate any identified hazards.

Communication and Collaboration

Effective communication is crucial during implementation. The nurse collaborates with other healthcare team members to ensure coordinated care. This step involves discussing the care plan with physicians, therapists, and other relevant professionals to gain their insights and support.

Initiation of Interventions

With the care plan in hand, the nurse initiates the planned interventions. This may include providing direct care to the patient, assisting with activities of daily living, administering medications, performing treatments, and providing education.

Monitoring and Evaluation

Throughout the implementation process, the nurse continuously monitors the patient's response to the interventions. Ongoing evaluation helps to determine the effectiveness of the interventions and whether adjustments to the care plan are needed.

Documentation

Accurate and timely documentation of the interventions performed, the patient's response, and any changes to the care plan are essential for maintaining continuity of care, legal purposes, and communication with other healthcare providers.

Closure and Follow-up

After the implementation phase, the nurse ensures proper handoff communication if the patient is transferred to another healthcare setting. Follow-up care and instructions are provided as needed to support the patient's ongoing health and recovery.

SKILLS REQUIRED FOR EFFECTIVE IMPLEMENTATION

During the implementation phase in nursing, various skills are essential to ensure the successful execution of nursing interventions and the provision of high-quality patient care. These skills can be broadly categorized into cognitive, psychomotor, and affective (emotional) skills:

Cognitive Skills

- **Critical thinking:** The ability to analyze information, make informed decisions, and solve problems based on evidence, clinical judgment, and patient assessments.
- **Clinical reasoning:** Applying knowledge and experience to assess patient needs, identify priorities, and determine appropriate nursing interventions.
- **Decision making:** Making timely and effective decisions in complex and dynamic healthcare situations to optimize patient outcomes.
- **Problem-solving:** Identifying and resolving challenges or issues that may arise during implementation to ensure safe and effective care.

Psychomotor Skills

- **Technical proficiency:** The competence to perform various nursing procedures, administer medications, and carry out treatments with precision and skill.

- **Hand-eye coordination:** The ability to coordinate hand movements with visual cues, necessary for performing delicate procedures and interventions.
- **Dexterity:** Having nimble and precise hand movements to ensure patient comfort and safety during procedures.

Affective (Emotional) Skills

- **Empathy:** Demonstrating empathy and understanding towards patients' feelings, concerns, and emotions, and providing compassionate care.
- **Communication:** Effectively conveying information and actively listening to patients, their families, and other healthcare team members with empathy and respect.
- **Emotional resilience:** Coping with the emotional challenges and stress that may arise during patient care, while maintaining a positive and supportive demeanor.
- **Cultural competence:** Being sensitive to diverse cultural backgrounds, beliefs, and values, and providing culturally appropriate care.
- **Patient advocacy:** Advocating for the patient's rights, preferences, and needs to ensure they receive the best possible care and treatment.

▮ EVALUATION

Introduction

Evaluation is the final (fifth) step in the nursing process, encompassing a comprehensive assessment of the patient's response to nursing interventions and the effectiveness of the care plan. As a crucial component of the nursing process, evaluation plays a pivotal role in determining the success of patient care, identifying areas for improvement, and ensuring the delivery of high-quality, patient-centered healthcare.

Throughout the nursing process, which consists of assessment, diagnosis, planning, implementation, and evaluation, nurses meticulously collect data, analyze patient needs, and develop tailored care plans to address health concerns effectively. However, the true efficacy of these interventions is revealed during the evaluation phase.

Definitions

- **Dorothy E Johnson (1968):** "Evaluation is the process by which the nurse determines the extent to which the patient's goals have been achieved."
- **Herbert A Simmons (1975):** "Evaluation is the process of determining the extent to which the patient's goals have been achieved and the effectiveness of the nursing care plan."
- **Margaret A Newman (1979):** "Evaluation is the process of determining the patient's progress toward achieving the goals of care."
- **Patricia Benner (1984):** "Evaluation is the process of determining whether the patient's goals have been met and whether the nursing care plan was effective."
- **Joyce J Fitzpatrick (1992):** "Evaluation is the process of determining the extent to which the patient's goals have been achieved and the effectiveness of the nursing care plan."

▮ PURPOSES

Evaluation in the nursing process serves several important purposes, all aimed at ensuring the delivery of high-quality, patient-centered care and improving patient outcomes. Some of the key purposes for evaluation in the nursing process include:

- **Assessing effectiveness:** The primary purpose of evaluation is to assess the effectiveness of the nursing interventions and care plan in achieving the desired patient outcomes. By comparing the achieved outcomes with the expected outcomes, nurses can determine whether the interventions were successful in addressing the patient's health needs.
- **Monitoring patient progress:** Through evaluation, nurses continuously monitor

the patient's progress and response to care. This ongoing assessment allows for early detection of any changes or complications, enabling prompt intervention and prevention of adverse events.

- **Identifying variations and deviations:** Evaluation helps nurses identify any variations or deviations from the expected outcomes. This enables them to recognize potential problems, analyze the reasons behind such variations, and take appropriate corrective actions to improve care.

- **Promoting evidence-based practice:** Evaluation is essential for promoting evidence-based practice in nursing. By evaluating the outcomes of different interventions, nurses can identify which approaches are most effective and align with the best available evidence.

- **Enhancing patient safety:** Through evaluation, nurses can identify any potential safety issues or risks associated with specific interventions. This allows for the implementation of preventive measures and ensures patient safety is prioritized.

- **Quality improvement:** Evaluation is a crucial component of the quality improvement process in healthcare. By regularly evaluating the effectiveness of care, nurses and healthcare organizations can identify areas for improvement and implement changes to enhance the overall quality of care.

- **Patient-centered care:** Evaluation reinforces a patient-centered approach to care. By regularly evaluating the patient's response to care, nurses can adapt their interventions to meet the individual needs, preferences, and values of each patient.

- **Enhancing communication and collaboration:** Evaluation facilitates communication and collaboration among the healthcare team members. Through the sharing of evaluation findings, the entire team can work together to optimize patient care and outcomes.

- **Resource utilization:** Evaluation helps in assessing the efficient utilization of resources, including time, personnel, and equipment. By evaluating the impact of interventions, nurses can allocate resources effectively to maximize patient benefits.

- **Empowering patients:** Evaluation involves engaging patients in their care process and discussing their progress and outcomes. This empowers patients to take an active role in their healthcare decisions and self-management.

EVALUATION PROCESS

The evaluation phase in the nursing process involves a systematic and comprehensive assessment of the patient's response to nursing interventions and the effectiveness of the care plan. It is a critical step that helps nurses determine the success of patient care, identify areas for improvement, and make evidence-based decisions to optimize patient outcomes. The steps of evaluation in the nursing process are as follows:

- **Establishing evaluation criteria and expected outcomes:** Before implementing the nursing interventions, the nurse collaborates with the patient, their family, and the healthcare team to establish clear and measurable criteria for evaluating the patient's progress. These criteria become the expected outcomes, representing the specific goals the patient is expected to achieve through the nursing interventions.

- **Collecting data:** During the implementation phase and afterward, the nurse collects relevant data related to the patient's response to the interventions. This data includes objective measurements (e.g., vital signs, lab results) and subjective information (e.g., patient reports of symptoms or feelings). Data collection may involve observations, physical assessments, patient interviews, and reviewing documentation.

- **Comparing achieved outcomes with expected outcomes:** The nurse compares the achieved outcomes with the expected outcomes established in the planning phase. This step involves analyzing the data collected during the evaluation process to determine whether the patient has met the predefined goals.

- **Identifying variance or deviations:** If there are differences between the achieved outcomes and the expected outcomes, the nurse identifies these variances or deviations. It is essential to explore the reasons behind these discrepancies, as they may indicate the need for adjustments to the care plan or interventions.
- **Analyzing the effectiveness of nursing interventions:** Based on the evaluation findings, the nurse critically analyzes the effectiveness of the nursing interventions. This analysis involves determining whether the chosen interventions were appropriate for the patient's condition and if they contributed to the achieved outcomes.
- **Determining the need for care plan modification:** If there are variations or deviations from the expected outcomes, the nurse assesses whether modifications to the care plan are necessary. This may involve revising nursing diagnoses, changing interventions, or setting new goals to better address the patient's needs.
- **Documenting evaluation findings:** The nurse documents the evaluation findings, including the achieved outcomes, identified variances, and any modifications made to the care plan. Accurate and timely documentation ensures the continuity of care and provides a basis for further assessments and decision-making.
- **Providing feedback and communication:** The nurse communicates the evaluation findings to the healthcare team, the patient, and their family. Feedback on the patient's progress and response to care is essential for fostering a collaborative approach to patient care and ensuring that everyone involved is informed about the patient's status.
- **Continuing monitoring and re-evaluation:** Evaluation is an ongoing process that continues throughout the patient's care journey. After making any necessary adjustments to the care plan, the nurse continues to monitor the patient's progress, reevaluate outcomes, and make further modifications as needed.

By following these steps of evaluation in the nursing process, nurses can ensure that care is patient-centered, evidence-based, and continuously tailored to meet the changing needs of the patient. The evaluation phase plays a crucial role in promoting optimal patient outcomes and delivering high-quality nursing care.

TYPES OF EVALUATION

In the nursing process, there are several types of evaluation that nurses use to assess the patient's response to care and the effectiveness of nursing interventions. These types of evaluation can be broadly categorized as follows:

- **Formative evaluation:** Formative evaluation occurs during the implementation phase and involves ongoing assessments and feedback to monitor the patient's progress and the effectiveness of nursing interventions. It helps nurses make real-time adjustments to the care plan, ensuring that the patient receives timely and tailored care.
- **Summative evaluation:** Summative evaluation takes place at the end of the nursing process, typically after the patient has completed the care plan or undergone a significant period of treatment. It assesses the overall outcomes achieved and the extent to which the patient's health goals have been met.
- **Process evaluation:** Process evaluation focuses on evaluating the process of care delivery rather than the outcomes. It assesses whether the nursing interventions were carried out as planned, the

adherence to protocols and guidelines, and the effectiveness of the healthcare team's collaboration.

- **Outcome evaluation:** Outcome evaluation measures the impact of nursing interventions on the patient's health status and well-being. It assesses whether the desired outcomes have been achieved and the effectiveness of the care plan in improving patient outcomes.
- **Concurrent evaluation:** Concurrent evaluation occurs simultaneously with the delivery of care. It involves ongoing monitoring of the patient's response to interventions, allowing for immediate adjustments to the care plan as needed.
- **Comprehensive evaluation:** Comprehensive evaluation entails a holistic assessment of the patient's response to care, considering all aspects of the patient's health and well-being, including physical, emotional, social, and spiritual dimensions.
- **Partial evaluation:** Partial evaluation focuses on specific aspects of the care plan or interventions. It may be used to evaluate the effectiveness of particular treatments or interventions without assessing the overall patient outcomes.

CHAPTER SUMMARY

1. After identifying nursing diagnoses and collaborative problems, develop a customized care plan that gives priority to the diagnoses and outlines nursing interventions, patient-centered goals, and expected outcomes.
2. In the planning phase, emphasize the importance of tailoring the care plan to address the patient's distinct requirements.
3. Rank nursing diagnoses and patient problems according to urgency and significance, establishing a preferred sequence for nursing actions.
4. Patient-centered goals and outcomes should reflect the specific behaviors desired from the patient, emphasizing the patient's needs rather than the nurse's own goals or interventions.
5. Outcomes indicate the desired responses in various aspects, signifying the resolution of the patient's health problems.
6. When crafting goals and outcomes, adhere to the SMART acronym: Specific, Measurable, Attainable, Realistic, and Timed, to ensure clarity and effectiveness.
7. During the planning phase, select interventions that aid the patient in progressing from their current health status to the level described in the goal, as measured by the expected outcomes.
8. Independent nursing interventions are actions that nurses autonomously initiate based on scientific rationale without supervision or direction from others, and they do not require an order from another healthcare provider. In contrast, healthcare provider-initiated interventions necessitate specific nursing responsibilities and technical knowledge.
9. Care plans promote communication among nurses and facilitate continuity of care between different nurses and healthcare settings.
10. The implementation phase in nursing involves formally putting the care plan into action after the development of relevant nursing diagnoses.
11. Interventions may encompass direct care measures, performed directly on the patient, and indirect care measures conducted for the benefit of the patient or a group of patients.
12. Several factors can influence the implementation phase, including the patient's condition, available resources, healthcare setting, and the nurse's knowledge and skills.
13. Proper preparation, including time management, personnel coordination, and patient engagement, is essential for a smooth implementation process.

14. Skills required for effective implementation include cognitive abilities such as critical thinking, clinical reasoning, and decision-making.
15. Evaluation is the final step in the nursing process and involves a comprehensive assessment of the patient's response to nursing interventions and the effectiveness of the care plan.
16. It plays a crucial role in determining the success of patient care, identifying areas for improvement, and ensuring high-quality, patient-centered health care.
17. The purposes of evaluation in the nursing process are multi-faceted and include assessing the effectiveness of interventions, monitoring patient progress, identifying variations, promoting evidence-based practice, enhancing patient safety, and supporting quality improvement efforts.
18. Nurses use various types of evaluation, such as formative, summative, process, outcome, concurrent, comprehensive, and partial evaluation, depending on the specific context and purpose.
19. By conducting thorough evaluations, nurses can adapt care plans to meet individual patient needs, continuously improve care quality, and achieve the best possible patient outcomes.

REVIEW QUESTIONS

1. Explain the key steps involved in the planning phase of the nursing process.
2. Discuss the importance of critical thinking and problem-solving skills during the planning phase of the nursing process.
3. Compare and contrast the three types of nursing interventions.
4. Define implementation and discuss the steps in the implementation process.
5. Explain the types of evaluation in context of nursing process.
6. Discuss the steps of the evaluation process.
7. Explain the skills required for effective implementation of a care plan.

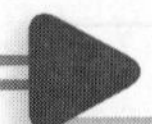 **BIBLIOGRAPHY** 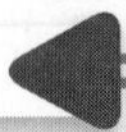

1. Riesenberg LA. Shift-to-shift handoff research: where do we go from here? J Grad Med Educ. 2012;4(1): 4-8.
2. Riesenberg LA, Leitzsch J, Cunningham JM. Nursing handoffs: a systematic review of the literature. Am J Nurs. 2010;110(4):24-34.
3. Jones TL. A holistic framework for nursing time: implications for theory, practice and research. Nurs Forum. 2010;45(3):185-96.
4. Potter P, Deshields T, Kuhrik M. Delegation practices between registered nurses and nursing assistive personnel. J Nurs Manag. 2010;18(2):157-65.
5. Tanner CA. Thinking like a nurse: a research-based model of clinical judgment in nursing. J Nurs Educ. 2006;45(6):204-11.
6. University of Iowa. Evidence-based practice guidelines, n.d., University of Iowa [cited Sep 27, 2014]. Available from: http://www.nursing.uiowa.edu/excellence/evidence-based-practice-guidelines.
7. Kalisch BJ, Landstrom GL, Hinshaw AS. Missed nursing care: a concept analysis. J Adv Nurs. 2009;65(7):1509-17.
8. Mamede S, Splinter TA, van Gog T, Rikers RM, Schmidt HG. Exploring the role of salient distracting clinical features in the emergence of diagnostic errors and the mechanisms through which reflection counteracts mistakes. BMJ Qual Saf. 2012;21(4):295-300.

9. Potter PA, Perry AG, Stockert PA, Hall AM. Fundamentals of nursing, 10th edition. Elsevier; 2021.

10. Wilkinson JM, Treas LS. Fundamentals of nursing, 3rd edition. FA Davis Company; 2019.

11. Bulechek GM, Butcher HK, Dochterman JMM, Wagner CM, editors. Nursing interventions classification (NIC), 6th edition. Elsevier Health Sciences; 2013.

12. Taylor C, Lillis C, Lynn P, LeMone P. Fundamentals of nursing: the art and science of person-centered care, 9th edition. Wolters Kluwer Health; 2018.

13. Carpenito LJ. Nursing diagnosis: application to clinical practice, 16th edition. Wolters Kluwer Health; 2019.

14. Doenges ME, Moorhouse MF, Murr AC. Diagnoses, prioritized interventions, and rationales, 14th edition. F A Davis Company; 2016. Nurse's pocket guide.

15. Black JM, Hawks JH. Medical-surgical nursing: clinical management for positive outcomes, 9th edition. Saunders; 2017.

16. Ackley BJ, Ladwig GB. Nursing diagnosis handbook: an evidence-based guide to planning care, 12th edition. Elsevier; 2019.

17. Gulanick M, Myers JL. Nursing care plans: diagnoses, interventions, and outcomes, 9th edition. Elsevier; 2019.

15

Documentation and Reporting

Learning Objectives

- Explain the purposes of maintaining a health care record.
- Explore the legal principles concerning documentation.
- Outline quality criteria for proper documentation.
- Elaborate on the diverse record-keeping methods utilized.
- Discuss the benefits and problems of using documentation forms.
- Investigate the different types of nursing reports.
- Discuss the purposes of reporting in nursing.
- Explain the advantages and disadvantages associated with nursing reports.

INTRODUCTION

Documentation is a crucial nursing action involving the recording of relevant patient data, nursing clinical decisions, interventions, and patient responses in a health record. It holds significant importance in nursing practice as it provides a detailed account of the care delivered. Accuracy and comprehensiveness are essential in nursing documentation. The systems used for nursing documentation should be flexible, allowing for easy retrieval of clinical data, promoting continuity of care, monitoring patient outcomes, and reflecting current nursing practice standards. Effective documentation contributes to continuity of care, time-saving, and error reduction. Considering the quality of care, regulatory standards, nursing practice guidelines, healthcare reimbursement structure, and legal requirements, documentation and reporting are critical nursing responsibilities.

DEFINITIONS

- "Documentation in nursing is the written and electronic recording of pertinent patient data, nursing clinical decisions and interventions, and patient responses to interventions." *(O'Toole, 2013)*
- "Nursing documentation is a critical component of nursing practice, involving the accurate and timely recording of patient information, care provided, and outcomes achieved."

  (American Nurses Association, 2018)
- "Documentation in nursing refers to the process of capturing patient data and healthcare activities to provide a clear picture of a patient's health status and the nursing care provided."

  (Muller-Staub, 2009)
- "Documentation is a means of communication between healthcare providers, ensuring continuity of care, and maintaining a legal record of the care provided."

  (JCAHO, 2018)

PURPOSES

Documentation in nursing serves several crucial purposes, playing a vital role in providing high-quality patient care, promoting effective communication, ensuring legal and regulatory compliance, and supporting research and quality improvement initiatives. Let's delve into each of these purposes in detail:

- **Communication:** A patient's medical record serves as a means for the healthcare team to exchange information regarding the patient's requirements and response to treatment, clinical decision-making, specific therapies, consultation details, patient education, and discharge planning. It stands as the most up-to-date and accurate continuous source of information about the patient's healthcare status, and it is crucial that the care plan is easily understandable for anyone accessing the record. The information shared in a patient's record enables healthcare providers to have a comprehensive understanding of the patient, thereby supporting safe, effective, timely, and patient-centered clinical decision-making. To promote effective communication and ensure patient safety, it is essential to promptly document assessment findings and patient information immediately after providing care, such as nursing interventions or completing a patient assessment.

- **Continuity of care:** In a healthcare setting, patients may receive care from multiple nurses or shift changes may occur. Documentation ensures the continuity of care, allowing nurses taking over the care of a patient to understand the patient's history, ongoing treatments, and any changes in the condition. This prevents important details from being overlooked, and the patient's needs are consistently met.

- **Legal and ethical protection:** Documentation serves as a legal record of the care provided and the patient's condition at specific points in time. In case of any adverse events, litigation, or medical-legal issues, comprehensive and accurate documentation can protect nurses and the healthcare facility by demonstrating that they provided appropriate care and followed established protocols.

- **Quality improvement and research:** Nursing documentation is valuable for quality improvement initiatives and research studies. Analyzing data from nursing records can identify patterns, trends, and areas for improvement in patient care. The information collected can be used to develop evidence-based practices and enhance patient outcomes.

- **Billing and reimbursement:** Proper documentation is essential for billing and reimbursement purposes. Accurate records of treatments, procedures, medications, and patient status are required for healthcare facilities to receive appropriate reimbursement from insurance providers and government agencies.

- **Monitoring patient progress:** Regular documentation of vital signs, symptoms, and responses to treatment allows nurses and other healthcare providers to monitor a patient's progress over time. This helps in assessing the effectiveness of interventions, identifying any deterioration or improvement in the patient's condition, and adjusting the treatment plan accordingly.

- **Patient safety:** Documentation is closely linked to patient safety. By documenting allergies, medications, and other relevant patient information, nurses can help prevent medication errors and adverse reactions. Comprehensive documentation also ensures that important details are not missed, reducing the risk of medical errors and improving patient safety.

- **Legal and regulatory compliance:** Healthcare facilities must adhere to various legal and regulatory requirements. Documentation provides evidence of compliance with these standards, including requirements set forth by accrediting bodies and government agencies. This is crucial for maintaining the facility's license and accreditation status.

- **Effective care planning:** Nursing documentation provides critical data for care planning and goal-setting. By understanding a patient's health history, current status, and potential risks, nurses can develop personalized care plans that address the specific needs of each patient.
- **Education and training:** Documentation serves as a valuable educational resource for nursing students, new healthcare professionals, and other members of the healthcare team. It allows them to review case studies, understand various patient conditions and treatments, and learn from past experiences.

CHARACTERISTICS OF GOOD RECORDING/DOCUMENTATION

Characteristics of good recording in nursing are specific attributes that contribute to accurate, comprehensive, and effective documentation of patient care. These characteristics ensure that nurses maintain high-quality records that support continuity of care, promote patient safety, and comply with legal and regulatory requirements. Here are some key characteristics of good recording in nursing:

- **Accuracy:** The information recorded should be precise and reflect the actual care provided, observations made, and assessments conducted. Avoid making assumptions or documenting information based on hearsay.
- **Completeness:** Ensure that all relevant and essential information is documented. This includes patient assessments, interventions, treatments, medications administered, and responses to interventions.
- **Relevance:** Record only information that is directly related to the patient's care and medical condition. Avoid including unnecessary or extraneous details.
- **Timeliness:** Record information as close to the time of the event or care delivery as possible. Delayed documentation can lead to errors and omissions.
- **Clarity:** Use clear and legible handwriting or electronic documentation. If others cannot read the records easily, it can lead to misinterpretations and potential harm to the patient.
- **Objectivity:** Document facts objectively, without personal biases or judgments. Use neutral language and avoid subjective statements.
- **Organized structure:** Follow a logical and consistent structure for recording information. This helps ensure that records are well-organized and easy to navigate.
- **Conciseness:** Be succinct in recording information without sacrificing essential details. Use concise and clear language to convey the necessary information effectively.
- **Chronological order:** Document events and care in chronological order to create a clear timeline of the patient's care and progress.
- **Standard terminology:** Use standardized terminology and medical abbreviations when appropriate. Avoid using jargon or acronyms that might not be universally understood.
- **Confidentiality:** Adhere to strict patient confidentiality guidelines and store records securely to prevent unauthorized access.
- **Evidence-based practice:** Base your documentation on evidence-based practices and guidelines, ensuring that care is provided according to the best available evidence.
- **Legibility of signatures:** When signing off on entries, ensure that your signature is legible and can be easily attributed to you.
- **Consistency:** Follow institutional policies and procedures consistently for documenting various aspects of patient care.
- **Integrity and accountability:** Take ownership of your documentation and be honest about any errors or omissions. Follow proper protocols for correcting mistakes.

- **Interprofessional collaboration:** Use documentation as a means of effective communication with other members of the healthcare team.
- **Patient-centered:** Focus on the patient's needs and individualize the documentation to reflect their unique care requirements.

Good recording in nursing plays a crucial role in ensuring safe and effective patient care, promoting communication among healthcare providers, and providing a comprehensive account of the patient's health status and treatment plan.

METHODS OF DOCUMENTATION

In nursing, various methods of documentation are used to record patient information, assessments, interventions, and outcomes. The choice of documentation method may depend on the healthcare facility's policies, available resources, and the level of technology adoption. Broadly, methods of documentation in nursing divided into Paper-based or traditional documentation and electronic documentation systems.

Paper-based or Traditional Documentation Systems

Paper-based or traditional documentation systems in nursing refer to the practice of recording patient information, assessments, care interventions, and other relevant data on physical paper forms, charts, or notebooks. Historically, this method was the primary means of documenting patient care before the advent of electronic health records (EHRs) and other digital documentation systems. Even with the rise of technology, some healthcare facilities may still utilize paper-based systems for certain aspects of patient care or in regions where electronic systems are not yet widely adopted.

Types of Paper-based or Traditional Documentation Systems

There are two common types of paper-based or traditional documentation systems in nursing are source-oriented records (SOR) and problem-oriented medical records (POMR). Let's look at each of these systems in more detail:

1. Source-oriented Records

Source-oriented records (SOR) is a traditional method of organizing and documenting patient information in nursing and healthcare settings. In this system, each discipline or healthcare professional creates and maintains their own separate section of the patient's medical record, containing relevant information related to their specific area of expertise. The record is divided into sections, with each section dedicated to a particular department or discipline involved in the patient's care. Here are some key features and characteristics of source-oriented records in nursing:

- **Multidisciplinary approach:** Source-oriented records allow different healthcare professionals, including nurses, physicians, therapists, and others, to document their assessments, observations, treatments, and interventions in their designated sections of the patient's medical record.
- **Sectioned format:** The record is divided into sections, each corresponding to a specific healthcare discipline or department, such as nursing notes, physician progress notes, laboratory reports, radiology reports, and more.
- **Focus on professional perspective:** Each section emphasizes the professional's perspective and area of expertise, making it easier for healthcare providers to find information relevant to their practice.

Advantages of Source-oriented Records

- **Easy to follow:** Each healthcare discipline has its own section, making it simple for professionals to find information relevant to their practice.
- **Specialized entries:** Professionals document information from their perspective, emphasizing their area of expertise.

- **Concurrent documentation:** Healthcare providers can document patient care concurrently, avoiding delays in recording information.
- **Multidisciplinary approach:** SOR allows different disciplines to contribute to the patient's record, enhancing collaboration.

Disadvantages of Source-oriented Records

- **Limited accessibility:** Information is scattered across sections, making it challenging to access a comprehensive patient profile quickly.
- **Data duplication:** The same patient information may be duplicated across multiple sections, leading to inefficiencies.
- **Communication challenges:** Interdisciplinary communication may suffer due to limited access to other disciplines' entries.
- **Potential incomplete information:** If a discipline fails to document relevant data, important patient information may be missing.

2. Problem-oriented Medical Record

Problem-oriented Medical Records (POMR) is an approach to documentation used in nursing and healthcare that focuses on organizing patient information around specific healthcare problems or issues. Developed by Dr. Lawrence Weed in the 1960s, POMR is designed to promote a systematic and comprehensive approach to patient care. This method encourages healthcare providers, including nurses, to collaborate and think critically about each patient's health concerns and develop individualized care plans.

POMR is considered an effective and systematic approach to documentation in nursing and healthcare because it focuses on problem resolution and individualized care planning. By identifying and addressing specific health concerns, healthcare providers can work together to provide targeted and comprehensive patient care.

Components of Problem-oriented Medical Records

Problem-oriented medical records consist of several key components that work together to organize patient information around specific healthcare problems or issues. These components help healthcare providers systematically document, manage, and evaluate patient care. The major components of POMR include:

- **Problem list:** The problem list is a crucial component of POMR and serves as a catalog of all the patient's health issues or concerns. Each problem is identified with a unique number or identifier. The list is continually updated as new problems arise or existing ones are resolved.
- **Database:** The database contains comprehensive and relevant patient information, including past medical history, laboratory results, diagnostic reports, and any other data relevant to the patient's current health status.
- **Initial problem-oriented note (IPN):** The IPN is the first progress note entered in the patient's medical record and serves as an introduction to the problem list and care plan. It provides a summary of the patient's presenting problems and initial management.
- **Progress notes:** Healthcare providers add progress notes to the POMR regularly to document changes in the patient's condition, responses to interventions, and any updates to the care plan.
- **Care plan:** Each problem identified on the problem list corresponds to a specific care plan. The care plan outlines the interventions and treatments recommended to address the patient's unique health concerns.
- **Discharge summary:** The discharge summary is a comprehensive document created when the patient is discharged from the healthcare facility. It includes an overview of the patient's course of

treatment, outcomes, and any follow-up recommendations.

- **Collaborative documentation:** POMR encourages interdisciplinary collaboration among healthcare providers. Different disciplines contribute to the problem list, progress notes, and care plans, ensuring coordinated and integrated patient care.
- **Continuity of care:** POMR promotes continuity of care by providing a unified and up-to-date patient record accessible to all healthcare providers involved in the patient's care.
- **Problem-solving approach:** The problem-oriented approach in POMR prompts healthcare providers to think critically and analytically in identifying, diagnosing, and managing patient problems.

Problem-oriented Medical Record Formats

In problem-oriented medical records, various formats can be used to organize patient information around specific healthcare problems or issues. These formats help healthcare providers structure their documentation and facilitate a comprehensive and systematic approach to patient care. Here are some common formats used in problem-oriented medical records:

- **SOAP format:** This is one of the most widely used formats in POMR. It stands for Subjective, Objective, Assessment, and Plan. Each progress note follows this format to address a specific problem or set of problems.
  - *Subjective*: This section includes information provided by the patient or their family, such as symptoms, concerns, and medical history.
  - *Objective*: The objective section contains measurable and observable data collected by healthcare providers, including physical assessments, test results, and vital signs.
  - *Assessment:* In this section, healthcare providers analyze and interpret the subjective and objective data to make clinical judgments or diagnoses related to the specific problem.
  - *Plan:* The plan outlines the proposed interventions, treatments, and ongoing management for the identified problem.
- **SOAPIER format:** This is an extension of the SOAP format, with additional components for Intervention and Evaluation.
  - *Intervention:* This section details the specific actions or treatments implemented to address the problem.
  - *Evaluation:* The evaluation section documents the patient's response to the interventions and the progress made towards resolving the problem.
- **PIE format:** PIE stands for Problem, Intervention, and Evaluation. This format organizes documentation around nursing care plans and interventions.
  - *Problem*: This section identifies the nursing problem or diagnosis.
  - *Intervention*: The intervention section outlines the nursing actions and care provided to address the problem.
  - *Evaluation:* The evaluation section assesses the patient's response to the nursing interventions and the effectiveness of the care provided.
- **Focus charting:** Focus charting is another format used in POMR, which centers on the patient's specific concerns or nursing diagnoses. It involves using a three-column format:
  - *Data:* This column contains the patient information, including subjective and objective data.
  - *Action*: The action column describes the nursing interventions or actions taken in response to the patient's needs or concerns.
  - *Response:* The response column documents the patient's outcomes or responses to the nursing interventions.
- **DAR format:** DAR stands for Data, Action, and Response. This format is similar to the PIE format and is commonly used in nursing documentation.

- *Data:* This section includes relevant patient data, both subjective and objective.
- *Action:* The action section details the nursing interventions or actions taken.
- *Response*: The response section documents the patient's response or outcome after the interventions were implemented.

Different healthcare facilities and professionals may use variations or combinations of these formats based on their specific needs and documentation preferences. The common thread among all these formats is their focus on organizing patient information around specific problems to enhance problem-solving, care planning, and evaluation in healthcare.

Advantages of Problem-oriented Medical Records

- **Comprehensive approach:** POMR promotes a systematic and comprehensive approach to patient care, focusing on resolving specific health problems.
- **Organized structure:** The problem list and SOAP format provide a structured way to document patient information, facilitating efficient information retrieval.
- **Collaboration:** POMR encourages interdisciplinary collaboration among healthcare providers, leading to coordinated and integrated patient care.
- **Individualized care plans:** Each problem is addressed with a tailored care plan, ensuring personalized treatment for the patient.
- **Continuity of care:** POMR enhances continuity of care as all healthcare providers have access to a unified and up-to-date patient record.

Disadvantages of Problem-oriented Medical Records

- **Time-consuming:** The process of creating and maintaining problem lists and SOAP notes may require more time compared to other documentation methods.
- **Learning curve:** Implementing POMR may require training and adjustment for healthcare providers to become proficient in the approach.
- **Duplication of information:** Similar information may be repeated across different problem-specific entries, leading to redundant documentation.
- **Limited standardization:** POMR may lack uniformity across different healthcare facilities, resulting in variations in documentation practices.
- **Technology integration:** Transitioning POMR to electronic health record (EHR) systems may present challenges in terms of data entry and retrieval.

Electronic Medical Records

Electronic Medical Records (EMRs) in nursing refer to digital systems used to store, manage, and access patient health information in a healthcare facility. EMRs have replaced traditional paper-based records in many healthcare settings due to their numerous advantages in terms of efficiency, accessibility, and data management. EMRs play a crucial role in nursing practice, facilitating better patient care, communication, and collaboration among healthcare providers. Here are the key details on electronic medical records in nursing:

Features and Characteristics of EMRs

- **Digital format:** EMRs are entirely digital, eliminating the need for paper-based documentation. All patient information, including medical history, test results, medications, treatment plans, progress notes, and nursing assessments, is stored electronically.
- **Accessibility:** EMRs enable authorized healthcare providers to access patient records from various locations within the healthcare facility or even remotely, facilitating real-time access to critical patient information.

- **Interoperability:** EMRs promote interoperability, allowing seamless information exchange between different departments and healthcare facilities. This enhances continuity of care and communication among healthcare providers.
- **Security and confidentiality:** EMRs are designed with robust security measures to protect patient data from unauthorized access or breaches. Access to patient records is restricted to authorized personnel only.
- **Data integration:** EMRs often integrate with other digital systems, such as laboratory information systems, radiology systems, and pharmacy systems. This integration allows for automatic updating of patient information and reduces the risk of errors.
- **Clinical decision support:** EMRs may include clinical decision support tools that provide healthcare providers with alerts, reminders, and best practice guidelines to enhance patient safety and improve care quality.
- **Electronic prescriptions:** EMRs support electronic prescribing, allowing nurses to send prescriptions directly to pharmacies, reducing errors and streamlining medication management.
- **Efficient documentation:** EMRs streamline nursing documentation, making it faster and more accurate. Nurses can use templates, prepopulated data, and standardized terminology for consistent and efficient documentation.
- **Data analytics and reporting:** EMRs can generate various reports and analyze patient data to identify trends, outcomes, and quality metrics. This information can be used to improve care processes and patient outcomes.
- **Patient engagement:** Some EMRs offer patient portals that enable patients to access their health records, communicate with healthcare providers, schedule appointments, and access educational materials.
- **Audit trail:** EMRs maintain an audit trail, recording any changes or access to patient records, providing a record of who accessed or modified patient data and when.

Benefits of EMRs

- **Improved efficiency:** EMRs streamline nursing workflows, saving time and reducing paperwork burden.
- **Enhanced patient safety:** EMRs support clinical decision support tools, reducing medication errors and adverse events.
- **Better communication and collaboration:** EMRs enable seamless communication and information sharing among healthcare providers, fostering collaboration in patient care.
- **Access to comprehensive patient information:** EMRs provide a centralized repository of patient data, allowing nurses to access comprehensive information at their fingertips.
- **Continuity of care:** EMRs promote continuity of care by facilitating the exchange of patient information among healthcare providers.

Disadvantages of HER

- **Cost and implementation:** Setting up and maintaining EMRs can be expensive and require significant initial investment.
- **Learning curve:** Nurses may require time to adapt to using electronic systems and may face challenges in navigating the new technology.
- **Technical issues:** EMRs are susceptible to technical problems, such as system downtime or slow response times, which can disrupt workflow.
- **Data security and privacy concerns:** EMRs store sensitive patient information, and maintaining data security and privacy is crucial to prevent breaches.
- **Copy-paste errors:** The ease of copying and pasting information in EMRs can lead to the propagation of incorrect or outdated data.
- **Loss of personal touch:** EMRs may reduce face-to-face interaction between nurses and patients, potentially impacting the patient-provider relationship.

- **Data overload:** EMRs may result in an abundance of information, making it challenging for nurses to find the most relevant data efficiently.

COMMON RECORD-KEEPING FORMS

In nursing and healthcare settings, various record-keeping forms are commonly used to document patient information and other relevant data. These forms help healthcare providers maintain accurate and organized records for each patient. The specific forms used may vary depending on the healthcare facility, specialty, and documentation requirements. Here are some common record-keeping forms in nursing:

- **Admission assessment form:** This form is used to document the initial assessment of a patient upon admission to the healthcare facility. It includes the patient's medical history, current health status, allergies, medications, and other relevant information.
- **Vital signs record:** Vital signs, such as blood pressure, heart rate, respiratory rate, and temperature, are recorded on this form at regular intervals to monitor the patient's physiological status.
- **Nursing care plan:** The nursing care plan outlines the individualized care and interventions required for each patient. It includes nursing diagnoses, goals, interventions, and evaluation of patient responses.
- **Medication administration record (MAR):** The MAR is used to document the administration of medications to patients. It includes details such as medication name, dosage, route of administration, time, and the signature of the administering nurse.
- **Intake and output (I&O) record:** This form records the patient's fluid intake and output, including oral intake, IV fluids, urine output, and other measurable outputs, which helps assess the patient's fluid balance.
- **Patient assessment forms:** Various assessment forms are used to document specific aspects of patient assessments, such as neurological assessment, pain assessment, skin assessment, etc.
- **Progress notes:** Progress notes are used to document daily observations, changes in the patient's condition, treatments provided, and any other relevant information related to the patient's care.
- **Incident report form:** This form is used to document any unexpected events, incidents, or accidents that occur during the patient's stay, such as falls, medication errors, or equipment malfunctions.
- **Discharge summary:** The discharge summary provides a summary of the patient's treatment, outcomes, and any follow-up instructions upon discharge from the healthcare facility.
- **Consent forms:** These forms are used to document informed consent for various procedures, treatments, or surgeries, ensuring that patients are fully aware of the risks and benefits before providing their consent.
- **Transfer form:** When a patient is transferred to another healthcare facility or unit, a transfer form is used to document essential patient information for a smooth transition of care.
- **Laboratory and diagnostic test result forms:** These forms are used to record the results of various laboratory tests, imaging studies, and other diagnostic procedures.
- **Consultation request forms:** When requesting consultations from other healthcare professionals, nurses use these forms to provide relevant patient information and the reason for the consultation.

The availability and usage of these record-keeping forms may vary depending on the healthcare facility's policies, electronic health record (EHR) systems, and other documentation practices. Proper documentation using these forms is essential for maintaining accurate, complete, and legally compliant patient records.

GENERAL GUIDELINES OF DOCUMENTATION

General guidelines for recording apply to various professional settings, including nursing, healthcare, education, research, and more. Effective and accurate recording is essential for maintaining clear communication, ensuring accountability, and preserving information for future reference. Here are some general guidelines for recording:

- **Accuracy:** The information recorded should be precise and reflect the actual care provided, observations made, and assessments conducted. Avoid making assumptions or documenting information based on hearsay.
- **Completeness:** Ensure that all relevant and essential information is documented. This includes patient assessments, interventions, treatments, medications administered, and responses to interventions.
- **Relevance:** Record only information that is directly related to the patient's care and medical condition. Avoid including unnecessary or extraneous details.
- **Timeliness:** Record information as close to the time of the event or care delivery as possible. Delayed documentation can lead to errors and omissions.
- **Clarity:** Use clear and legible handwriting or electronic documentation. If others cannot read the records easily, it can lead to misinterpretations and potential harm to the patient.
- **Organized structure:** Follow a logical and consistent structure for recording information. This helps ensure that records are well-organized and easy to navigate.
- **Use objective language:** Record facts and observations objectively without personal biases or opinions. Stick to the information that can be objectively verified.
- **Use standard terminology:** Utilize standardized terminology and acronyms that are widely accepted in your field. Avoid using local or nonstandardized abbreviations.
- **Date and time stamp:** Always include the date and time of each entry to establish a chronological record.
- **Legibility:** Ensure that your handwriting or typed text is easily readable. Illegible records can lead to misunderstandings and potential errors.
- **Sign and authenticate entries:** Sign each entry with your full name or initials and include any necessary authentication details (e.g., employee number).
- **Avoid blank spaces:** Do not leave any blank spaces in the record. If a section does not apply, mark it as "N/A" or "Not Applicable."
- **Cross-referencing:** When necessary, refer to other related documents or records for additional context or information.
- **Confidentiality:** Adhere to strict confidentiality guidelines when recording sensitive information. Store records securely and only share them with authorized personnel.
- **Use corrections appropriately:** If an error is made, draw a single line through the mistake, write "error" above it, and then provide the correct information. Do not erase or use correction fluid.
- **Include signature and credentials:** Sign and add your professional credentials (e.g., RN for registered nurse) to verify your entries.
- **Consistency:** Follow consistent recording practices and adhere to the guidelines established by your organization or profession.
- **Review and validate:** Regularly review your records to ensure accuracy and completeness. Validate information with patients when appropriate.
- **Be nondiscriminatory:** Avoid recording any information that may be discriminatory or offensive.
- **Secure record storage:** Store physical records in secure locations with limited access. For electronic records, ensure proper security measures are in place to protect against unauthorized access.

- **Training and education:** Stay updated on record-keeping practices and participate in training sessions to improve your recording skills.

Following these general guidelines for recording will help maintain accurate, comprehensive, and reliable documentation in various professional settings, fostering effective communication and supporting quality outcomes.

REPORTING

Introduction

In nursing, reports are written or verbal accounts that provide essential information about a patient's condition, care, and treatment to other members of the healthcare team. These reports play a crucial role in promoting effective communication, collaboration, and continuity of care among healthcare providers. Different types of reports are used in nursing, each serving a specific purpose.

Definitions

- The American Nurses Association defines a report in nursing as "a communication of information about a patient's condition and care plan from one nurse to another."
- The Royal College of Nursing defines a report in nursing as "a concise and accurate summary of a patient's condition, care needs, and progress."
- Patricia A. Benner defines a report in nursing as "a way of transferring knowledge and responsibility for care from one nurse to another."

PURPOSES OF REPORTING

Reporting serves various essential purposes in nursing and healthcare settings. The accurate and timely communication of information through reports is crucial for patient care, safety, and effective collaboration among healthcare providers. Some of the primary purposes of reporting in nursing include:

- **Continuity of care:** Reporting, especially during nursing handoffs and shift changes, ensures continuity of care as nurses transfer patient information to their colleagues. This helps maintain a consistent approach to patient care and minimizes the risk of errors or omissions during transitions.
- **Patient safety:** Reporting adverse events, incidents, and changes in a patient's condition helps identify potential safety issues. Incident reports, e.g., play a key role in investigating and addressing safety concerns, contributing to enhanced patient safety and the prevention of future incidents.
- **Interdisciplinary collaboration:** Reports facilitate effective collaboration among healthcare disciplines. Consultation reports allow nurses to seek input from physicians, specialists, or other healthcare professionals, ensuring a comprehensive and well-coordinated approach to patient care.
- **Documentation of care:** Reporting serves as legal documentation of the care provided to patients. Comprehensive and accurate reports document patient assessments, interventions, and responses, providing evidence of the nursing care delivered and supporting the healthcare facility's legal and regulatory compliance.
- **Evidence-based practice:** Quality improvement reports and outcome reports provide data and findings that support evidence-based practice. Analyzing trends and outcomes can inform the development and implementation of evidence-based interventions to improve patient care.
- **Patient education and discharge planning:** Discharge reports play a vital role in patient education and discharge planning. They provide patients and their families with essential information about their health status, medications, follow-up care, and self-management, promoting better patient outcomes after leaving the healthcare facility.
- **Quality improvement:** Reporting data on clinical outcomes, incident rates, and process measures is integral to quality

improvement initiatives. Regular analysis of these reports helps healthcare organizations identify areas for improvement and implement changes to enhance care quality and patient outcomes.

- **Communication with healthcare providers:** Reports serve as a means of communication between healthcare providers who are not physically present at the same time. They facilitate the sharing of essential patient information and updates among team members, enhancing collaboration and patient care.
- **Research and education:** Reports contribute to nursing research and education. They provide valuable data and insights for research studies, academic papers, and educational programs, advancing nursing knowledge and practice.

Reporting in nursing is a fundamental aspect of patient care and healthcare management. It supports effective communication, continuity of care, patient safety, interdisciplinary collaboration, and quality improvement. By documenting and sharing critical patient information, reports play a pivotal role in ensuring optimal patient outcomes and enhancing the overall quality of healthcare services.

METHODS OF REPORTING

Methods of reporting refer to the different ways in which information, data, or findings are presented and communicated to specific audiences. The choice of reporting method depends on the nature of the information, the target audience, and the purpose of the report. Here are some common methods of reporting:

- **Written reports:** Written reports are formal and structured documents that present information in a clear and organized manner. They include text, tables, charts, graphs, and other visual aids to convey data and findings effectively. Written reports can be in the form of research papers, business reports, progress reports, or policy briefs.

- **Oral reports:** Oral reporting involves presenting information verbally, typically in meetings, presentations, or interviews. Oral reports may be accompanied by visual aids, such as slides or handouts, to enhance understanding. This method allows for real-time interaction and feedback from the audience.
- **Email reports:** Email reports are brief reports sent via email to communicate important updates, summaries, or data to recipients.
- **Mobile apps and reporting tools:** With advancements in technology, mobile apps and reporting tools have become popular methods for reporting. These tools enable users to access and share information on-the-go, facilitating real-time reporting and decision-making.
- **Online reports and web-based portals:** Online reports and web-based portals provide a platform for sharing data and information with a broader audience. They allow for easy access to reports and enable data sharing across different locations.
- **Video reports:** Video reports use video recordings or presentations to communicate information. They are effective for visually demonstrating processes, interviews, or fieldwork.

TYPES OF REPORT IN NURSING

In nursing, various types of reports are used to communicate essential patient information, document care interventions, and ensure effective collaboration among healthcare providers. Each type of report serves a specific purpose and is critical for maintaining accurate and comprehensive patient records. Here are details about different types of reports commonly used in nursing:

Nursing Handoff Report

- **Description:** The nursing handoff report is a crucial communication tool used during shift changes when one nurse transfers the care of patients to another nurse. It can take the form of face-to-face communication, written documentation, or electronic handoff tools.

- **Purpose:** The primary purpose of the nursing handoff report is to provide an overview of each patient's current condition, recent interventions, upcoming treatments, and any changes in the patient's status that require attention.
- **Importance:** The nursing handoff report ensures continuity of care by facilitating the transfer of critical patient information between nurses. It reduces the risk of errors during care transitions and promotes effective teamwork among healthcare providers.

Incident Report

- **Description:** An incident report is used to document any unexpected or adverse events that occur during patient care, such as falls, medication errors, or equipment malfunctions.
- **Purpose:** The primary purpose of an incident report is to identify and investigate the cause of incidents, implement corrective actions, and improve patient safety and care quality.
- **Importance:** Incident reports provide valuable data for quality improvement initiatives and help prevent future incidents. They also contribute to the development of evidence-based practices to enhance patient safety.

Patient Assessment Report

- **Description:** The patient assessment report provides a comprehensive summary of the patient's assessment, including physical, psychological, and social aspects of their health.
- **Purpose:** The primary purpose of the patient assessment report is to document subjective and objective data, vital signs, and any notable findings that aid in formulating care plans and making clinical decisions.

- **Importance:** The patient assessment report is crucial for accurate diagnosis, individualized care planning, and ongoing evaluation of patient progress. It serves as the foundation for providing appropriate and effective nursing interventions.

Discharge Report

- **Description:** The discharge report provides a summary of a patient's healthcare journey and treatment outcomes upon discharge from the healthcare facility.
- **Purpose:** The primary purpose of the discharge report is to communicate the patient's condition at the time of discharge, medications, follow-up care instructions, and any relevant patient education.
- **Importance:** The discharge report ensures a smooth transition of care from the healthcare facility to the patient's home or another healthcare setting. It plays a significant role in promoting patient understanding of post-discharge care plans and reducing the risk of readmissions.

Consultation Report

- **Description:** A consultation report documents the process of seeking expert advice or opinion from other healthcare professionals, such as physicians, specialists, or therapists.
- **Purpose:** The primary purpose of the consultation report is to outline the reason for the consultation, relevant patient information, and the recommendations received from the consultant.
- **Importance:** The consultation report supports interdisciplinary collaboration and helps in formulating comprehensive care plans that consider inputs from various healthcare disciplines.

Quality Improvement Report

- **Description:** A quality improvement report documents data and findings related to a specific quality improvement initiative in nursing.

- **Purpose:** The primary purpose of the quality improvement report is to outline the objectives, methodologies, outcomes, and recommendations for enhancing care quality and patient safety.
- **Importance:** The quality improvement report supports evidence-based practice and fosters a culture of continuous improvement in healthcare. It helps healthcare organizations identify areas for improvement and implement evidence-based interventions to enhance patient outcomes and care processes.

ADVANTAGES OF REPORTING IN NURSING

- **Facilitates communication:** Reporting allows nurses to share critical patient information with other healthcare providers, ensuring continuity of care and effective collaboration.
- **Promotes patient safety:** Incident reporting helps identify and address safety issues, leading to improved patient safety and a reduction in adverse events.
- **Supports evidence-based practice:** Reporting outcomes and quality improvement data contribute to evidence-based decision-making and the implementation of best practices.
- **Enhances accountability:** Documentation and reporting provide a legal record of care, promoting accountability and adherence to standards of practice.
- **Improves patient outcomes:** Comprehensive and accurate reporting leads to better care planning and patient outcomes.

DISADVANTAGES OF REPORTING IN NURSING

- **Time-consuming:** Nurses may find reporting time-consuming, especially in busy clinical settings with a heavy workload.
- **Risk of errors:** Inaccurate or incomplete reporting can lead to errors in patient care and decision-making.
- **Privacy concerns:** Maintaining patient confidentiality and privacy in reporting requires careful handling of sensitive information.
- **Duplication of efforts:** In some cases, nurses may need to duplicate information in multiple reports, leading to inefficiencies.

CHAPTER SUMMARY

1. Documentation in nursing is a crucial nursing action involving the recording of relevant patient data, nursing clinical decisions, interventions, and patient responses in a health record.
2. It serves several purposes, including effective communication, continuity of care, legal and ethical protection, quality improvement, billing and reimbursement, monitoring patient progress, and patient safety.
3. Good recording in nursing should be accurate, comprehensive, relevant, timely, clear, and objective.
4. Methods of documentation in nursing include paper-based or traditional documentation systems and electronic medical records (EMRs).
5. Paper-based systems include source-oriented records (SOR) and problem-oriented medical records (POMR).
6. The progress notes in SOAP, SOAPIE, PIE, or DAR charting formats are structured to align with the nursing process.
7. EMRs are digital systems that provide numerous advantages, such as improved efficiency, enhanced patient safety, better communication, and access to comprehensive patient information.

8. Reporting provides essential information about a patient's condition, care, and treatment to other healthcare team members.
9. Types of reports include nursing handoff report, incident report, patient assessment report, discharge report, consultation report, and quality improvement report.
10. Reporting promotes effective communication, patient safety, interdisciplinary collaboration, documentation of care, evidence-based practice, patient education, and quality improvement.
11. Reporting methods include written reports, oral reports, email reports, mobile apps, online reports, and video reports.

REVIEW QUESTIONS

1. Define documentation and discuss the crucial purposes of documentation in nursing.
2. Explain the characteristics of good recording in nursing.
3. Describe the various methods of documentation in nursing.
4. Discuss the guidelines for effective documentation in nursing.
5. Define reports and discuss the various types of reports in nursing.
6. Explain various method of reporting in nursing and elaborate the advantages and disadvantages of reporting in nursing.

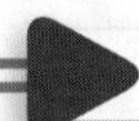 **BIBLIOGRAPHY** 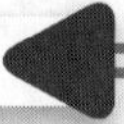

1. American Nurses Association (ANA). Nursing documentation: Know the facts. Retrieved from: https://www.nursingworld.org/practice-policy/workforce/what-is-nursing/the-essentials-of-nursing-documentation/[2020].
2. American Nurses Association (ANA). Nursing informatics: Scope and standards of practice. Silver Spring, MD; 2018.
3. Baker SK. Minimizing litigation risk: Documentation strategies in the occupational health setting. AAOHN J. 2000;48(2):100-5.
4. Bastable SB. Registered nurse as educator: Principles of teaching and learning for nursing practice. Sudbury, MA: Jones and Bartlett Publishers; 2003.
5. Blegen MA, Charns MP. Assessing the context of healthcare quality and safety improvement interventions: Clinical vignettes and evidence from the field. BMJ Quality and Safety. 2012;21(4):287-94.
6. Cahill J. Patient's perceptions of bedside handovers. J Clin Nurs. 1998;7(4):351-9.
7. Englebright J, Aldrich K, Taylor CR. Defining and incorporating basic nursing care actions into the electronic health record. J Nurs Scholarsh. 2014;46(1):50-7.
8. Hurley JS, Franklin MJ, Hamilton GA. Analysis of incident reports in nursing: A longitudinal study. J Nurs Educ Pract. 2018;8(3):54-60.
9. Jensen SA, Lippincott M. Nursing health assessment: A best practice approach. Wolters Kluwer Health; 2017.
10. Mitchell PH. Patient safety and quality: An evidence-based handbook for nurses. Agency for Healthcare Research and Quality (US); 2018.
11. Murphy JF, Maisto M. The nursing process in the age of electronic health records: Implications for critical care nursing practice. Crit Care Nurs Q. 2018;41(1):32-44.

12. Potter PA, Perry AG, Stockert PA, Hall, A. Fundamentals of nursing. Elsevier Health Sci. 2016.
13. Saleem JJ, Flanagan ME, Wilck NR, Demetriades J, Doebbeling BN. The next-generation electronic health record: perspectives of key leaders from the US Department of Veterans Affairs. J Am Med Inform Assoc. 2013;20(e1):e175-7.
14. Schuster PM, Gjerde CL. Nursing consultation: A framework for action. Springer Publishing Company; 2017.
15. The Joint Commission (TJC). Comprehensive accreditation manual for hospitals: The official handbook, Oak Brook, IL, The Joint Commission; 2015.
16. Wager KA, Lee FW, Glaser JP. Health care information systems: A practical approach for health care management. John Wiley & Sons; 2017.
17. Weis JM, Levy PC. Copy, paste, and cloned notes in electronic health records. Chest.2014;145(3):632.

5 Section

Ensuring Quality in Nursing Practice

Section Outline

16

Quality Management

CHAPTER 16

Learning Objectives

- Understand the significance of quality and quality assurance in nursing.
- Define quality assurance in nursing.
- Identify the key components of quality assurance in nursing.
- Examine the various definitions of total quality management (TQM) in nursing.
- Differentiate between quality control and quality improvement in nursing.
- Recognize the purposes of quality management in nursing.
- Explore the key principles of quality management in nursing.
- Discuss the various models of quality assurance/management in nursing.
- Explain the various methods of quality assessment in nursing.

INTRODUCTION

In today's increasingly competitive and globalized world, the pursuit of quality has become a fundamental aspect of success for any organization, industry, or individual. Whether in the manufacturing of goods, the delivery of services, or the development of software, the quest for excellence drives innovation, customer satisfaction, and overall organizational performance. At the heart of this pursuit lies the principles of quality and quality assurance.

Quality in nursing encompasses much more than just clinical competence; it is a holistic approach that involves delivering compassionate, patient-centered care that addresses both physical and emotional needs. We will delve into the multifaceted nature of quality nursing care, examining the importance of empathy, communication, evidence-based practice, and continuous learning in achieving excellence.

QUALITY ASSURANCE

Quality assurance is the systematic and proactive approach that empowers nurses and healthcare organizations to deliver consistent and safe care. We will explore how quality assurance processes and protocols are integrated into nursing practice, focusing on monitoring, evaluation, and continuous improvement initiatives that enhance patient safety and overall care quality.

DEFINITIONS

- **Marquis and Huston (2019):** "Quality assurance in nursing refers to the ongoing, systematic, and comprehensive activities implemented to evaluate and improve the quality and safety of patient care. It involves the development of standards, the monitoring of performance against these standards, and the implementation of corrective actions to enhance patient outcomes."

- **Finkelman (2016):** "Quality assurance in nursing is the process of consistently examining nursing practices, identifying potential areas for improvement, and implementing evidence-based strategies to enhance the effectiveness and efficiency of nursing care. It encompasses the assessment of clinical competence, patient satisfaction, and the integration of best practices into daily nursing routines."

- **Sherman and Pross (2018):** "In nursing, quality assurance refers to the organized and systematic efforts to ensure that nursing care consistently meets established standards of excellence. It involves a commitment to continuous quality improvement, the measurement of key performance indicators, and the implementation of quality enhancement initiatives to provide optimal patient outcomes."

- **Hughes and Parker (2015):** "Quality assurance in nursing involves a multifaceted approach to delivering patient-centered care that is safe, effective, and efficient. It includes the evaluation of nursing processes, the identification of potential risks, and the implementation of evidence-based guidelines to minimize errors and improve the overall quality of care."

COMPONENTS OF QUALITY ASSURANCE IN NURSING

Quality assurance in nursing involves several key components that work together to ensure the highest standards of patient care and safety. These components are designed to systematically evaluate nursing practices, identify areas for improvement, and implement evidence-based strategies to enhance the overall quality of care. The key components of quality assurance in nursing include:

- **Standards and guidelines:** Establishing clear and evidence-based standards and guidelines is fundamental to quality assurance in nursing. These standards serve as a reference for nurses to follow best practices, protocols, and procedures in various clinical situations. They ensure consistency in care delivery and help maintain a high level of quality across different healthcare settings.

- **Performance monitoring and measurement:** Regularly monitoring and measuring nursing performance is essential for identifying variations from established standards. This component involves the collection and analysis of data related to nursing care, patient outcomes, and other relevant metrics. Performance indicators may include patient satisfaction scores, clinical outcomes, adherence to protocols, and infection rates.

- **Clinical audits and reviews:** Conducting clinical audits and reviews allows for a thorough examination of nursing practices and processes. These audits assess whether care provided aligns with established standards and guidelines. The findings from audits help identify areas for improvement and enable corrective actions to be taken to enhance the quality of care.

- **Continuous professional development:** Quality assurance in nursing emphasizes the importance of continuous professional development. Nurses are encouraged to stay updated with the latest evidence-based practices, attend relevant workshops, conferences, and training sessions, and engage in self-assessment to enhance their clinical competence and knowledge.

- **Risk management:** Identifying and mitigating potential risks in nursing care is a critical component of quality assurance. This involves proactive measures to prevent errors, adverse events, and patient harm. Nurses play an active role in reporting incidents, near misses, and potential hazards to promote a culture of safety and quality improvement.

- **Interdisciplinary collaboration:** Quality assurance in nursing extends beyond the individual nurse and requires collaboration with other healthcare professionals. Interdisciplinary teamwork ensures that nursing care is integrated into the overall patient care plan and that communication and coordination among healthcare providers are optimized.

- **Feedback and communication:** Encouraging open and transparent communication is essential for quality assurance in nursing. Regular feedback loops, peer reviews, and constructive feedback from patients and colleagues contribute to continuous improvement and foster a culture of excellence.

- **Implementing evidence-based practices:** Ensuring that nursing care is based on the best available evidence is a cornerstone of quality assurance. Nurses are encouraged to apply evidence-based practices in their decision-making, incorporating the latest research findings and clinical guidelines into their care plans.

- **Compliance with regulations and standards:** Adhering to relevant regulations, professional standards, and accreditation requirements is vital for maintaining quality in nursing practice. Compliance with these guidelines ensures that nursing care meets the highest standards of safety and effectiveness.

By integrating these key components into their practice, nurses can contribute significantly to the delivery of high-quality care and continuously improve patient outcomes, safety, and satisfaction. Quality assurance in nursing is an ongoing commitment that requires collaboration, dedication, and a commitment to excellence from all healthcare professionals involved in patient care.

TOTAL QUALITY MANAGEMENT

In the ever-evolving landscape of healthcare, the pursuit of excellence in patient care stands as the core objective of nursing professionals worldwide. Total quality management (TQM) has emerged as a powerful framework that seeks to revolutionize nursing practices, placing patient well-being and safety at the heart of the healthcare ecosystem.

Total Quality Management is a holistic and all-encompassing approach that aims to achieve excellence in every aspect of nursing practice. Drawing inspiration from the business world, TQM's core principles, such as customer focus, continuous improvement, and data-driven decision-making, find profound application in nursing. We delve into the foundational principles of TQM and explore how they can be tailored to address the unique challenges and complexities of nursing practice.

DEFINITIONS

- Total quality management (TQM) in Nursing is a philosophy that places the patient at the center of all nursing activities. It involves a commitment to ongoing improvement, a focus on preventing errors, and the implementation of best practices to deliver high-quality care and ensure patient safety.

- Total quality management (TQM) in Nursing is a transformative approach that empowers nurses to deliver the best possible care by incorporating continuous improvement principles, fostering a culture of teamwork and open communication, and embracing evidence-based practices to achieve optimal patient outcomes.

- Total quality management (TQM) in Nursing is a comprehensive system that aims to enhance patient care and safety by promoting a culture of excellence, involving all healthcare professionals in quality improvement initiatives, and using data and feedback to drive positive change.

- Total quality management (TQM) in Nursing is a patient-centered philosophy that seeks to provide the highest quality of care by continuously assessing and improving nursing practices, fostering collaboration among healthcare teams, and maintaining a strong focus on patient satisfaction and safety.

■ COMPONENTS OF QUALITY MANAGEMENTS

Quality control and quality improvement are two essential components of quality management. While they share the common goal of ensuring product or service quality, they have distinct roles and approaches in achieving that objective.

Quality Control

Quality control (QC) is the process of monitoring and inspecting products or services to identify defects, errors, or deviations from the established quality standards. Its primary focus is on detecting and addressing issues during or after the production or service delivery process. Here are some key aspects of quality control:

- **Inspection:** QC involves conducting inspections, tests, and measurements to check whether the output meets the predefined quality criteria.
- **Reactive approach:** Quality control is a reactive approach, as it identifies and deals with issues after they have occurred.
- **Defect detection:** The main purpose of quality control is to identify defects or non-conformities and take corrective actions to prevent further occurrences.
- **Conformance to standards:** Quality control ensures that products or services conform to the established quality standards and specifications.
- **Control charts:** Control charts are often used in quality control to monitor process performance and identify any variations that may indicate potential issues.

Quality Improvement

Quality improvement is a proactive and continuous process focused on enhancing processes, products, and services to achieve better outcomes and customer satisfaction. It involves analyzing data, identifying areas for enhancement, and implementing changes to achieve higher quality levels. Key aspects of quality improvement include:

- **Continuous improvement:** Quality improvement is an ongoing effort to make incremental and significant advancements in quality over time.
- **Data analysis:** Improvement initiatives rely on data analysis to identify trends, patterns, and opportunities for enhancement.
- **Root cause analysis:** Quality improvement efforts often involve conducting root cause analysis to determine the underlying reasons behind issues or deficiencies.
- **Process optimization:** Quality improvement aims to optimize processes and eliminate waste to enhance efficiency and effectiveness.
- **Quality management tools:** Various quality management tools, such as Six Sigma, Lean, and total quality management (TQM), are employed to drive improvement efforts.

■ DIFFERENCES BETWEEN QUALITY CONTROL AND QUALITY IMPROVEMENT

In nursing, quality control focuses on ensuring that patient care adheres to established standards and guidelines. It involves activities such as monitoring patient care processes, auditing medical records, and conducting compliance checks to identify and correct any deviations from the protocols. On the other hand, quality improvement in nursing aims to proactively enhance patient care processes and outcomes. It involves data analysis to identify areas for improvement, root cause analysis to understand the underlying issues, and implementation of evidence-based practices to enhance healthcare delivery. **Table 16.1** highlighting the key differences between quality control and quality improvement in nursing.

■ PURPOSES OF QUALITY MANAGEMENT

- Enhance patient safety and reduce medical errors.
- Improve the overall quality of patient care and outcomes.

Table 16.1: Differences between quality control and quality improvement.

Aspect	Quality control	Quality improvement
Focus	Ensuring adherence to established standards and guidelines	Proactively enhancing patient care processes and outcomes
Approach	Reactive—detects and addresses issues after they occur	Proactive—constantly seeks to identify areas for improvement
Purpose	Identifying and correcting deviations from established protocols	Achieving better patient outcomes and enhancing healthcare practices
Timing	During or after patient care delivery	Continuous and ongoing process
Primary activities	Monitoring, auditing, and compliance checks	Data analysis, root cause analysis, and process optimization
Goal	Preventing errors and ensuring patient safety	Improve healthcare efficiency, effectiveness, and patient experience
Key characteristics	Use of checklists and audits for compliance	Data-driven decision-making and implementation of evidence-based practices

- Ensure compliance with established healthcare standards and guidelines.
- Implement evidence-based practices to enhance healthcare delivery.
- Continuously monitor and evaluate healthcare processes to identify areas for improvement.
- Increase patient satisfaction and experience.
- Optimize resource utilization and minimize wastage.
- Foster a culture of continuous learning and improvement among healthcare professionals.
- Enhance communication and collaboration among healthcare teams.
- Promote accountability and responsibility in patient care.
- Reduce healthcare costs through efficiency and effectiveness improvements.
- Improve risk management and patient risk assessment processes.

PRINCIPLES OF QUALITY MANAGEMENT

The principles of quality management in nursing guide healthcare professionals in delivering safe, effective, and patient-centered care. These principles are essential for maintaining high standards of nursing practice and ensuring positive patient outcomes. Here are the key principles of quality management in nursing:

- **Patient-cantered care:** The patient's needs, preferences, and values are at the center of all care decisions. Nurses prioritize the individual patient's well-being and actively involve them in their care planning and decision-making.
- **Evidence-based practice:** Nursing care is based on the best available evidence, including research findings, clinical guidelines, and expert consensus. Nurses continuously update their knowledge and practices to provide the most effective and up-to-date care.
- **Continuous quality improvement:** Nurses engage in ongoing efforts to identify opportunities for improvement, monitor performance, and implement changes to enhance the quality of care provided.
- **Teamwork and collaboration:** Effective communication and collaboration among healthcare teams are essential to ensure seamless and coordinated patient care. Nurses work collaboratively with other healthcare professionals to optimize patient outcomes.
- **Safety first:** Patient safety is paramount. Nurses adhere to safety protocols, identify

potential risks, and actively work to prevent errors, infections, and adverse events.

- **Ethical practice:** Nurses adhere to ethical standards and maintain patient confidentiality while ensuring that care decisions align with ethical principles.
- **Accountability and responsibility:** Nurses take responsibility for their actions and are accountable for the care they provide. They strive to deliver care in a manner consistent with professional standards and best practices.
- **Patient education and empowerment:** Nurses educate patients and their families about their conditions, treatment options, and self-care management. Empowering patients with knowledge enables them to participate actively in their care.
- **Cultural competence:** Nurses respect and consider patients' cultural backgrounds, beliefs, and values while delivering care. They recognize and respond to the unique healthcare needs of diverse patient populations.
- **Efficiency and resource utilization:** Nurses strive to provide efficient and cost-effective care without compromising quality. They optimize resource utilization to achieve the best possible outcomes for patients.
- **Communication and information sharing:** Effective communication is essential to convey critical information accurately and promptly among healthcare teams. Nurses ensure that important patient information is communicated clearly and comprehensively.
- **Regulatory compliance:** Nurses adhere to all applicable laws, regulations, and standards governing nursing practice to ensure quality and safety in healthcare delivery.

MODELS FOR QUALITY MANAGEMENT/ QUALITY ASSURANCES IN NURSING

In nursing, there are several models and frameworks used for quality management and quality assurance. Here are some prominent ones:

The Donabedian's Model of Quality Care

One of the commonly used quality management models in nursing is the Donabedian's Model of Quality Care. Developed by Avedis Donabedian, a prominent healthcare quality expert, this model provides a framework for assessing and improving healthcare quality. The Donabedian's Model consists of three interrelated components: structure, process, and outcomes. Let's explore each component:

1. Structure

The "structure" component of the Donabedian's Model refers to the underlying foundation and resources of the healthcare system. It includes the physical, organizational, and human resources that support the delivery of healthcare. Some aspects of structure that are evaluated in nursing include:

- Facilities and physical environment of the healthcare setting.
- Availability and qualification of healthcare staff, including nurses and other healthcare professionals.
- Adequacy of medical equipment, technology, and supplies.
- Policies, protocols, and guidelines in place to govern care delivery.
- Management and leadership practices within the healthcare organization.

2. Process

The "process" component of the model focuses on the actual delivery of healthcare and how care is provided to patients. This aspect assesses the methods, procedures, and interactions involved in delivering care. For nursing, the process component includes:

- Adherence to evidence-based practice guidelines and standards of care.
- The effectiveness and efficiency of nursing interventions and treatments.
- Communication and collaboration among healthcare team members.

- Patient education and engagement in their care.
- Documentation and record-keeping practices.

3. Outcomes

The "outcomes" component evaluates the impact of healthcare on patients' health status and overall well-being. It includes measures of the results of care and the achievement of desired patient outcomes. In nursing, outcome measures include:

- Patient satisfaction with nursing care.
- Improvement in the patient's health status and symptoms.
- Reduced rates of complications and adverse events.
- Length of hospital stay and readmission rates.
- Patient-reported quality of life and functional outcomes.

The American Nurses Association (ANA) Model for Quality Management

The American Nurses Association (ANA) model for quality management is a comprehensive framework designed to guide nurses and healthcare organizations in delivering high-quality care. It emphasizes the importance of nursing practice in ensuring patient safety, improving outcomes, and enhancing the overall healthcare system. The ANA Model for Quality Management incorporates principles of patient-centered care, evidence-based practice, and continuous quality improvement.

The ANA Model for Quality involves a systematic process that includes the eight steps presented in **Figure 16.1**.

Identify Value

- Assess patient/client needs and rights from various perspectives (economic, social, psychological, and spiritual).
- Recognize the values and philosophy of the healthcare organization and nursing service providers.

Identify Structure, Process, and Outcome Standards and Criteria

- Establish structural standards based on the organization's philosophy and objectives.
- Evaluate the agency's structural standards using internal or external groups.
- Define process standards by referencing professional organization standards or agency-specific procedures.
- Evaluate process standards through peer review committees and client satisfaction surveys.
- Determine outcome standards by assessing changes in the client's health status due to nursing care.
- Evaluate outcome standards using research studies, client satisfaction surveys, and client classification.

Select Measurement Needed to Determine Degree of Attainment of Criteria and Standards

- Choose appropriate measurement tools based on the selected standards and criteria.
- Utilize techniques like nursing audits, utilization reviews, direct observations, questionnaires, and interviews for evaluation.

Make Interpretations

- Evaluate the level of compliance with criteria to identify program strengths and weaknesses.
- Compare the compliance rate with the expected level of criteria accomplishment.

Identify Course of Action

- If compliance exceeds expectations, provide positive feedback and reinforcement.
- If compliance falls below expectations, identify the causes of deficiency and various solutions to address the problems.

Choose Action

- Consider different alternative courses of action, weighing pros and cons while considering the environmental context and resource availability.

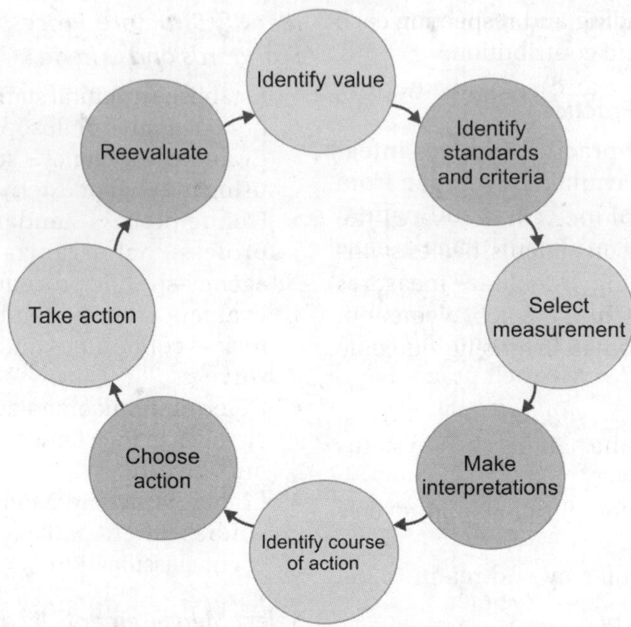

Fig. 16.1: The basic components of ANA model.

- Address each contributing factor if multiple causes of deficiency are identified.

Take Action

- Establish accountability for the proposed actions, defining responsibilities and timelines.
- Implement the chosen courses of action.

Reevaluate

- Evaluate the results of the actions taken.
- Reassess in the same manner as the original assessment, initiating a new cycle of the quality assurance process.
- Offer positive reinforcement for successful improvements and decide when to reevaluate aspects of care that still require attention.

The Quality and Safety Education for Nurses (QSEN) Model

The Quality and Safety Education for Nurses (QSEN) Model is a widely recognized framework that aims to prepare nurses with the knowledge, skills, and attitudes necessary to deliver safe, high-quality care. Developed in response to the Institute of Medicine's landmark report "To Err Is Human," which highlighted the need for improving patient safety in healthcare, the QSEN Model was launched in 2005 by a collaborative effort of nursing educators and leaders.

The QSEN Model incorporates six core competencies that guide nursing education and practice:

1. Patient-centered Care

- Patient-centered care involves recognizing the patient as the source of control and full partner in their healthcare decisions.
- Nurses should communicate effectively with patients and their families, respect their preferences and values, and provide compassionate and coordinated care.

2. Teamwork and Collaboration

- Effective communication and collaboration among healthcare professionals are essential for providing safe and efficient care.
- Nurses need to work collaboratively with other members of the healthcare

team, understanding and respecting each member's role and contribution.

3. Evidence-based Practice

- Evidence-based practice involves integrating the best available evidence from research, clinical expertise, and patient preferences to make informed care decisions.
- Nurses should continually update their knowledge and skills based on the latest evidence and apply it to their practice.

4. Quality Improvement

- Quality improvement focuses on continuously monitoring and evaluating healthcare processes to identify areas for improvement.
- Nurses should actively participate in quality improvement initiatives, using data to drive changes and enhance patient outcomes.

5. Safety

- Patient safety is paramount in nursing practice, aiming to prevent harm to patients and healthcare providers.
- Nurses should identify and mitigate risks, adhere to safety protocols, and contribute to a culture of safety in their healthcare setting.

6. Informatics

- Informatics involves using information and technology to improve patient care and healthcare delivery.
- Nurses should be competent in using health information systems, electronic health records, and other informatics tools to support safe and efficient care.

The QSEN Model has significantly influenced nursing education curricula, promoting the integration of these competencies into nursing programs. It encourages the use of simulation, case studies, and experiential learning to prepare nurses for real-world challenges in delivering safe and quality care.

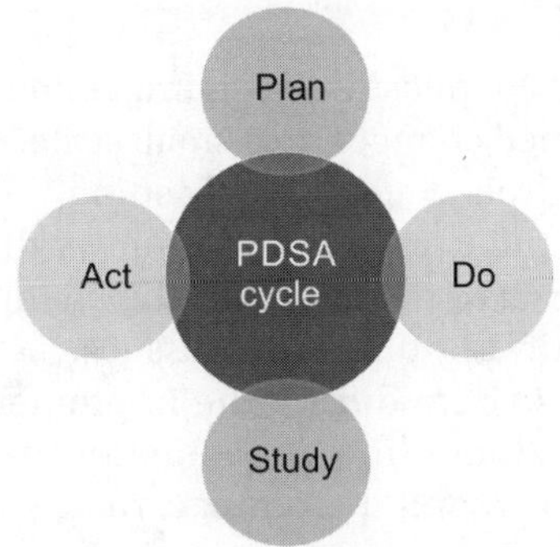

Fig. 16.2: Components of the Plan-Do-Study-Act (PDSA) cycle.

The Plan-Do-Study-Act (PDSA) Cycle

The Plan-Do-Study-Act (PDSA) Cycle, also known as the Deming Cycle or the Shewhart Cycle, is a continuous improvement framework widely used in various industries, including healthcare. It was developed by Walter A. Shewhart in the 1920s and popularized by W. Edwards Deming in the 1950s. The PDSA Cycle provides a structured approach to implementing and testing changes to improve processes, solve problems, and achieve better outcomes. The cycle consists of four iterative steps: Plan, Do, Study, and Act depicted in **Figure 16.2**.

1. Plan

- In the "Plan" phase, the team identifies a problem or an opportunity for improvement and develops a plan for change.
- Define the objectives and goals of the improvement initiative and establish specific, measurable, achievable, relevant, and time-bound (SMART) aims.
- Conduct a thorough analysis of the current process, collect relevant data, and identify potential barriers or challenges.
- Formulate a detailed plan for change, including the proposed interventions, strategies, and resources required for implementation.
- Develop a prediction or hypothesis about the expected outcomes of the change.

2. Do

- The "Do" phase involves implementing the planned changes on a small scale, often in a controlled and limited setting.
- This pilot or test phase allows the team to observe the effects of the changes and identify any unexpected issues.
- Collect data during the implementation to evaluate how the changes are being executed and their impact on the process and outcomes.
- Document the process of implementation, including any modifications made during the test.

3. Study

- The "Study" phase involves analyzing the data collected during the implementation to assess the results of the change.
- Compare the actual outcomes with the predicted or hypothesized outcomes to determine if the change has been successful in achieving the desired objectives.
- Consider the impact of the change on different aspects, such as quality, efficiency, safety, and patient satisfaction.
- Identify patterns or trends in the data and evaluate the effectiveness of the change in addressing the identified problem or opportunity.

4. Act

- In the "Act" phase, the team decides whether to adopt, modify, or abandon the change based on the findings from the Study phase.
- If the change was successful and achieved the desired outcomes, it is implemented on a broader scale and integrated into the standard practice.
- If the change did not produce the expected results, the team reviews the data to understand the reasons for the failure and makes necessary adjustments or iterations to improve the change.

- Once the adjustments are made, the PDSA Cycle starts again, repeating the Plan-Do-Study-Act process to continually improve and refine the process or intervention.

The PDSA Cycle promotes a culture of continuous improvement by encouraging teams to test small changes, learn from the results, and make data-driven decisions. It is a flexible and adaptable model that allows healthcare organizations to address complex challenges and achieve sustained improvements in patient care, safety, and operational efficiency. The PDSA Cycle is widely used in quality improvement initiatives, research studies, and process improvement projects across healthcare settings to achieve better patient outcomes and enhance the overall delivery of care.

QUALITY ASSESSMENT METHODS IN NURSING

Quality assessment methods in nursing are used to evaluate and measure the quality of healthcare services and patient outcomes. These methods aim to identify areas for improvement and ensure that nursing care meets established standards and best practices. Several quality assessment methods are employed in nursing, including:

Nursing Audits

- Nursing audits involve systematic and objective reviews of nursing practices, processes, and documentation to assess compliance with standards and guidelines.
- These audits can be conducted internally within the healthcare organization or by external accrediting bodies.

Patient Satisfaction Surveys

- Patient satisfaction surveys collect feedback from patients regarding their experiences with nursing care and overall healthcare services.

- The information gathered helps identify areas of strength and areas that may need improvement to enhance patient satisfaction.

Clinical Indicators and Benchmarking

- Clinical indicators are measurable variables used to monitor the quality of care and patient outcomes.
- Benchmarking involves comparing an organization's performance against established standards or best-performing healthcare institutions to identify opportunities for improvement.

Peer Review

- Peer review involves healthcare professionals evaluating the performance of their colleagues to ensure adherence to standards of care and ethical principles.
- This method encourages a culture of accountability and continuous improvement.

Root Cause Analysis (RCA)

- RCA is a structured approach used to investigate adverse events, errors, or sentinel events to identify their underlying causes.
- The findings from RCA help implement corrective actions to prevent similar occurrences in the future.

Direct Observation

- Direct observation involves a qualified observer monitoring and assessing nursing practices and patient interactions in real-time.
- This method provides valuable insights into the actual delivery of care and adherence to best practices.

Chart Reviews

- Chart reviews involve the assessment of patient records and documentation to ensure accuracy, completeness, and compliance with standards of care.
- This method helps identify potential issues related to documentation and care delivery.

Readmission and Length of Stay Analysis

- Analyzing readmission rates and length of hospital stays can provide valuable information on the quality and effectiveness of nursing care.
- Higher readmission rates may indicate potential gaps in care or patient education.

Clinical Pathways and Care Protocols

- Clinical pathways and care protocols are evidence-based guidelines that outline best practices for specific conditions or procedures.
- Following standardized pathways can improve care consistency and patient outcomes.

Patient Outcome Measures

- Patient outcome measures assess specific aspects of patient health and functional status to evaluate the effectiveness of nursing interventions.
- Examples include pain scores, wound healing rates, and patient mobility assessments.

By employing these quality assessment methods, nursing professionals and healthcare organizations can continuously improve the quality of nursing care and ultimately enhance patient outcomes and safety.

CHAPTER SUMMARY

1. In nursing, quality encompasses more than just clinical competence; it involves delivering compassionate and patient-centered care that addresses physical and emotional needs.
2. Quality assurance is a systematic and proactive approach that empowers nurses and healthcare organizations to deliver consistent and safe care.
3. Total quality management (TQM) is a holistic approach that aims to achieve excellence in every aspect of nursing practice.
4. Quality control and quality improvement are two essential components of quality management in nursing.
5. Quality control focuses on monitoring and inspecting products or services to identify defects and address issues, while quality improvement proactively enhances processes and outcomes through data analysis, root cause analysis, and process optimization.
6. The purposes of quality management in nursing include enhancing patient safety, improving the overall quality of care, ensuring compliance with standards, implementing evidence-based practices, enhancing collaboration, and reducing healthcare costs.
7. The principles of quality management in nursing guide healthcare professionals to deliver safe, effective, and patient-centered care.
8. The Donabedian's Model of Quality Care, which consists of three components: structure, process, and outcomes.
9. The American Nurses Association (ANA) Model for Quality Management, which emphasizes patient-entered care, evidence-based practice, and continuous quality improvement.
10. The Quality and Safety Education for Nurses (QSEN) Model is focusing on its six core competencies that prepare nurses to provide safe and quality care.
11. The QSEN Model's influence on nursing education curricula and its role in promoting a culture of continuous improvement are highlighted.
12. The Plan-Do-Study-Act (PDSA) Cycle is presented as a continuous improvement framework widely used in various industries, including healthcare. The four iterative steps of the PDSA Cycle are—Plan, Do, Study, and Act
13. The quality assessment methods in nursing, including nursing audits, patient satisfaction surveys, clinical indicators, peer reviews, root cause analysis, and others. These methods are essential in evaluating the quality of nursing care and identifying areas for improvement.

REVIEW QUESTIONS

1. Define quality and explain the importance of quality assurance in nursing.
2. Explain the multifaceted nature of quality nursing care and why it encompasses much more than just clinical competence.
3. Define quality assurance in nursing and analyze the key components of quality assurance in nursing.
4. Discuss the concept of Total Quality Management (TQM) in nursing and explore the purposes of quality management in nursing.
5. Examine the key principles of quality management in nursing.
6. Discuss the American Nurses Association (ANA) Model for Quality Management in nursing.
7. Explain the quality assessment methods in nursing.

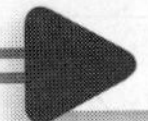 **BIBLIOGRAPHY** 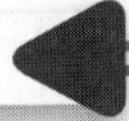

1. Donabedian A. Criteria and standards for quality assessment and monitoring. Qual Rev Bull. 1986;12(3):99-108. Http://Www.Ncbi.Nlm.Nih.Gov/Pubmed/3085044

2. Donabedian A. Quality of care: problems of measurement. II. Some issues in evaluating the quality of nursing care. Am J Public Health Nations Health. 1969;59(10):1833-6.

3. Donabedian A. The quality of care: How can it be assessed? JAMA. 1988;260(12):1743-8.

4. George ML, Rowlands D, Price M, Maxey, J. The Lean Six Sigma Pocket Toolbook: A Quick Reference Guide to 100 Tools for Improving Quality and Speed. McGraw-Hill Education; 2005.

5. Joint Commission on Accreditation of Health Care Organizations. An introduction to quality improvement in health care. Chicago; 1991.

6. Oakland JS. Total Quality Management and Operational Excellence: Text with Cases. Routledge; 2003.

7. Reddy BK, Arundhathy M, Acharyulu GVRK. A strategy for successful TQM in a corporate hospital—a study using six sigma. J Acad Hosp Adm. 2002;14(2):7-14.

8. Sherman JJ, Malkmus MA. Integrating quality assurance and total quality management/ quality management. J Nurs Adm. 1994;24(3):37-41. Http://Www.Ncbi.Nlm.Nih.Gov/Pubmed/8133323

9. Toussaint JS, Berry LL. The promise of lean in health care. Mayo Clinic Proceedings. 2013;88(1): 74-82.

17

Nursing Standard and Audit

- Define nursing standards and their significance in guiding and evaluating nursing practice.
- Understand the purpose of nursing standards.
- Describe the process of setting quality standards in nursing practice.
- Identify the key elements involved in developing evidence-based and patient-centered nursing standards.
- Explain the methods and tools used to measure and assess nursing quality standards.
- Describe the different types of nursing practice standards, including ethical, professional, and clinical standards.
- Recognize the role of nursing practice standards in guiding ethical decision-making, professional conduct, and clinical interventions.
- Define nursing audit and its purpose in evaluating the adherence to nursing standards and identifying areas for improvement.
- Identify the steps involved in conducting a nursing audit and utilizing audit findings to enhance nursing practice.
- Understand the role and function of nursing councils and professional bodies in establishing and enforcing nursing standards.
- Recognize the significance of regulatory bodies in ensuring the competence and accountability of nursing professionals.

INTRODUCTION

In the dynamic and rapidly evolving field of healthcare, nursing standards play a crucial role in guiding nurses through the complexities of their roles. Nursing standards serve as the foundation of quality and compassionate patient care, ensuring that nursing practice aligns with the highest levels of professionalism, ethics, and evidence-based approaches. These standards are essential guidelines that govern the delivery of nursing services and are designed to uphold the safety, well-being, and dignity of patients while promoting the development and maintenance of competent nursing professionals.

DEFINITIONS

- The American Nurses Association defines nursing standards as "the authoritative statements of the duties that all registered nurses, regardless of role, population, or specialty, are expected to perform competently". *(ANA, 2015)*
- The International Council of Nurses defines nursing standards as "the criteria or norm

against which behavior or performance can be measured". **(ICN, 2009)**

- The Nursing and Midwifery Board of Australia defines nursing standards as "the benchmark for assessing nursing practice and performance". **(NMBA, 2016)**
- The National League for Nursing defines nursing standards as "the authoritative statements that describe the responsibilities for which nurses are accountable". **(NLN, 2000)**

SIGNIFICANCE OF NURSING STANDARDS

The significance of nursing standards lies in their crucial role in shaping and maintaining the quality, safety, and professionalism of nursing practice. Here are the key points that highlight the significance of nursing standards:

- Ensures consistent and high-quality patient care
- Provides a clear framework for nursing practice
- Promotes patient safety and well-being
- Guides ethical decision-making and professional conduct
- Enhances patient outcomes and satisfaction
- Facilitates effective communication and collaboration among healthcare professionals
- Supports evidence-based practice and continuous improvement
- Establishes accountability and responsibility in nursing practice
- Fosters a culture of professionalism and lifelong learning
- Ensures compliance with regulatory and accreditation requirements
- Contributes to the credibility and reputation of the nursing profession.

PURPOSES FOR NURSING STANDARDS

The purposes of nursing standards are multifaceted and serve to guide, enhance, and maintain the quality and professionalism of nursing practice. Here are some of the key purposes for nursing standards:

- **Ensuring patient safety and quality of care:** Nursing standards provide guidelines and benchmarks that promote safe and high-quality patient care, reducing the risk of errors and adverse events.
- **Guiding ethical practice:** Nursing standards outline ethical principles and professional behaviors expected of nurses, ensuring that ethical considerations are integrated into nursing care.
- **Establishing professional accountability:** Nursing standards define the roles and responsibilities of nurses, promoting professional accountability and fostering a culture of excellence in nursing practice.
- **Supporting evidence-based practice:** Nursing standards encourage the use of evidence-based practice, integrating the best available evidence with clinical expertise and patient preferences to optimize patient outcomes.
- **Facilitating interdisciplinary collaboration:** Standardized nursing practices enable effective collaboration with other healthcare professionals, enhancing teamwork and promoting seamless patient care.
- **Promoting continuous professional development:** Nursing standards encourage ongoing learning and professional development, ensuring that nurses stay updated with the latest advancements in healthcare.
- **Guiding education and training:** Nursing standards provide a foundation for nursing education curricula and training programs, ensuring that future nurses are equipped with the necessary knowledge and skills.
- **Ensuring regulatory compliance:** Nursing standards are essential for regulatory and licensing purposes, ensuring that nurses meet the required competencies and maintain professional standards.
- **Supporting research and innovation:** Adherence to nursing standards contributes to research efforts and the advancement of

nursing science, driving innovation and improvements in patient care.

- **Enhancing patient satisfaction:** By adhering to nursing standards, nurses provide consistent, competent, and patient-centered care, leading to increased patient satisfaction.
- **Facilitating quality improvement:** Nursing standards serve as a basis for evaluating and improving nursing practices, fostering a culture of continuous quality improvement in healthcare settings.
- **Strengthening the nursing profession:** Nursing standards elevate the credibility and professionalism of the nursing profession, emphasizing its critical role in the healthcare system.

QUALITY STANDARD PROCESS

The process of setting quality standards in nursing practice involves several steps to ensure that the standards are evidence-based, achievable, and aligned with the overall goals of providing safe and effective patient care. Here is a description of the process:

- **Identify the need for quality standards:** The process begins by recognizing the need for quality standards in nursing practice. This may arise from a desire to improve patient outcomes, enhance patient safety, comply with regulatory requirements, or align with best practices in the healthcare industry.
- **Review existing literature and guidelines:** Next, a comprehensive review of existing literature, evidence-based guidelines, and best practices related to nursing care is conducted. This step helps identify established standards and evidence supporting effective nursing interventions and patient care.
- **Involve stakeholders:** Stakeholders, including nurses, nursing leaders, healthcare administrators, patient representatives, and other healthcare professionals, are involved in the process. Their input and perspectives are essential to ensure that the quality standards reflect the needs and expectations of all stakeholders.

- **Establish a quality standards committee:** A committee or task force is formed to oversee the development of quality standards. This committee may consist of subject matter experts, nursing leaders, educators, researchers, and representatives from different nursing specialties.
- **Define the scope and objectives:** The committee defines the scope and objectives of the quality standards. This includes identifying the specific areas of nursing practice to be covered by the standards and setting measurable goals for improvement.
- **Draft the quality standards:** Based on the literature review, stakeholder input, and committee expertise, the quality standards are drafted. These standards should be specific, measurable, achievable, relevant, and time-bound (SMART).
- **Pilot testing:** Before finalizing the quality standards, they are pilot tested in a clinical setting to assess their feasibility and effectiveness. Feedback from nurses and other stakeholders is gathered to refine the standards as needed.
- **Seek expert review and approval:** The draft quality standards are submitted for expert review to ensure that they are evidence-based and align with best practices. Once reviewed and approved by experts, the standards are ready for implementation.
- **Implement and monitor:** The approved quality standards are implemented across nursing practice settings. Nursing staff is educated and trained on the new standards to ensure consistent adherence. Regular monitoring and evaluation of compliance with the standards are conducted.
- **Continuous quality improvement:** The process of setting quality standards does not end with implementation. A continuous quality improvement process is established to review the effectiveness of the standards, identify areas for improvement, and make necessary revisions based on feedback and emerging evidence.

- **Communicate and disseminate:** Effective communication and dissemination of the quality standards are essential to ensure that all nurses and healthcare professionals are aware of the standards and their importance in providing high-quality care.
- **Reassess and update:** As healthcare practices evolve and new evidence emerges, the quality standards should be regularly reassessed and updated to remain current and relevant to the changing healthcare landscape.

DEVELOPMENT OF EVIDENCE-BASED AND PATIENT-CENTERED NURSING STANDARDS

Developing evidence-based and patient-centered nursing standards involves considering several key elements to ensure that the standards are grounded in the best available evidence and focused on meeting the unique needs and preferences of patients. Here are the key elements involved in this process:

- **Evidence-based practice:**
  - Conduct a comprehensive literature review to gather the best available evidence related to nursing interventions and patient care.
  - Ensure that the standards are aligned with evidence-based guidelines, protocols, and recommendations from reputable sources, such as professional nursing organizations and healthcare regulatory bodies.
  - Involve nurse researchers and experts in the development process to incorporate the latest research findings into the standards.
- **Clinical expertise:**
  - Engage experienced and knowledgeable nurses with expertise in different nursing specialties to contribute their clinical insights to the development of the standards.
  - Recognize and incorporate the valuable insights gained from years of practical experience and patient interactions.

- **Patient and family input:**
  - Involve patients and their families as active partners in the development of nursing standards to ensure that the standards are patient-centered and address patients' unique needs, preferences, and concerns.
  - Gather feedback from patients and families through focus groups, surveys, or advisory councils to incorporate their perspectives into the standards.
- **Holistic approach:**
  - Embrace a holistic approach to patient care that considers the physical, emotional, social, and spiritual aspects of patients' well-being.
  - Develop standards that address the whole person and focus on promoting health and well-being, rather than merely treating symptoms.
- **Ethical considerations:**
  - Ensure that the nursing standards adhere to ethical principles and respect patients' autonomy, confidentiality, and dignity.
  - Address ethical challenges that may arise in nursing practice and outline guidelines for ethical decision-making.
- **Cultural competence:**
  - Recognize the diversity of patients and their cultural backgrounds.
  - Develop standards that promote cultural competence in nursing care, respecting patients' cultural beliefs and values.
- **Interdisciplinary collaboration:**
  - Foster collaboration among healthcare professionals to develop comprehensive and coordinated care plans that address the complex needs of patients.
  - Ensure that the nursing standards complement and align with the standards of other healthcare disciplines.
- **Continuous quality improvement:**
  - Establish a framework for continuous quality improvement to monitor the effectiveness of the nursing standards and make necessary revisions based on feedback and evaluation data.

- Encourage a culture of learning and openness to change and improvement.
- **Communication and education:**
  - Effectively communicate the nursing standards to all nursing staff and healthcare professionals involved in patient care.
  - Provide education and training on the standards to ensure consistent implementation.
- **Regulatory and accreditation compliance:** Ensure that the nursing standards align with relevant regulatory and accreditation requirements to maintain compliance with healthcare standards and guidelines.

By considering these key elements, nursing organizations and healthcare institutions can develop nursing standards that are evidence-based, patient-centered, and aligned with best practices in nursing care, leading to improved patient outcomes and enhanced nursing practice.

QUALITY STANDARD MEASUREMENT METHODS OR TOOLS

Measuring and assessing nursing quality standards is essential to ensure that nursing practices meet established benchmarks and provide high-quality, safe, and effective care to patients. Various methods and tools are used for this purpose. Here are some commonly used methods and tools:

- **Nursing quality indicators:** Nursing quality indicators are specific measures or metrics used to assess the performance of nursing care. These indicators may include patient outcomes, safety measures, patient satisfaction scores, nursing-sensitive indicators (e.g., pressure ulcers, falls, medication errors), and adherence to evidence-based nursing practices. Regularly monitoring and analyzing these indicators help identify areas for improvement and track the effectiveness of nursing interventions.
- **Audits and chart reviews:** Conducting audits and chart reviews is a method to evaluate the compliance of nursing care with established standards and protocols. Audits involve systematically reviewing patient records, nursing documentation, and processes to ensure adherence to best practices, policies, and guidelines. Chart reviews help identify potential gaps in care and areas for improvement.
- **Patient and family feedback:** Gathering feedback from patients and their families through surveys, focus groups, or interviews is a valuable tool to assess nursing quality from the patient's perspective. Patient satisfaction surveys and patient-reported outcome measures (PROMs) provide insights into the patient's experience and the impact of nursing care on their well-being.
- **Clinical pathways and care bundles:** Clinical pathways and care bundles are standardized, evidence-based care plans designed to guide nurses in delivering consistent and high-quality care for specific patient conditions or procedures. By adhering to these pathways and bundles, nurses can ensure that best practices are consistently applied.
- **Nursing peer review:** Nursing peer review involves nurses evaluating the care provided by their colleagues to ensure it meets established standards. Peer review can be conducted through regular peer evaluations, case presentations, or peer-led discussions about challenging cases. This process promotes continuous learning and fosters a culture of excellence.
- **Healthcare quality improvement frameworks:** Using established quality improvement frameworks, such as the Plan-Do-Study-Act (PDSA) cycle or the Six Sigma approach, enables nurses to systematically identify areas for improvement, implement changes, measure outcomes, and sustain positive changes in nursing care.
- **National and international quality reporting systems:** National and international healthcare organizations often develop and maintain quality reporting

systems that collect and analyze data on various quality indicators in nursing care. These reports can provide benchmarks and comparisons to assess nursing care performance on a broader scale.

- **Clinical simulation and skills assessment:** Clinical simulation and skills assessment allow nurses to practice and demonstrate their clinical competencies in a controlled environment. Utilizing simulation-based assessments ensures that nurses are proficient in critical nursing skills and can deliver safe and effective care.
- **Nursing dashboards and scorecards:** Nursing dashboards and scorecards provide a visual representation of key performance indicators and nursing quality metrics. They offer an easy-to-read overview of nursing performance, facilitating quick identification of areas that need improvement.
- **Continuous professional development:** Nursing education and professional development play a vital role in maintaining nursing quality standards. Nurses can participate in workshops, conferences, and continuing education programs to enhance their knowledge and skills and stay updated with best practices in nursing care.

TYPES OF NURSING PRACTICE STANDARDS

Nursing practice standards encompass various types of standards that guide the professional conduct and clinical performance of nurses. These standards provide a framework for delivering safe, competent, and ethical nursing care. The different types of nursing practice standards include:

- **Ethical standards:** Ethical standards in nursing outline the moral principles and values that guide nurses' behavior and decision-making in their interactions with patients, families, colleagues, and the broader healthcare community. Ethical standards address issues of respect for autonomy, beneficence, nonmaleficence, justice, confidentiality, and integrity. Nurses are expected to uphold these ethical standards to ensure patient safety, protect patient rights, and maintain the trust of the public in the nursing profession.
- **Professional standards:** Professional standards in nursing define the expectations for nurses in terms of their competence, responsibilities, and professional conduct. These standards cover areas such as professional development, continuing education, maintaining licensure, adherence to regulatory requirements, and participation in quality improvement initiatives. Professional standards set the bar for the level of knowledge, skills, and accountability expected of nurses throughout their careers.
- **Clinical standards:** Clinical standards in nursing pertain to the delivery of patient care and encompass evidence-based guidelines, best practices, and established protocols for various nursing interventions and procedures. These standards ensure that nursing care is consistent, safe, and based on the latest evidence. Clinical standards cover areas such as medication administration, wound care, infection control, pain management, patient assessment, and documentation. Adherence to clinical standards helps nurses provide high-quality care and achieve positive patient outcomes.
- **Scope of practice standards:** The scope of practice standards defines the range of activities, procedures, and responsibilities that a nurse is authorized and competent to perform within their specific role and level of licensure. Scope of practice standards vary among different types of nurses (e.g., registered nurses, licensed practical nurses) and across different practice settings (e.g., hospitals, clinics, home care). Adhering to the scope of practice ensures that nurses work within their competencies and avoid performing tasks beyond their training and qualifications.

- **Educational standards:** Educational standards in nursing set the requirements for nursing education and training programs. These standards govern the curriculum, faculty qualifications, clinical experiences, and learning outcomes of nursing programs. Meeting educational standards ensures that nurses receive a comprehensive and rigorous education that prepares them to meet the demands of professional nursing practice.
- **Documentation standards:** Documentation standards in nursing outline the guidelines for accurate and comprehensive documentation of patient care. Nurses are required to record patient assessments, interventions, and outcomes in a timely and organized manner. Documentation standards promote effective communication among healthcare providers and support continuity of care for patients.

ROLE OF NURSING PRACTICE STANDARDS

Nursing practice standards play a crucial role in guiding ethical decision-making, professional conduct, and clinical interventions for nurses. These standards provide a framework and set of principles that help nurses navigate complex situations, uphold ethical values, and deliver safe and competent patient care. Here's how nursing practice standards influence these aspects of nursing practice:

- **Ethical decision-making:** Nursing practice standards include ethical principles and values that guide nurses in making morally sound decisions when faced with ethical dilemmas. By adhering to these standards, nurses are better equipped to recognize ethical issues, consider the implications of various courses of action, and choose the most ethically justifiable approach. Ethical standards help nurses prioritize patient autonomy, beneficence, nonmaleficence, and justice, ensuring that patient rights and well-being remain at the forefront of decision-making.

- **Professional conduct:** Nursing practice standards define the expectations for professional conduct and behavior in the nursing profession. They outline the importance of honesty, integrity, and accountability in interactions with patients, families, colleagues, and the healthcare team. By following these standards, nurses maintain a high level of professionalism and build trust with patients and their families. They also foster a positive work environment and contribute to the overall reputation of the nursing profession.
- **Clinical interventions:** Nursing practice standards encompass evidence-based guidelines and best practices for clinical interventions. By following these standards, nurses ensure that their clinical interventions are based on the latest research and proven effective. Adhering to clinical standards enhances the quality and safety of nursing care and contributes to improved patient outcomes. It also helps nurses avoid unnecessary variations in care and ensures a consistent and standardized approach to clinical practice.
- **Patient safety and quality of care:** Nursing practice standards focus on patient safety and the delivery of high-quality care. By adhering to these standards, nurses contribute to reducing the risk of adverse events, errors, and complications during patient care. Standardized practices and evidence-based interventions help nurses deliver consistent, effective, and safe care across various healthcare settings. This commitment to patient safety and quality care is at the core of nursing practice standards.
- **Professional development:** Nursing practice standards emphasize the importance of ongoing professional development and continuing education. Nurses are encouraged to stay updated with advancements in healthcare, evidence-based practices, and new technologies. Continuous learning enables nurses to provide the best possible care, enhance

their clinical skills, and adapt to changing healthcare needs.

- **Legal and regulatory compliance:** Nursing practice standards also align with legal and regulatory requirements governing nursing practice. By adhering to these standards, nurses ensure compliance with applicable laws and regulations, protecting themselves and their patients from potential legal liabilities.

NURSING AUDIT

Nursing audit is a systematic and critical examination of nursing practices, procedures, and processes within a healthcare setting to evaluate adherence to nursing standards and identify areas for improvement. It is a quality improvement method that helps assess the effectiveness and efficiency of nursing care delivery and ensures that nursing practices align with established standards and guidelines.

DEFINITIONS

- **Audu BG, and Okafor JO (2015):** "Nursing audit is a systematic and critical examination of nursing care outcomes, nursing procedures, and nursing processes within a healthcare organization to ensure adherence to established nursing standards and identify areas for improvement in the quality of care."
- **Rana RK, and Chauhan SR (2016):** "Nursing audit is a process of evaluating and verifying nursing care delivery, nursing documentation, and nursing practices in a healthcare setting to assess the level of compliance with nursing standards, identify deviations, and facilitate quality improvement."
- **Oktay Ş., and Çıtlak GS (2020):** "Nursing audit is a comprehensive and objective review of nursing care practices, nursing documentation, and nursing outcomes in a healthcare organization, aimed at evaluating adherence to nursing standards, identifying opportunities for improvement, and optimizing patient care."

PURPOSES OF NURSING AUDIT

The purposes of nursing audit include:

- **Evaluating adherence to nursing standards:** To assess whether nursing practices, procedures, and documentation comply with established nursing standards and guidelines.
- **Identifying areas for improvement:** To pinpoint areas where nursing care can be enhanced, ensuring consistent and high-quality patient care.
- **Monitoring patient safety:** To promote patient safety by identifying potential risks, errors, and deviations from best practices.
- **Enhancing quality of care:** To ensure that nursing care is evidence-based, effective, and meets the needs of patients.
- **Promoting professional accountability:** To hold nursing staff accountable for their actions and decisions in patient care.
- **Supporting evidence-based practice:** To encourage the use of current evidence-based guidelines and best practices in nursing care.
- **Facilitating continuous quality improvement:** To drive ongoing improvement initiatives within the nursing department and healthcare organization.
- **Ensuring regulatory compliance:** To ensure that nursing practices align with legal and regulatory requirements.
- **Improving documentation:** To enhance the accuracy and completeness of nursing documentation for effective communication and continuity of care.
- **Optimizing resource utilization:** To identify areas where resources can be allocated more efficiently to improve patient care outcomes.
- **Strengthening interprofessional collaboration:** To foster effective collaboration and communication among healthcare team members.
- **Facilitating benchmarking:** To compare nursing care practices with external benchmarks and standards for performance improvement.

- **Promoting ethical practice:** To ensure that nursing care is delivered with integrity, respect for patient rights, and ethical considerations.
- **Enhancing staff development:** To identify opportunities for training, education, and professional growth for nursing staff.
- **Improving patient outcomes:** To contribute to better patient outcomes and overall healthcare quality.

TYPES OF NURSING AUDIT

Nursing audits are essential tools for assessing and improving the quality of nursing care provided to patients. Various types of nursing audits are conducted to evaluate different aspects of nursing practice and performance. Some common types of nursing audits include:

Based on Agency

Nursing audits can be categorized based on the agency or organization conducting the audit and the specific areas of focus. Some common types of nursing audits based on the agency or organization include:

- **Internal nursing audit:** This type of audit is conducted by the healthcare facility's internal quality improvement or nursing department. It focuses on evaluating and improving nursing care practices, adherence to standards, and patient outcomes within the organization.
- **External nursing audit:** External audits are conducted by external accrediting bodies or regulatory agencies to assess the quality of nursing care and overall performance of the healthcare facility. These audits ensure compliance with national or international standards and guidelines.
- **State or government nursing audit:** Government health departments or state healthcare regulatory agencies may conduct nursing audits to assess the quality of care in healthcare facilities within their jurisdiction. These audits aim to ensure patient safety and regulatory compliance.
- **Accreditation nursing audit:** Accrediting bodies, such as The Joint Commission or the commission on accreditation of rehabilitation facilities (CARF), conduct nursing audits as part of the accreditation process. These audits assess the facility's compliance with accreditation standards.
- **Professional nursing association audit:** Professional nursing associations may conduct audits to evaluate the practice standards and professional development of their members. These audits aim to ensure that nurses meet the association's standards of practice.

Based on Methodology

Nursing audits can also be categorized based on the methodology or approach used to conduct the audit. Different methodologies are employed to assess various aspects of nursing care and performance. Some common types of nursing audits based on methodology include:

- **Retrospective nursing audit:** In a retrospective audit, data is collected from past nursing records and documentation to assess the quality of care provided during a specific period. This type of audit allows for an in-depth review of nursing practices and patient outcomes over time.
- **Concurrent nursing audit:** Concurrent audits are conducted in real-time as patient care is delivered. Nursing staff and auditors work together to assess adherence to standards, identify issues, and make immediate improvements to care processes.
- **Prospective nursing audit:** In a prospective audit, auditors plan and set criteria for nursing care in advance. The audit then assesses the implementation of these planned criteria during patient care delivery.
- **Focused nursing audit:** Focused audits concentrate on specific aspects of nursing care, such as medication administration, infection control, or patient assessment. These audits target particular areas of concern or improvement.
- **Process-based nursing audit:** Process-based audits focus on evaluating nursing

processes and procedures, such as hand hygiene compliance, medication administration protocols, or patient assessment procedures.

- **Outcome-based nursing audit:** Outcome-based audits assess patient outcomes resulting from nursing care. They evaluate the effectiveness of nursing interventions and their impact on patient health and well-being.

NURSING AUDIT PROCESS

The nursing audit process is a systematic and objective examination of nursing practices, processes, and outcomes to evaluate the quality of nursing care provided to patients. It involves the collection, analysis, and interpretation of data related to nursing care to identify strengths, areas for improvement, and opportunities for enhancing patient outcomes. The nursing audit process typically consists of the following steps:

- **Planning:** The first step in the nursing audit process involves planning and defining the objectives of the audit. The audit team identifies the specific aspects of nursing care to be assessed, sets audit criteria, and establishes a timeline for conducting the audit.
- **Data collection:** In this step, data related to nursing care are collected from various sources, such as patient records, nursing documentation, observation, and interviews with nursing staff. The data collected may include patient assessments, care plans, medication records, infection control practices, and adherence to nursing standards.
- **Data analysis:** Once the data is collected, it is analyzed to evaluate the quality and effectiveness of nursing care. The audit team compares the collected data with established audit criteria, nursing standards, and evidence-based practices to identify areas of compliance and non-compliance.

- **Identification of deviations:** During data analysis, deviations or discrepancies from nursing standards and best practices are identified. These deviations may include medication errors, incomplete documentation, lapses in infection control measures, or other issues affecting patient care.
- **Findings and recommendations:** The audit team presents the findings of the audit, including both strengths and areas for improvement. Based on the audit findings, recommendations for enhancing nursing care quality and patient safety are proposed.
- **Action plan:** An action plan is developed to address the identified areas for improvement. The action plan outlines specific steps, responsibilities, and timelines for implementing the recommended changes in nursing practice.
- **Implementation:** Nursing staff, along with relevant stakeholders, implement the action plan. This may involve training sessions, process improvements, policy updates, or other interventions aimed at enhancing nursing care quality.
- **Monitoring and evaluation:** After implementation, the progress and effectiveness of the action plan are monitored and evaluated. Follow-up audits may be conducted to assess whether the recommended changes have been successfully integrated into nursing practice.
- **Feedback and continuous improvement:** Feedback on the audit results and the effectiveness of the action plan is provided to nursing staff and other stakeholders. Continuous improvement is emphasized as nursing care processes are continually evaluated and refined.

ADVANTAGES OF NURSING AUDIT

- **Quality improvement:** Nursing audits help identify areas for improvement in nursing care, leading to enhanced patient outcomes and overall quality of care.

- **Patient safety:** Audits contribute to the identification and correction of potential patient safety issues, reducing the risk of adverse events and medical errors.
- **Compliance and standards:** Audits ensure adherence to nursing standards, guidelines, and regulatory requirements, promoting consistency and compliance in nursing practice.
- **Accountability:** Nursing audits promote accountability among nursing staff, encouraging them to take responsibility for their actions and performance.
- **Professional development:** Audits provide opportunities for continuous learning and professional development for nursing staff.
- **Data-driven decision making:** Audits provide objective data and insights that can be used for evidence-based decision-making and resource allocation.
- **Team collaboration:** Nursing audits involve collaboration among healthcare professionals, fostering teamwork and communication.
- **Risk management:** Audits help identify potential risks and vulnerabilities in nursing practice, enabling proactive risk management strategies.

DISADVANTAGES OF NURSING AUDIT

- **Time-consuming:** Conducting nursing audits can be time-consuming and may require significant resources.
- **Resistance to change:** Nursing staff may resist changes or improvements suggested by the audit findings.
- **Subjectivity:** The audit process may involve subjective judgments, leading to potential bias in the assessment.
- **Data accuracy:** The accuracy and reliability of data collected during audits may be influenced by documentation practices or data entry errors.
- **Resource constraints:** Limited resources, such as staffing or technology, may impact the thoroughness and frequency of nursing audits.
- **Emotional impact:** The audit process may create stress and anxiety among nursing staff, especially if perceived as punitive rather than constructive.
- **Overemphasis on compliance:** Focusing solely on compliance may overlook other important aspects of nursing care and patient outcomes.
- **Lack of standardization:** Inconsistencies in audit methodologies or criteria may affect the comparability of audit results.
- **Privacy concerns:** Auditing patient records may raise privacy and confidentiality concerns, necessitating careful handling of sensitive information.

ROLE OF COUNCIL AND PROFESSIONAL BODIES IN MAINTENANCE OF STANDARDS

The role and function of nursing councils and professional bodies in establishing and enforcing nursing standards are critical in ensuring the quality, safety, and professionalism of nursing practice. These organizations play a pivotal role in shaping the landscape of nursing care, education, and ethics. Let's delve into their roles and functions in more detail:

Role of Nursing Councils

Nursing councils, often established by governmental or regulatory bodies, are responsible for overseeing the nursing profession at a national or regional level. Their primary role is to regulate and ensure the quality of nursing education, practice, and professional conduct. Here's a closer look at their functions:

- **Setting standards:** Nursing councils develop comprehensive standards of practice that outline the expectations for nurses' knowledge, skills, and behavior. These standards cover various aspects, including clinical practice, ethical conduct, continuing education, and patient safety.

- **Accreditation and regulation:** They accredit nursing schools and programs to ensure they meet predefined educational standards. They also regulate licensing and registration of nurses, ensuring that only qualified individuals are allowed to practice.
- **Code of ethics:** Nursing councils establish and enforce a code of ethics that guides nurses' ethical behavior and interactions with patients, colleagues, and the healthcare system.
- **Continuous professional development:** They promote lifelong learning and continuing education for nurses, encouraging them to stay updated with advancements in healthcare and nursing practices.
- **Addressing complaints and disciplinary actions:** Nursing councils investigate complaints against nurses and take disciplinary actions when necessary, upholding professional standards and patient safety.

Function of Professional Nursing Bodies

Professional nursing bodies are organizations created by and for nurses to represent their interests, promote professional development, and uphold the integrity of the nursing profession. Their functions include:

- **Advocacy:** Professional nursing bodies advocate for nurses' rights, better working conditions, and fair compensation. They also engage in healthcare policy discussions to influence decisions that impact nursing practice and patient care.
- **Education and training:** These bodies offer educational resources, workshops, conferences, and certification programs to help nurses enhance their skills and knowledge.
- **Networking and collaboration:** They provide a platform for nurses to connect, share experiences, and collaborate on research and best practices, fostering a sense of community within the profession.
- **Research and innovation:** Professional nursing bodies support research initiatives that contribute to evidence-based practice, driving improvements in patient care outcomes.
- **Quality improvement:** They contribute to the development of nursing practice standards, guidelines, and protocols that align with current healthcare trends and research.
- **Influencing policy:** These bodies engage in policy discussions and lobbying efforts to shape healthcare policies and regulations that impact nursing practice and patient care.
- **Synergy and collaboration:** Nursing councils and professional nursing bodies often work in synergy. While nursing councils establish regulatory standards, professional bodies advocate for nurses and facilitate their professional growth. This collaboration ensures that nursing standards remain current, relevant, and reflective of the evolving healthcare landscape.

In conclusion, nursing councils and professional nursing bodies are integral components of the nursing profession. Their roles encompass setting and enforcing standards, advocating for nurses' interests, facilitating education and professional development, and contributing to the overall improvement of patient care and healthcare systems. Their combined efforts uphold the high standards of nursing practice and ensure that nurses provide safe, ethical, and quality care to individuals and communities.

CHAPTER SUMMARY

1. In the rapidly evolving landscape of healthcare, nursing standards hold a pivotal role in guiding nurses through their multifaceted responsibilities.
2. Nursing standards act as the bedrock for delivering high-quality, compassionate patient care, ensuring that nursing practice is steeped in professionalism, ethics, and evidence-based approaches.
3. Nursing standards serve as authoritative benchmarks that govern the delivery of nursing services, safeguarding patient safety, well-being, and dignity, while cultivating a cadre of skilled and competent nursing professionals.
4. The importance of nursing standards is illuminated through their role in ensuring consistent, high-quality patient care, offering a clear framework for practice, promoting patient safety, guiding ethical decisions, and fostering professionalism.
5. The process of setting quality nursing standards is depicted as a comprehensive journey involving stakeholder engagement, expert input, scope definition, drafting, pilot testing, implementation, and continuous improvement.
6. Measurement methods for nursing quality standards encompass a range of tools, including nursing quality indicators, audits, patient feedback, clinical pathways, and simulation-based assessments.
7. Various types of nursing practice standards are elucidated, including ethical, professional, clinical, scope of practice, educational, and documentation standards.
8. Nursing audit is a systematic evaluation of nursing practices, procedures, and processes within healthcare settings to ensure adherence to established nursing standards and identify opportunities for improvement.
9. The multifaceted purposes of nursing audit, ranging from evaluating adherence to nursing standards and identifying improvement areas to enhancing patient safety.
10. The nursing audits classified based on the agency conducting the audit (internal, external, government, accreditation and professional association) and the methodology employed (retrospective, concurrent, prospective, focused, process-based and outcome-based).
11. The nursing audit process is elucidated as a systematic journey encompassing planning, data collection, analysis, identification of deviations, findings and recommendations, action plan implementation, monitoring, evaluation, and continuous improvement.
12. The advantages of nursing audit, including its role in quality improvement, patient safety enhancement, compliance with standards, fostering accountability and enabling professional development.
13. The potential drawbacks of nursing audit include time-consuming nature, potential resistance to change, subjectivity, etc.

REVIEW QUESTIONS

1. What are nursing standards, and how do they contribute to the overall quality of nursing care?
2. Explain the underlying objectives of nursing standards and how they align with providing patient-centered care.
3. Outline the steps involved in developing and establishing effective nursing quality standards.
4. Describe various methods used to assess adherence to nursing quality standards.
5. Describe the different types of nursing practice standards.

6. Define nursing audit and elaborate on its role in promoting quality assurance in nursing practice.
7. Outline the sequential steps of conducting a nursing audit, from planning to implementing changes based on audit results.
8. Explain the purpose of nursing councils and professional bodies in the context of setting and maintaining nursing practice standards.

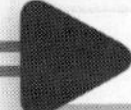 # BIBLIOGRAPHY 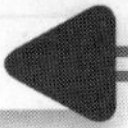

1. American Association of Colleges of Nursing. Accreditation. Available from: https://www.aacnnursing.org/CCNE-Accreditation; 2021.
2. American Nurses Association (ANA). Nursing: Scope and standards of practice, 3rd edition. Silver Spring, MD; 2015.
3. Audu BG, Okafor JO. An appraisal of nursing audit in a tertiary hospital in Nigeria. Ann Afr Med. 2015;14(1):11-7.
4. Canadian Nurses Association (CNA). Code of ethics for registered nurses. Available from: https://www.cna-aiic.ca/~/media/cna/page-content/pdf-en/code-of-ethics-2017-edition-secure-interactive; 2017.
5. Instefjord MH, Aasekjær K, Espehaug B, Graverholt B. Assessment of quality in psychiatric nursing documentation—a clinical audit. BMC Nurs. 2014;13:32.
6. Melnyk BM, Fineout-Overholt E (Eds). Evidence-based practice in nursing and healthcare: A guide to best practice, 4th edition. Philadelphia: Wolters Kluwer; 2019.
7. National Council of State Boards of Nursing (NCSBN). Transition to practice study. Available from: https://www.ncsbn.org/2015_TransitiontoPracticeStudy.pdf; 2015.
8. National League for Nursing (NLN). NLN core competencies for nurse educators. Available from: https://www.nln.org/docs/default-source/default-document-library/core-competencies.pdf; 2015.
9. National League for Nursing (NLN). Outcomes and competencies for graduates of practical/vocational. Available from: https://www.nln.org/docs/default-source/about/nln-vision-series-%28position-statements%29/outcomes-and-competencies-for-graduates-of-practicalvocational-diploma-baccalaureate-master-s-practice-doctorate-and-research-doctorate-programs-in-nursing.pdf?sfvrsn=2 [diploma], baccalaureate, master's practice doctorate, and research doctorate programs in nursing; 2000.
10. Nursing and Midwifery Board of Australia (NMBA). Registered nurse standards for practice. Available from: https://www.nursingmidwiferyboard.gov.au/Codes-Guidelines-Statements/Professional-standards/registered-nurse-standards-for-practice.aspx; 2016.
11. Nursing and Midwifery Board of Australia. Professional standards. Nursing and Midwifery Board of Australia. Available from: https://www.nursingmidwiferyboard.gov.au/Codes-Guidelines-Statements/Professional-standards.aspx; 2020.
12. Nursing and Midwifery Board of Ireland. Requirements for renewal of registration. Available from: https://www.nmbi.ie/Registration/Requirements-for-Renewal-of-Registration; 2020.
13. Nursing and Midwifery Council. NMC standards for education. Available from: https://www.nmc.org.uk/standards-for-education/; 2021.
14. Oktay Ş, Çıtlak GS. Evaluation of nursing audits performed in a training and research hospital in Turkey. J Caring Sci. 2020;9(1):13-9.
15. Royal College of Nursing. Continuing professional development. Available from: https://www.rcn.org.uk/professional-development/cpd; 2021.
16. Royal College of Nursing. Nursing standards and guidance. Available from: https://www.rcn.org.uk/professional-development/nursing-standards-and-guidance; 2018.
17. Sigma Theta Tau International Honor Society of Nursing (STTI). Nursing research: A resource for students, clinicians, and nurse educators. Available from: https://www.sigmarepository.org/sigma-landing-pages/research-landing-page; 2018.
18. World Health Organization (WHO). Framework for action on interprofessional education and collaborative practice. Available from: https://www.who.int/hrh/resources/framework_action/en/; 2010.

Nursing Care Concept

Learning Objectives

♦ Define the concept of primary health care and its essential components.
♦ Describe the role and responsibilities of a nurse in providing comprehensive nursing care.
♦ Identify the core principles and values that guide primary healthcare practices.
♦ Identify and describe the key principles that guide primary healthcare delivery.
♦ Define the concept of community-oriented nursing and its core components.
♦ Explain the holistic nursing approach and its holistic view of patient care.
♦ Discuss the significance of addressing physical, emotional, psychological, and spiritual aspects of patient well-being.
♦ Define the primary nursing model and its characteristics.
♦ Identify and discuss the advantages of the primary nursing model in patient care.
♦ Analyze the team nursing approach and its collaborative nature.
♦ Discuss the benefits of team nursing in terms of patient care, resource utilization, and diverse skillsets.
♦ Define family-oriented nursing and its principles.
♦ Discuss how involving families in patient care contributes to improved patient outcomes.
♦ Define progressive patient care and its role in patient care continuum.
♦ Identify and discuss the challenges faced in managing patients in progressive care units.

PRIMARY HEALTH CARE CONCEPT

Introduction

Primary health care (PHC) is a fundamental approach to healthcare that serves as the cornerstone of a well-functioning and equitable healthcare system. It encompasses a wide range of essential healthcare services, focusing on the prevention, treatment, and management of common health issues, as well as addressing the social determinants of health. The concept of PHC was first introduced in the Alma-Ata Declaration of 1978, and it has since evolved to become a central component of global health strategies.

Definitions

- **World Health Organization (WHO):** "PHC is essential health care based on practical, scientifically sound and socially acceptable methods and technology made universally accessible to individuals and families in the community through their full participation and at a cost that the community and the country can afford."
- **Pan American Health Organization (PAHO):** "PHC is a comprehensive approach to health care that provides for the needs of the whole person, from birth to death, and that emphasizes prevention and early intervention. It is also community-

based, with a focus on empowering people to take control of their own health."

- **American Public Health Association (APHA):** "PHC is an approach to health care that emphasizes prevention and early intervention, and that is accessible to everyone, regardless of their ability to pay. It is also community-based, with a focus on empowering people to take control of their own health."

Key Principles of Primary Health Care

- **Accessibility:** PHC aims to provide accessible and affordable healthcare services to all individuals and communities, regardless of their socioeconomic status or geographic location. This is achieved by establishing healthcare facilities in close proximity to people's homes and ensuring that services are affordable and culturally sensitive.
- **Comprehensiveness:** PHC offers a wide range of essential healthcare services, including preventive, promotive, curative, and rehabilitative care. These services cover a broad spectrum of health needs, from vaccinations and maternal care to chronic disease management and mental health support.
- **Holistic approach:** PHC takes into consideration not only physical health but also mental, emotional, and social well-being. It recognizes that health is influenced by a complex interplay of factors, including socioeconomic conditions, education, environment, and lifestyle.
- **Community engagement:** PHC encourages active participation and collaboration between healthcare providers, individuals, families, and communities. Local communities are involved in identifying health priorities, planning services, and implementing health interventions that are tailored to their specific needs.
- **Empowerment and education:** PHC emphasizes health education and empowerment, enabling individuals to make informed decisions about their health and adopt healthier lifestyles. Education also extends to healthcare providers, ensuring they are equipped with the knowledge and skills to deliver effective care.
- **Equity:** PHC seeks to eliminate health disparities and promote health equity by addressing the root causes of health inequalities. This includes tackling social determinants of health such as poverty, inequality, and discrimination.

Components of Primary Health Care

- **Promotion and prevention:** PHC focuses on preventing health issues before they arise through activities like immunizations, health education, nutrition programs, and lifestyle interventions. By promoting healthy behaviors and providing early interventions, PHC reduces the burden of disease.
- **Treatment and management:** PHC offers timely diagnosis, treatment, and management of common health conditions such as infections, chronic diseases, and injuries. Basic curative services are provided by healthcare professionals at the primary care level, reducing the need for more specialized care.
- **Maternal and child health:** PHC plays a crucial role in ensuring safe pregnancies, childbirth, and early childhood development. Services include prenatal care, childbirth assistance, neonatal care, and child immunizations.
- **Mental health:** PHC integrates mental health services to address the growing burden of mental health issues. It provides counseling, support, and early detection of mental health disorders.
- **Health promotion:** PHC promotes healthy lifestyles, disease prevention, and health education through community outreach, awareness campaigns, and partnerships with local organizations.
- **Essential medicines:** PHC ensures access to essential medicines and basic medical technologies, making them available

and affordable to all members of the community.

Role of Nurse in Primary Health Care

The role of nurses in primary health care is pivotal, as they play a crucial and multifaceted role in delivering comprehensive and patient-centered healthcare services to individuals and communities. Nurses are often at the forefront of primary health care, working in various settings such as clinics, community health centers, schools, and homes. Their roles encompass a wide range of responsibilities that contribute to promoting health, preventing illness, and managing various health conditions. Here are some key aspects of the role of nurses in primary health care:

- **Health promotion and education:** Nurses are instrumental in educating individuals and communities about healthy behaviors, disease prevention, and health promotion. They provide information on topics such as nutrition, exercise, immunizations, family planning, and hygiene, empowering people to make informed decisions about their health.
- **Preventive care:** Nurses are involved in preventive healthcare activities such as administering vaccinations, conducting screenings for various health conditions, and promoting early detection of diseases. They also work to identify risk factors and provide counseling to mitigate health risks.
- **Patient assessment and diagnosis:** Nurses perform thorough assessments of patients' health status, including physical, mental, and emotional well-being. They gather information, conduct physical examinations, and contribute to the diagnosis of health issues in collaboration with other healthcare professionals.
- **Treatment and management:** Nurses are responsible for implementing treatment plans, administering medications, and providing care for patients with acute and chronic health conditions. They monitor patients' progress, educate them about their conditions, and offer support for self-management.
- **Care coordination and collaboration:** Nurses play a central role in coordinating care for patients, ensuring that they receive the appropriate services from different healthcare providers. They collaborate with physicians, pharmacists, social workers, and other team members to create integrated and holistic care plans.
- **Chronic disease management:** Nurses are involved in managing patients with chronic diseases such as diabetes, hypertension, and asthma. They educate patients on disease management, medication adherence, lifestyle modifications, and monitor their progress over time.
- **Maternal and child health:** Nurses provide maternal and child health services, including prenatal care, postnatal care, childbirth assistance, and pediatric care. They support expectant mothers and families throughout the pregnancy journey and early childhood development.
- **Health counseling and support:** Nurses offer emotional support and counseling to patients and families, addressing their concerns, fears, and questions related to their health conditions. They also provide guidance on coping strategies and ways to improve overall well-being.
- **Health advocacy:** Nurses advocate for patients' rights, health equity, and access to healthcare services. They work to ensure that individuals and communities receive appropriate and timely care, especially those who may be marginalized or underserved.
- **Community engagement:** Nurses actively engage with communities to assess health needs, develop health programs, and foster partnerships with local organizations. They participate in health education campaigns, workshops, and outreach activities to improve community health.
- **Data collection and research:** Nurses contribute to data collection, research,

and quality improvement initiatives in primary health care settings. They help gather valuable information to monitor health trends, assess the effectiveness of interventions, and enhance healthcare delivery.

Benefits and Importance of Primary Health Care

- **Cost-effectiveness:** PHC is a cost-effective approach that focuses on prevention and early intervention, reducing the overall healthcare expenditure by minimizing the need for expensive treatments and hospitalizations.
- **Equity and accessibility:** PHC helps bridge the gap in healthcare access, particularly for vulnerable and underserved populations, ensuring that everyone has access to essential services.
- **Improved health outcomes:** By addressing health issues at an early stage and promoting healthier lifestyles, PHC contributes to improved health outcomes and overall well-being.
- **Reduced health disparities:** PHC's focus on equity and social determinants of health helps reduce health disparities and promote equal access to healthcare services.
- **Community empowerment:** PHC encourages community participation, empowerment, and ownership of health initiatives, fostering a sense of responsibility and accountability for health outcomes.
- **Strong health systems:** A robust PHC system serves as the foundation for a strong and resilient healthcare system, allowing for efficient referral to higher levels of care when necessary.

Challenges and Future Directions

While PHC offers numerous benefits, its effective implementation can be hindered by various challenges, including inadequate funding, workforce shortages, lack of infrastructure, and limited community engagement. To strengthen PHC, governments and stakeholders must invest in health systems, prioritize training and capacity-building, and address systemic barriers to access.

In the future, PHC will continue to evolve to meet the changing health needs of populations. Innovations in technology, telemedicine, and community engagement strategies will play a significant role in enhancing PHC delivery and expanding its reach.

■ COMMUNITY-ORIENTED NURSING

Introduction

Community-oriented nursing is a nursing approach that focuses on the health and well-being of populations and communities rather than just individual patients. It emphasizes the importance of understanding and addressing the health needs of communities, promoting preventive care, and collaborating with various stakeholders to improve the overall health of the population. This approach recognizes that many health issues are influenced by social, economic, and environmental factors that extend beyond the clinical setting.

Definitions

- Margaret A. Newman defined CON as "a practice of nursing that is directed toward the achievement of optimal health for individuals, families, and communities through the application of social and preventive as well as clinical nursing."
- Madeline Leininger defined CON as "a collaborative process of assessment, planning, intervention, and evaluation of the health care needs of individuals, families, groups, and communities."
- The American Nurses Association defined CON as "a synthesis of nursing practice and public health practice applied in promoting and preserving the health of populations."

Key Principles

- **Population focus:** Community-oriented nursing centers on the health needs of entire populations or specific communities rather than isolated individuals. Nurses work to identify common health problems, risk factors, and trends within these groups.

- **Preventive care:** Prevention is a cornerstone of community-oriented nursing. Nurses aim to prevent health problems before they occur by promoting healthy behaviors, offering health education, and addressing risk factors. This proactive approach helps reduce the burden of disease.
- **Community engagement:** Collaboration with community members is central to this approach. Nurses work alongside community leaders, organizations, and residents to understand the unique health challenges and co-create solutions that are culturally sensitive and tailored to the community's needs.
- **Holistic approach:** Community-oriented nursing considers the interconnectedness of physical, emotional, social, and environmental factors that contribute to health. Nurses assess not only medical conditions but also social determinants of health like income, education, housing, and access to healthcare.
- **Empowerment:** The aim is to empower individuals and communities to take control of their health. Nurses provide education, resources, and support, enabling people to make informed decisions and actively participate in their own well-being.

Nurses Role in Community-oriented Nursing

- **Community assessment:** Nurses conduct thorough assessments of the community's health status, identifying prevalent health issues, risk factors, and available resources. This assessment informs the development of targeted interventions.
- **Health promotion:** Nurses engage in health promotion and education activities to raise awareness about healthy lifestyles, disease prevention, and the importance of regular health screenings. These efforts empower individuals to make informed choices.

- **Disease prevention:** Community-oriented nursing focuses on preventing diseases by identifying at-risk populations and implementing measures to reduce their susceptibility. Immunization campaigns, screenings, and health education are commonly used strategies.
- **Collaboration:** Nurses collaborate with community leaders, local organizations, public health agencies, and other healthcare providers to create a comprehensive approach to addressing community health needs.
- **Policy advocacy:** Nurses play a role in advocating for policies that support community health. They can voice the needs and concerns of the community to influence decisions that impact healthcare services, resources, and social determinants of health.
- **Data collection and analysis:** Nurses collect and analyze data to monitor health trends, evaluate the effectiveness of interventions, and make evidence-based decisions to improve community health outcomes.

Benefits and Challenges

Benefits

- Improved health outcomes at the community level.
- Greater emphasis on preventive care, leading to reduced healthcare costs.
- Culturally sensitive interventions that address the unique needs of diverse populations.
- Increased community engagement and empowerment.
- Enhanced collaboration among healthcare providers and community stakeholders.

Challenges

- Limited resources and funding for community-oriented programs.
- Balancing individual patient care with community-focused initiatives.

- Addressing cultural and language barriers in diverse communities.
- Navigating complex political and social dynamics within communities.
- Measuring the long-term impact of interventions on population health.

■ HOLISTIC NURSING

Introduction

Holistic nursing is a patient-centered approach to healthcare that recognizes and emphasizes the interconnectedness of the physical, emotional, social, and spiritual aspects of an individual's well-being. This approach goes beyond treating only the symptoms of a medical condition; it aims to address the whole person and their unique experiences within the context of their environment and life circumstances. Holistic nurses consider all dimensions of a person's health and work to promote healing, balance, and overall wellness.

Definitions

- **American Holistic Nurses Association (AHNA):** "Holistic nursing is the practice of nursing that recognizes the wholeness of the person. It is based on the belief that the physical, mental, emotional, and spiritual aspects of a person are interconnected and that all aspects must be considered in order to achieve optimal health."
- **Margaret Newman:** "Holistic nursing is a way of being with people that honors their uniqueness and wholeness. It is a way of seeing people as more than the sum of their parts, and of appreciating their capacity for self-healing."
- **Jean Watson:** "Holistic nursing is a caring-healing praxis that promotes and facilitates health and well-being through the creation of a caring-healing environment."

Key Principles

- **Holism:** Holistic nursing views individuals as complex beings with interconnected dimensions. It acknowledges that physical health is influenced by emotional, social, spiritual, and environmental factors, and all these aspects must be considered to provide truly effective care.
- **Individualization:** Holistic nursing recognizes that each person is unique and has their own health goals, values, and experiences. Care plans are personalized to meet the individual's specific needs and preferences.
- **Empowerment:** The approach seeks to empower patients by involving them in their care decisions, providing education, and encouraging self-care practices. Holistic nurses believe that patients should be active participants in their healing journey.
- **Wellness promotion:** Holistic nursing places a strong emphasis on prevention and wellness promotion. It seeks to not only address illness but also to enhance overall well-being and quality of life.
- **Holistic assessment:** Holistic nurses use comprehensive assessment tools that go beyond physical symptoms. They assess emotional states, social support systems, spirituality, lifestyle factors, and more to gain a complete picture of the patient's health.
- **Therapeutic relationships:** Building strong therapeutic relationships is crucial in holistic nursing. Nurses provide a compassionate and non-judgmental presence, fostering trust and open communication.

Nurses Role in Holistic Nursing

- **Mind-body-spirit connection:** Holistic nursing recognizes that the mind, body, and spirit are interconnected. Emotional and spiritual well-being can impact physical health and vice versa. Nurses support patients in achieving balance and harmony in these aspects.
- **Complementary and integrative therapies:** Holistic nurses often integrate complementary therapies such as acupuncture, aromatherapy, yoga, meditation, and other alternative practices alongside convention-

al medical treatments to enhance healing and alleviate symptoms.

- **Patient education:** Holistic nurses educate patients about their health conditions, treatment options, and the importance of lifestyle choices. This empowers patients to actively participate in their care and make informed decisions.
- **Nutrition and lifestyle:** The approach emphasizes the role of nutrition, exercise, sleep, and stress management in overall health. Holistic nurses guide patients in adopting healthier lifestyles to support their well-being.
- **Environmental considerations:** Holistic nursing takes into account the physical environment and its impact on health. Creating healing and supportive environments contributes to patients' comfort and recovery.
- **Spiritual care:** Addressing patients' spiritual needs is a crucial component of holistic nursing. Nurses respect and support patients' individual beliefs and practices, recognizing the role of spirituality in healing.

Benefits and Challenges

Benefits

- Improved patient satisfaction due to individualized and patient-centered care.
- Enhanced patient engagement and empowerment in the healing process.
- A more comprehensive understanding of patients' health and well-being.
- Potential for improved treatment outcomes and overall quality of life.
- Greater focus on prevention and wellness promotion.

Challenges

- Integrating holistic practices within conventional healthcare settings.
- Ensuring that holistic care is evidence-based and safe.
- Overcoming skepticism and resistance from some healthcare professionals.

- Balancing holistic approaches with evidence-based medical treatments.
- Addressing diverse cultural and spiritual beliefs in a sensitive manner.

▮ PRIMARY NURSING

Introduction

Primary nursing is a patient care delivery model that focuses on providing personalized and continuous care by assigning a primary nurse to oversee the patient's care throughout their healthcare journey. This model places the patient at the center of care and ensures that a designated nurse takes responsibility for coordinating, planning, and advocating for the patient's needs. Primary nursing aims to enhance communication, continuity, and quality of care while fostering strong nurse-patient relationships.

Definitions

- **Marie Manthey:** "Primary nursing is a method of providing nursing care in which one nurse is responsible for the total care of a patient from admission to discharge."
- **American Nurses Association (ANA):** "Primary nursing is a patient care delivery system in which one nurse is the responsible professional for the planning, coordination, delivery, and evaluation of care to a specific patient or group of patients over a period of time."
- **World Health Organization (WHO):** "Primary nursing is a nursing care delivery system in which a qualified nurse is responsible for the total care of a patient or group of patients for a period of time."

Key Principles

- **Continuity of care:** In the primary nursing model, a specific nurse is responsible for the patient's care from admission to discharge, creating a consistent and seamless care experience.
- **Patient-centered care:** Primary nursing prioritizes the individual needs, preferences, and goals of the patient. The

nurse collaborates closely with the patient to develop a personalized care plan.

- **Nurse-patient relationship:** The primary nurse develops a strong therapeutic relationship with the patient, fostering trust, open communication, and a sense of partnership in the care process.
- **Holistic approach:** Primary nursing takes into account not only the patient's medical needs but also their emotional, psychological, and social well-being. The nurse addresses the patient as a whole person.
- **Collaboration:** While the primary nurse takes a lead role, collaboration with other members of the healthcare team is essential to ensure comprehensive and coordinated care.

Core Components

- **Assignment:** A primary nurse is assigned to each patient upon admission. This nurse conducts a comprehensive assessment, gathers information about the patient's history, needs, and preferences, and collaborates with the patient to establish goals.
- **Care planning:** Based on the assessment, the primary nurse develops an individualized care plan that addresses the patient's specific needs, medical conditions, and goals. The plan is continuously updated as the patient's condition changes.
- **Coordination:** The primary nurse coordinates all aspects of the patient's care, including medical treatments, medications, tests, therapies, and consultations with other healthcare providers.
- **Advocacy:** The primary nurse advocates for the patient's preferences, needs, and rights within the healthcare system. They ensure that the patient's voice is heard and respected.
- **Education:** The primary nurse provides patient education about their medical conditions, treatments, medications, and self-care strategies. This empowers patients to actively participate in their own care.

- **Communication:** The primary nurse serves as the main point of contact for the patient and their family. They provide regular updates, answer questions, and facilitate communication with other members of the healthcare team.

Role of Nurse in Primary Nursing

- Conduct comprehensive patient assessments considering physical, emotional, social, and psychological aspects.
- Collaborate with patients to set personalized care goals and create individualized care plans.
- Coordinate all aspects of patient care, including treatments, medications, therapies, and consultations.
- Advocate for patient preferences, needs, and rights within the healthcare system.
- Develop a strong therapeutic relationship with patients, built on trust and open communication.
- Provide emotional support and address patient fears and concerns.
- Deliver patient education about medical conditions, treatments, medications, and self-care strategies.
- Monitor patient progress, evaluate treatment effectiveness, and make necessary adjustments.
- Serve as the main point of contact for patients and families, ensuring regular updates and addressing questions.
- Collaborate with other healthcare team members to ensure seamless and coordinated care.
- Consider holistic aspects of patient well-being, including emotional, social, and spiritual needs.
- Encourage patient empowerment and involvement in care decisions.
- Facilitate smooth transitions of care as patients move between different healthcare settings.
- Maintain accurate documentation of patient care and progress.
- Incorporate complementary and integrative therapies if appropriate and desired by the patient.

- Foster patient engagement and ownership of their health and well-being.
- Address changes in the patient's condition promptly and initiate appropriate interventions.

Benefits and Challenges

Benefits

- Improved patient satisfaction due to personalized and consistent care.
- Enhanced nurse-patient relationships built on trust and communication.
- Increased patient engagement and empowerment in the care process.
- Improved coordination and continuity of care.
- Potential for better clinical outcomes and reduced hospital stays.

Challenges

- Staffing challenges, as assigning a primary nurse to each patient requires proper staffing levels.
- Ensuring effective communication and collaboration among primary nurses and other healthcare team members.
- Balancing the primary nurse's workload with the need for collaboration and teamwork.
- Adapting the model to various healthcare settings and patient populations.
- Addressing situations where the primary nurse is unavailable due to schedule changes or emergencies.

▌ TEAM NURSING

Introduction

Team nursing is a care delivery model that involves a team of healthcare professionals working collaboratively to provide comprehensive care to a group of patients. In this model, the responsibility for patient care is shared among various team members, each contributing their expertise to ensure the holistic well-being of the patients. Team nursing emphasizes effective communication, collaboration, and coordinated efforts to meet patients' medical, emotional, and social needs.

Definitions

- **Hildegard Peplau:** "Team nursing is a method of providing nursing care in which a team of nurses is responsible for the care of a group of patients."
- **American Nurses Association (ANA):** "Team nursing is a method of providing nursing care in which a team of nurses is responsible for the care of a group of patients, with each nurse having a specific role and responsibility."
- **World Health Organization (WHO):** "Team nursing is a method of providing nursing care in which a group of nurses work together to provide care for a group of patients."

Key Principles

- **Collaboration:** Team nursing emphasizes teamwork and cooperation among healthcare professionals, including registered nurses, licensed practical nurses, nursing assistants, and other allied healthcare workers.
- **Shared responsibility:** Care responsibilities are distributed among team members based on their skills and competencies. The primary nurse often coordinates care, while other team members contribute according to their roles.
- **Patient-centered care:** The model focuses on individualized patient care, ensuring that patients' unique needs and preferences are considered in the care planning and delivery process.
- **Efficiency:** By distributing tasks based on skill level, team nursing aims to optimize workflow and ensure that care is provided in a timely manner.

Core Components

- **Primary Nurse:** The primary nurse takes on the role of care coordinator. They assess the patients' needs, develop care plans, and oversee the overall care delivery. They also serve as the main point of contact for patients and families.

- **Team members:** The care team includes licensed practical nurses, nursing assistants, and other healthcare professionals who work under the direction of the primary nurse. They perform tasks such as administering medications, assisting with activities of daily living, and providing basic nursing care.
- **Collaboration:** Effective communication and collaboration are crucial in team nursing. Team members work together to ensure that patients' needs are met comprehensively and efficiently.
- **Continuity:** The primary nurse and the team members collaborate to ensure continuity of care as patients move through different shifts or stages of treatment.

Role of a Nurse in Team Nursing

- Organize and oversee care provided by the healthcare team.
- Delegate tasks based on team members' skills and competencies.
- Ensure effective communication among team members.
- Conduct initial and ongoing patient assessments.
- Collaborate with the team to develop individualized care plans.
- Continuously adapt care plans based on changing patient needs.
- Provide information about conditions, treatments, medications, and self-care.
- Offer emotional support and active listening to patients and families.
- Administer medications safely and accurately.
- Perform clinical interventions and procedures as needed.
- Maintain accurate patient records and document care interventions.
- Communicate patient information and changes to the care team.
- Advocate for patient preferences, needs, and rights.

- Collaborate with families and involve them in care decisions.
- Analyze complex situations and make informed decisions.
- Address urgent situations with quick and accurate responses.
- Work closely with various healthcare professionals.
- Ensure effective communication among team members.
- Advocate for patient needs and safety.
- Encourage patient participation in care decisions.
- Facilitate smooth care transitions between shifts or settings.
- Convey essential information to incoming team members.

Benefits and Challenges

Benefits

- **Efficiency:** The workload is distributed among team members, which can lead to more efficient care delivery.
- **Holistic care:** Different team members contribute their expertise, addressing various aspects of patients' physical, emotional, and social well-being.
- **Collaboration:** Effective teamwork fosters better communication, knowledge sharing, and problem-solving.
- **Workforce utilization:** Team nursing allows for optimal utilization of healthcare professionals' skills and competencies.

Challenges

- **Communication:** Effective communication is essential for successful team nursing. Miscommunication can lead to misunderstandings and errors in care.
- **Consistency:** Varied staffing levels and changing team compositions can affect the consistency of care.
- **Leadership:** Clear leadership and communication of roles are necessary to avoid confusion and ensure that care plans are followed.

- **Patient preferences:** Patients might prefer more personalized care from the same nurse rather than multiple caregivers.

FAMILY-ORIENTED NURSING

Introduction

Family-oriented nursing, also referred to as family-centered care or family nursing, is an approach to healthcare that recognizes the importance of the family unit in the well-being and care of the individual patient. It involves healthcare professionals actively involving and collaborating with the patient's family to provide comprehensive and holistic care. This approach goes beyond just treating the patient's medical condition and takes into account the family's beliefs, values, and dynamics.

Definitions

- **Friedemann (1995):** Family oriented nursing is a philosophy of care that recognizes the family as the unit of care. It is based on the belief that the family is the most important source of support for its members, and that nurses should work in partnership with families to promote health and well-being.
- **McFarlane (1983):** Family oriented nursing is a holistic approach to care that considers the needs of the whole family, not just the individual patient. It is focused on promoting family health and preventing illness, and on providing support to families during times of crisis.
- **Wright and Leahey (2000):** Family oriented nursing is a way of thinking about and providing care that recognizes the family as a system. It is based on the belief that the family's health and well-being are interconnected, and that nurses should work with families to address the needs of all members.

Key Principles of Family-oriented Nursing

- **Holistic care:** Family-oriented nursing recognizes that an individual's health and well-being are interconnected with their family's health and functioning. It considers the physical, emotional, psychological, and social aspects of both the patient and the family members.
- **Family as a unit of care:** In this approach, the family is viewed as a unit of care, rather than just a group of individuals. The family's support system, communication patterns, cultural background, and coping mechanisms all play a significant role in the patient's recovery and overall health.
- **Collaboration and partnership:** Healthcare professionals work in partnership with families, involving them in the decision-making process regarding the patient's care plan. This collaboration helps to create a care plan that aligns with the family's preferences, values, and goals.
- **Family assessment:** Nursing professionals conduct thorough assessments of the family's dynamics, structure, strengths, and challenges. This assessment guides the development of an individualized care plan that considers the family's resources and potential stressors.
- **Communication:** Effective communication is crucial in family-oriented nursing. Healthcare providers need to communicate openly with both the patient and the family, explaining medical terms, treatment options, and potential outcomes in a way that is easily understood.
- **Education and support:** Families are educated about the patient's condition, treatment options, and care needs. They are also provided with information on how to support the patient's recovery at home. Providing emotional support and counseling to the family members is also a significant aspect of family-oriented nursing.
- **Cultural competence:** Understanding and respecting the cultural beliefs and values of the family is important for providing culturally sensitive care. Healthcare professionals should be aware of cultural differences that might affect the patient's

and family's decision-making and care preferences.

- **Transition of care:** Family-oriented nursing extends beyond the hospital setting. It considers the transition of care from the hospital to home or other healthcare settings. Providing resources and guidance for the family to continue care at home is crucial.

Role of a Nurse in Family-oriented Nursing

- Conduct thorough assessments of both the patient and their family, considering dynamics, strengths, and challenges.
- Establish trust and open lines of communication with family members.
- Provide clear and understandable information about the patient's condition and care plan.
- Offer emotional support and address family members' concerns and anxieties.
- Collaborate with families to develop personalized care plans aligned with their preferences and goals.
- Act as a liaison between patients, families, and the healthcare team, ensuring effective communication.
- Advocate for patients' and families' rights and address conflicts that may arise.
- Demonstrate cultural competence and tailor care plans to align with diverse cultural backgrounds.
- Empower families to actively participate in the patient's care and decision-making.
- Assist families in navigating ethical dilemmas and end-of-life decisions.
- Facilitate smooth transitions of care from hospital to home, ensuring family preparedness.
- Continuously gather feedback and adjust care plans based on changing patient and family needs.
- Set an example for family-entered care, promoting its importance among healthcare professionals.

Benefits and Challenges

Benefits of Family-oriented Nursing

- **Improved patient outcomes:** Involving families in care decisions can lead to better adherence to treatment plans, improved patient outcomes, and reduced hospital readmissions.
- **Enhanced patient experience:** Patients often feel more supported and cared for when their families are actively involved in their care journey.
- **Holistic care:** By considering the family's dynamics and needs, healthcare professionals can provide more holistic care that addresses both the medical and emotional aspects of the patient's well-being.
- **Shared decision-making:** Collaborative decision-making between healthcare professionals, patients, and families can lead to decisions that are more aligned with the patient's values and preferences.
- **Cultural sensitivity:** Family-oriented care promotes cultural competence and respectful care that aligns with the family's cultural background.

Challenges and Considerations

- **Privacy and consent:** Healthcare professionals need to ensure that patients and families are comfortable with sharing medical information and involving the family in care decisions.
- **Conflicts and dynamics:** Family dynamics can sometimes lead to conflicts or disagreements about the patient's care. Healthcare providers need to mediate and navigate these situations sensitively.
- **Balancing autonomy:** While involving families, it is important to respect the patient's autonomy and ensure their wishes are prioritized.
- **Communication barriers:** Effective communication can be challenging when there are language barriers or differing levels of health literacy within the family.

- **Cultural differences:** Understanding and addressing cultural differences requires ongoing education and sensitivity.

■ PROBLEM-ORIENTED NURSING

Introduction

Problem-oriented nursing is an approach to nursing care that focuses on identifying, addressing, and resolving specific health-related issues or problems that patients are experiencing. This method is rooted in the nursing process, which involves systematic assessment, diagnosis, planning, implementation, and evaluation of care. Problem-oriented nursing aims to provide targeted and individualized care by focusing on the unique problems that each patient faces. Here's a detailed discussion of problem-oriented nursing.

Definitions

- **Gordon (1976):** Problem-oriented nursing is a method of nursing care that focuses on the patient's problems, rather than on their diagnoses. It is a systematic approach to care that involves assessment, identification of problems, planning, implementation, and evaluation.
- **Horsley and Rogers (1983):** Problem-oriented nursing is a problem-solving approach to nursing care that is based on the patient's individual needs. It is a holistic approach to care that considers the physical, emotional, social, and spiritual dimensions of the patient's health.
- **McFarland (1983):** Problem-oriented nursing is a method of nursing care that is organized around the patient's problems. It is a systematic approach to care that uses a problem list, a database, and a plan of care.

Components of Problem-oriented Nursing

- **Problem identification:**
  - Nurses assess the patient's condition to identify both medical and psychosocial issues that need attention.

- The assessment involves gathering information from the patient, medical history, diagnostic tests, and consultations with other healthcare professionals.
- **Problem diagnosis:**
  - Nurses analyze the collected data to identify nursing diagnoses, which are clinical judgments about the patient's actual or potential health problems.
  - Nursing diagnoses are distinct from medical diagnoses and focus on the patient's response to health issues.
- **Problem planning:**
  - Based on identified nursing diagnoses, nurses collaboratively develop care plans that outline goals, interventions, and expected outcomes.
  - The plan is individualized and takes into account the patient's preferences, cultural considerations, and resources.
- **Problem implementation:**
  - Nurses execute the planned interventions, which may include administering medications, performing treatments, providing education, and offering emotional support.
  - Interventions are directed toward addressing the identified nursing problems and promoting the patient's overall well-being.
- **Problem evaluation:**
  - Nurses assess the effectiveness of the interventions and evaluate whether the patient's responses and outcomes align with the goals.
  - If necessary, adjustments are made to the care plan to ensure optimal outcomes.

Role of a Nurse in Family-oriented Nursing

- Gather comprehensive patient data to identify health problems.
- Analyze physical, emotional, and social aspects to form a holistic understanding.
- Formulate nursing diagnoses based on assessed data.
- Administer medications, perform treatments, and provide emotional support.

- Continuously assess patient responses to interventions.
- Maintain accurate and up-to-date records of assessments, diagnoses, plans, interventions, and evaluations.
- Educate patients about their health problems, interventions, and self-care strategies.
- Empower patients to actively participate in their care.
- Collaborate with interdisciplinary teams to coordinate care.
- Share insights and contribute to patient-entered discussions.
- Adjust care plans based on changing patient conditions or responses.
- Prioritize interventions to address evolving priorities.
- Advocate for patients' needs, preferences, and goals within the healthcare team.
- Ensure patients' voices are heard during decision-making.
- Effectively manage time and resources to address multiple patient problems.
- Prioritize tasks based on the severity and impact of problems.
- Analyze complex patient situations to make informed clinical judgments.
- Problem-solve and adapt interventions as needed.
- Address ethical dilemmas that may arise in managing patient problems.
- Uphold patient autonomy while ensuring their safety and well-being.
- Consider cultural beliefs and practices when assessing and managing problems.
- Provide culturally sensitive care that respects patients' values.
- Maintain accurate and detailed records of interventions and patient responses.
- Ensure that the care provided is well-documented for continuity and legal purposes.
- Stay updated on evidence-based practices and advancements to improve problem-solving skills.
- Enhance knowledge and skills for better problem assessment and management.

Benefits and Challenges

Benefits of Problem-oriented Nursing

- **Individualized care:** This approach tailors care to the specific needs and problems of each patient, promoting personalized treatment.
- **Focused interventions:** By targeting specific issues, problem-oriented nursing helps to prioritize interventions and resources effectively.
- **Efficient resource allocation:** Resources such as time, manpower, and equipment are allocated based on identified problems, reducing waste and improving efficiency.
- **Holistic perspective:** While addressing individual problems, nurses consider the patient's holistic well-being, including physical, emotional, social, and psychological aspects.
- **Collaboration:** Problem-oriented care requires collaboration among healthcare professionals, enhancing communication and patient outcomes.
- **Goal-driven:** The approach sets clear goals and outcomes, allowing for objective evaluation of the effectiveness of interventions.

Challenges and Considerations

- **Complexity:** Patients often have multiple problems that interconnect. Nurses need to prioritize and manage these complexities effectively.
- **Dynamic nature:** Patient conditions can change rapidly, necessitating ongoing assessment and adaptation of care plans.
- **Comprehensive assessment:** Thorough assessment is crucial for accurate problem identification. Lack of information can lead to inaccurate diagnoses.
- **Balancing priorities:** Nurses need to balance addressing urgent problems with providing preventive care and patient education.
- **Interdisciplinary collaboration:** Effective communication and collaboration with other healthcare professionals are essential for comprehensive care.

PROGRESSIVE PATIENT CARE

Introduction

Progressive patient care, also known as progressive care or step-down care, refers to a level of healthcare provided to patients who require a higher intensity of monitoring, assessment, and treatment than what is typically provided on a general medical-surgical unit, but who do not require the same level of care as patients in an intensive care unit (ICU). This intermediate level of care is designed to bridge the gap between general inpatient care and critical care, ensuring that patients receive appropriate monitoring and interventions while optimizing the utilization of healthcare resources. Here's a detailed discussion of progressive patient care.

Definitions

- **Scribner (1971):** Progressive patient care is a system of patient care that provides for the progressive movement of patients through a variety of levels of care, from the most intensive to the least intensive.
- **Kramer (1974):** Progressive patient care is a system of patient care that is based on the principle of patient classification. Patients are classified according to their needs, and they are then assigned to a unit that can meet those needs.
- **Lynaugh (1987):** Progressive patient care is a system of patient care that is designed to improve the quality of care and the efficiency of care delivery. It does this by grouping patients together according to their needs, and by providing them with the level of care that they require.

Characteristics of Progressive Patient Care

- **Patient acuity:** Progressive care units accommodate patients who have complex medical conditions, require frequent monitoring, or are recovering from high-risk surgeries. These patients may have unstable vital signs, require specialized medications, or have potential complications.
- **Nursing ratio:** Nursing care in progressive patient care units is typically provided at a lower nurse-to-patient ratio compared to general medical-surgical units, allowing nurses to closely monitor and intervene as needed.
- **Equipment and monitoring:** Patients in progressive care often require advanced monitoring equipment, such as telemetry for continuous cardiac monitoring, pulse oximetry, and non-invasive blood pressure monitoring.
- **Interventions:** Nursing care in progressive care units includes administering intravenous medications, managing complex wound care, and providing respiratory support as needed.
- **Patient education:** Progressive care nurses educate patients and their families on the patient's condition, medications, and self-care techniques to facilitate a smooth transition to a lower level of care.
- **Transition of care:** Progressive care units are often used as a stepping stone for patients transitioning from critical care to general care. Patients move to progressive care units when they no longer require the intense monitoring of an ICU but still need more specialized care than what a general unit can provide.

Role of Nurses in Progressive Patient Care

- **Assessment:** Nurses assess patients' conditions, vital signs, and responses to treatments. They identify changes that might indicate deteriorating health and intervene promptly.
- **Monitoring:** Nurses closely monitor cardiac rhythms, oxygen levels, blood pressure, and other physiological parameters using advanced monitoring technology.
- **Medication administration:** Nurses administer medications, including intravenous medications, titrate doses as needed, and monitor for any adverse reactions.
- **Interventions:** Nurses manage wound care, provide respiratory support, and assist

with procedures such as the removal of chest tubes or drains.

- **Collaboration:** Progressive care nurses collaborate with interdisciplinary teams, including physicians, respiratory therapists, and physical therapists, to ensure comprehensive care.
- **Patient advocacy:** Nurses advocate for patients' needs and ensure their voices are heard during care decisions.
- **Patient education:** Nurses educate patients and families about the patient's condition, treatment plan, and self-care techniques to promote recovery.
- **Transition planning:** Nurses help prepare patients for discharge by providing information about follow-up appointments, medications, and lifestyle modifications.

Benefits and Challenges

Benefits of Progressive Patient Care

- **Optimized resource utilization:** Progressive care units help hospitals efficiently allocate resources by providing care to patients who need more monitoring and interventions than general care but not the intensity of an ICU.
- **Smooth transition:** Patients benefit from a gradual transition from critical care to general care, which can improve outcomes and reduce the risk of complications.
- **Expert nursing care:** Nurses with specialized training in progressive care deliver focused and comprehensive care to patients with specific needs.
- **Early intervention:** The close monitoring in progressive care units allows for early detection and intervention in case of complications.
- **Reduced ICU admissions:** Effective progressive care management can poten-

tially reduce the need for patients to be admitted to the ICU, freeing up critical care resources.

Challenges of Progressive Patient Care

- **Patient complexity:** Patients in progressive care units often have complex medical conditions and require advanced monitoring and interventions.
- **Variable acuity:** Patients in progressive care units can have varying levels of acuity, making it challenging to prioritize care and allocate resources effectively.
- **Staffing ratios:** Maintaining appropriate nurse-to-patient ratios can be a challenge due to the specialized care required by patients.
- **Resource allocation:** Balancing the allocation of advanced monitoring equipment, specialized medications, and other resources among patients with different needs requires careful planning and coordination.
- **Transitional care:** The transition from critical care to progressive care and eventually to general care can sometimes lead to gaps in communication and care continuity. Ensuring a seamless transition can be complex.
- **Skills and training:** Nurses and other healthcare professionals in progressive care units need specific training to manage the complex needs of patients. Ongoing education and skill development are essential to providing high-quality care.
- **High patient turnover:** Patients in progressive care units are often in a state of transition, which can lead to higher patient turnover rates. This frequent turnover can impact the workload and potentially affect the quality of care.

CHAPTER SUMMARY

1. In essence, nurses in primary health care settings are the linchpin connecting patients to a wide range of healthcare services.
2. Their holistic approach, dedication to patient care, and focus on health promotion make them essential contributors to achieving the goals of primary health care – improving health outcomes, enhancing access to care, and promoting overall well-being within communities.
3. Community-oriented nursing embodies a proactive and holistic approach to healthcare that recognizes the complex interplay of factors that influence health.
4. By focusing on prevention, collaboration, and community engagement, nurses can contribute significantly to improving the health and well-being of populations in various settings.
5. Holistic nursing embodies a deep understanding of the multi-dimensional nature of health and wellness.
6. By incorporating mind, body, spirit, and environment into patient care, holistic nurses aim to provide comprehensive and compassionate support that promotes healing and enhances the overall quality of life for their patients.
7. Primary nursing is a patient-centered care model that emphasizes continuity, individualized care, and strong nurse-patient relationships.
8. By assigning a dedicated nurse to oversee the patient's care, this model aims to improve patient experiences, outcomes, and overall quality of care.
9. Team nursing is a care delivery model that emphasizes collaboration, efficiency, and patient-centered care.
10. Team nursing requires effective communication, clear role delineation, and a coordinated approach among healthcare professionals.
11. While team nursing has benefits in terms of utilizing skills and delivering holistic care, it also comes with challenges that need to be addressed for successful implementation.
12. Problem-oriented nursing combines clinical expertise with a patient-centered approach to deliver efficient, effective, and individualized care.
13. Problem-oriented nursing ensures that nursing interventions are targeted toward resolving specific health problems, ultimately leading to improved patient outcomes and satisfaction.
14. Progressive patient care serves as an important intermediate level of care that meets the needs of patients requiring more than general care but less than intensive care.
15. Progressive patient care plays a vital role in patient recovery, resource utilization, and ensuring optimal patient outcomes.

REVIEW QUESTIONS

1. Explain the concept of primary health care and its significance in promoting community well-being.
2. Discuss the key principles and strategies that underpin effective primary health care delivery.
3. Define community-oriented nursing and elaborate on its role in addressing health disparities and improving population health.

4. Discuss the holistic nursing approach, highlighting its focus on treating the whole person rather than just their medical condition.
5. Describe the primary nursing and highlighting its advantages and challenges.
6. Analyze the team nursing approach to patient care. Discuss the benefits of this approach, potential challenges, and strategies to enhance effective teamwork.
7. Explain the principles of family-oriented nursing and its significance in patient care.
8. Define progressive patient care. Discuss the challenges and benefits of progressive patient care units and their impact on patient outcomes.

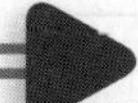 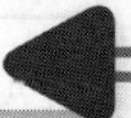

BIBLIOGRAPHY

1. Bell JM, Wright LM. The Calgary family assessment model: how to apply in clinical practice. Nurs Sci Q. 2018;31(2):117-20.
2. Benner PA, Tanner SJ. Nursing management: concepts and practice. New York: Pearson Education; 2011.
3. Chotchoungchatchai S, Marshall AI, Witthayapipopsakul W, Panichkriangkrai W, Patcharanarumol W, Tangcharoensathien V. Primary health care and sustainable development goals. Bull World Health Organ. 2020;98(11):792-800.
4. De Geest S, Moons P. Improving patient adherence to integrated care pathways. J Nurs Sch. 2008;40(4):309-14.
5. Dossey BM, Keegan L, Barrere C. Holistic nursing: A handbook for practice. Jones and Bartlett Publishers Learning; 2019.
6. Dracup KM, Jones JB. Nursing leadership and management. Philadelphia: F A Davis Company; 2013.
7. Feetham SL, Thomson BN. Conceptual models for family nursing. J Adv Nurs. 1984;9(5):491-7.
8. Finkelman AW. Case management for nurses: integrating the care plan. Springer Publishing Company; 2017.
9. Hall JE, Weaver EJ. A comparison of primary nursing and team nursing. Nurs Res. 1977;26(1):32-7.
10. Halloran JA. Team nursing: a review of the literature. J Nurs Admin. 1978;8(8):31-7.
11. Huber D. Leadership and nursing care management. Elsevier Health Sciences; 2017.
12. Kaakinen JR, Coehlo DP, Steele R, Tabacco A, Hanson SMH. Family Health care nursing: theory, practice, and research. F A Davis Company; 2014.
13. Koithan M, Cohen MZ. The role of the advanced practice nurse in integrative nursing: an emerging specialty. J Prof Nurs. 2012;28(4):197-203.
14. Kramer BL, Schmalenberg KS. The effects of primary nursing and team nursing on patient outcomes: A meta-analysis. Res Nurs Health. 1988;11(1):1-2.
15. Langlois EV, McKenzie A, Schneider H, Mecaskey JW. Measures to strengthen primary health-care systems in low- and middle-income countries. Bull World Health Organ. 2020;98(11):781-91.
16. Lee TH, Weinstein MC. The case for capitation. N Engl J Med. 2010;363(15):1393-5.
17. Leon DA, Adair H, Bhutta ZA, et al. Primary health care: a review of conceptual models and their relevance to global health. Health Policy Plan. 2016;31(2):171-81.
18. MacDonald C, MacLaren J. Problem-based learning in nursing education: A process for scenario development. Nurse Educ Pract. 2010;10(1):10-4.
19. Manthey M. Primary nursing: A handbook for nurses. St. Louis: Mosby; 1980.
20. McSherry W, Ross L. Dilemmas of Holistic, Spiritual Care: an exploratory investigation of the views of patients and staff. J Clin Nurs. 2002;11(1):48-57.
21. Pan American Health Organization. Primary health care: the foundation of universal health coverage. Washington, DC: Pan American Health Organization; 2017.

22. Radwin MA, Dracup KM. Nursing care delivery models: a review of the literature. New York: Springer Publishing Company; 2003.

23. Rantz MJ, Fleishman JS, Owen DM. The use of primary nursing and team nursing in nursing homes: A comparison of effects on patient outcomes. J Am Geriatr Soc. 1991;39(12):1309-16.

24. Smith MR, Bass PR. Primary nursing: a review of the literature. J Adv Nurs. 1987;12(7):683-91.

25. Tilley DS, Cameron RG. Understanding problem-based learning in nursing education. Springer; 2017.

26. United Nations Children's Fund. Primary health care: A promise to keep. New York: United Nations Children's Fund; 2018.

27. Weaver R. Problem-based learning in nursing: A new model for a new context. Nurse Educ Today. 2014;34(6):958-63.

28. White LK, Duncan G, Baumle WH. Foundations of nursing. Cengage Learning; 2018.

29. World Health Organization. Alma-Ata Declaration on primary health care. Geneva: World Health Organization; 1978.

30. World Health Organization. Primary health care: now more than ever. Geneva: World Health Organization; 2021.

31. Wright LM, Leahey M. Nurses and families: A guide to family assessment and intervention. FA. Davis Company; 2018.

O

Q